WORK LIFE BODY®

Fiona Slade

Cartoons by

Sally Artz

published by Walk-On
www.walk-on.info

The information given in this book is intended solely for education and personal interest and should not be taken as medical advice. Every effort has been made to ensure that such information is thoroughly researched and accurate. Neither the author nor the publisher accept any legal responsibility for any personal injury or other damage or loss arising from the use or misuse of the information given.

ISBN 978-0-9563246-0-3

Cover design: Fiona Slade

Typeset by Andrew Buchanan Communications
www.buchanan-communications.co.uk

Printed in the UK by Doveton Press
www.dovetonpress.co.uk

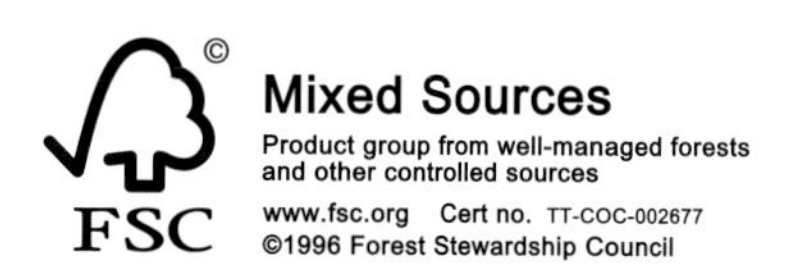

to Mum and Dad

Acknowledgements

So many people have been fantastically supportive; supportive, patient, long-suffering, generous, inspirational and wonderful. Andrew Buchanan, Robert Lee, Helen Cranston, Paul Clayton, Patrick Holford, Jane Sen, Mike Stroud, Jane Plant, Marianne, Sally Artz, Richard Bandler, Margot Charlton, Jeremy Holt, Martin Bazen, Liz Cook, Gavin Savage, all my family and so many more. Simply can't tell you how grateful I am. Thank you.

Contributions from Helen Cranston BSc, DNMed, Nutritional Therapist,
Registered Member of the British Association of Nutritional Therapists.

Contents

Errata:
p203 footnote; for *Poitics* read *Politics*
p292, last paragraph; for *Metal* Health read *Mental* Health

THEY SAY TO LEAD A HAPPY AND HEALTHY LIFE
WE NEED TO EAT FIVE PORTIONS OF FRUIT A DAY!

I FIND FIVE CHOCOLATE ORANGES WORK BEST!

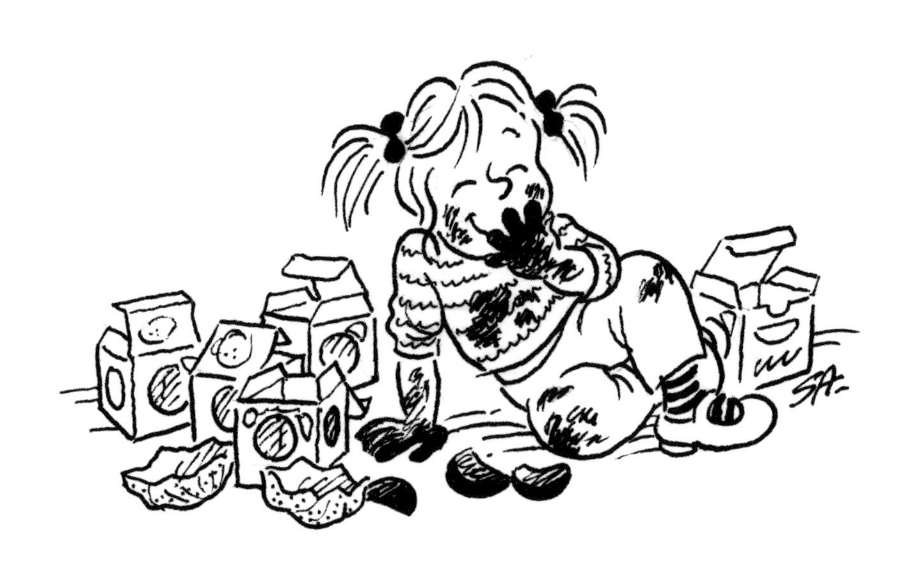

The Beginning

I suppose my philosophy was that this is the information I would have found useful, all collected and assembled in one place. To find the information I had to research 18+ books, 4 training courses, umpteen seminars and conferences and papers. It's what I wanted to know but never had the time to find out.

There is so much to know about us, about how we work, what makes us feel good and have energy – and the more I started to look into it, I was very struck by what we didn't know. The majority of us don't do Biology or Bio-Chemistry for O level or GCSE and so stop learning about ourselves and how we work by age 15 or 16 and go through life hoping it all hangs together.

I had pushed and pushed myself and my body, since school, through 24 years of long hours, hard work and a reasonable amount of achievement. For 13 of those, I had been aware that everything probably wasn't quite as it should be but the best solution was not to stop and think about it.

When I finally had the opportunity to stop and think about it, in 2001, my body and my health all took the opportunity together. I had, for the first time, reached a stage where I had to stop and do some serious thinking about what I was doing and my body had reached the stage where it wasn't going to put up with me any longer.

I studied courses and generally indulged myself in finding out more about things that had interested me all my life; health, fitness, nutrition, anatomy, physiology, allergies, energy levels, the immune system – study that had just kept being sidelined for another time.

The information I found out would have been so useful to know about 23 years earlier. Fortunately a general knowledge of health and a generally good diet had been enough to see me through.

The point at which many of us learn about our health and our bodies is when we become ill – even seriously ill. I prefer the approach of learning about health and staying healthy – without having to become ill to find out.

This is everything we should know anyway. This isn't something we should put off until one day when we have time, have nothing else to do.

It's about feeling good, being healthy, looking after yourself, your work, your life, your body.

It's about knowing more about your body and making the most sense of all the information that seems to be coming our way on health, nutrition, exercise and lifestyle.

It's about having less headaches, colds and flu, tiredness, aches and pains and more energy, better memory and concentration – better moods.

It's about what keeps us well and working well.

Many of us know more about computers or cars than we do about our own body. Some people probably know more about programming their central heating system or operating their music or TV systems.

We are surrounded by all sorts of theories and advice and people telling us what to do - a lot of which, I have to say, I find very fragmented and not necessarily consistent. People stand a much greater chance of making sense of all this information if there is a better understanding of how it applies to them.

It's very easy to go through life with very, very little knowledge of the workings and requirements of our anatomy, physiology, chemistry and bio-chemistry. At the moment there seems to be a growing trend for us to adopt all sorts of different health messages although these may be coming across in a fairly random, pick 'n mix sort of style. The enthusiasts can immerse themselves in endless information and make of it what they will - but more worryingly, far more people just seem to be switching off altogether - the information isn't consistent, we can't make sense of it, it involves stuff we don't want to do or don't want to eat, and it's just easier to have nothing to do with it.

Plus there is always someone whose granny smoked 40 a day and downed a bottle of whisky a day and lived till 99 - so why should they worry about anything?

In my business consultancy work - looking at health crept in in a sort of under the radar kind of way. Although the business brief may have been business development, or team working, or recruitment, or sales, or presentation, or whatever - in doing this I was becoming increasingly aware that there was no point trying to hang new skills off something that is falling apart. How people were was key to what we were trying to do. Just taking some time to look at how people felt, how they came across to other people, encouraging people to get into the right state, physically and mentally and remembering the importance of being fit and well came to be a recurring theme.

Work Life Body is non-discriminatory - this is for everyone - all individuals, at home and at work: board members, management, department staff, people who sit at pcs, people who drive lorries or forklift trucks, freelance professionals, medical teams, teachers, mums, dads, singles, carers, students, old, young - everyone - no discrimination, no place to hide.

It does seem to be much easier to do things if we are well. Life is easier if we are well.

How well we are can have significant influence on our effectiveness, what we can do, how we are with other people and their reactions and responses to us. Especially in relationships and teams, it is usually much easier for others to respond well to someone who seems well in themselves.

And I would especially mention here, people with disability or other long term conditions. Some of the people who are often best at all of this are disabled people. You can be extremely well even if you are disabled - and many disabled people have the respect of others as being exceptional because they do have disabilities and despite that they look after themselves and often have very good health and out-perform colleagues and are already paying a lot more attention to health than everyone else.

This is also a very practical, realistic, simple way of looking at these things - it isn't an academic piece of work. I know what it's like not having time to eat the right things, or anything at all, or drink the right things, or anything at all, or giving the marbles a chance to catch up with themselves, or breathing correctly, or getting the shoulders down out of the ears, or relaxing or switching off - I know what that's like. Extreme working hours and workload and busy lives are normal for many people.

We can work very hard at getting ill - and the great news is, that relatively, it can be quite easy to be well.

Speaking to people about health and how the body works and nutrition - people are usually very interested - it does seem to be one of those areas in which everyone has some kind of personal and/or general interest.

This isn't about being told off - it's about explanations and choices - establishing the ground so that we can make decisions for ourselves, make sense of things, create the interest that it is worth looking after ourselves and appreciate how fantastic we are. Explain how the brain, heart, lungs, liver and kidneys work and why they need nutrients and how they get them.

This is a shared responsibility. Health teams, families and employers need to be responsible for health and providing healthy environments and information and advice and support - and it's also our responsibility to look after ourselves.

Typically the point at which we receive information, or have the chance to stop to learn about ourselves is when something goes wrong. Until then, our bodies are just supposed to function and they aren't supposed to go wrong - and fortunately, a great deal of the time they don't.

But as a strategy, that isn't great. 'Let's not find out about something until it goes wrong and we have to'.

According to cumulative cancer research, currently 1 in 4 people die of cancer in the UK, and 2 in 4 of heart disease.

Both these diseases are over 75% lifestyle-related and are strongly protected against by healthy lifestyle. This would include strong networks, support, team spirit and community. Risk factors for both illnesses are typically smoking, poor diet, obesity, alcohol, lack of exercise, stress, unhappiness and isolation.

Fortunately the body can often be put right and has remarkable powers of recovery

– but it is very, very significantly influenced by how it is looked after and treated.

All day and all night, whatever we were doing to it, the body will try and survive. It can't help itself, it's pre-programmed – whatever we do to it, it will still try and survive, in whatever way it can, for as long as it can . . . and that's why we need to meet it halfway, at least . . . and eventually of course, if things don't change, body parts and systems will start to malfunction and pack in. To protect vital functions, the body will compromise, wherever it can – and all the ways in which the body has compromised, in order to keep going, can gradually start to have their side-effects. Some of us, of course, get away with more than others. There can be a macho image aspect to this, to punishing and stressing ourselves and defying nature – but it is a strange thing to be proud of – and it's not so great if and when you don't get away with it.

If we are ill – it is very striking how many more people we meet or find we know who have also had illnesses and people who have learned things about themselves and perhaps now do things differently – made changes. How about the idea of doing away with the being really ill bit? Cutting out the step of being unwell – to find out how we can look after ourselves.

And for the avoidance of doubt, we are talking about looking after our health, what we can do for ourselves. We aren't talking about DIY doctors. Wherever necessary you work with the GP or other qualified health professionals and perhaps even know more about when to do that.

There is also the stark discovery of how many people think it is normal to have headaches or migraines, to have back pain, always to feel tired, often to have colds or recurring colds, to struggle with lack of energy or concentration, poor sleep. It isn't normal. These are all things that are trying to tell us something and symptoms that we don't have to have.

What we cover here is very easy to cope with anatomy and physiology – and then the wonders of the gastro-intestinal tract – and all things to do with digestion. Then we look at the cell, then nutrition and eating and food labels and salt and detox and energy and hormones – followed by stress, exercise, breathing, bones, joints, muscles, teeth, eyes, ears, feet – sleep, mental health and lifestyle. We are our bodies, we should know about them – they shouldn't be a disassociated thing that is too complicated for us to be bothered to find out about.

This lays the ground for making sense of things. Doing the whole big picture thing explains why. Why everything is to do with everything else. Enabling us to step back into the loop. Why what we do affects us.

All the work involved in digestion is going on, whatever we are eating – and the reason good stuff, is good stuff is that it suits the system, doesn't hammer it too hard and we get comparatively high benefit from what we eat. Poor food hammers the system a lot harder and provides much less nutrition or energy - a very bad pay-back arrangement (and tends to leave gunk behind too).

What we eat and the health of our colon can have direct links to recurring headaches, tiredness and a weakened immune system. In turn a weakened immune system may lead to increased susceptibility to minor infections such as colds and flu, etc - and what are today's most common ailments? - headaches, tiredness, minor and recurring infections, colds and flu. If the colon is well and operating properly, we may be able to avoid a number of ailments.

Digestion and metabolism[1] are creating waste products and toxins in our body all the time. These have to be eliminated. We need our cellular elimination to work well and all our main routes of elimination to carry waste and toxins away.

There are explanations of which food groups foods come into, the best proportions in which to eat foods, which nutrients come from which foods, which are more easily digestible and so give most energy for less work and vice versa, foods that take more out of us than they have to offer to us. Nutrition is the food we eat as fuel to keep our bodies alive and well. There is nothing alternative about nutrition, we all have to eat.

Energy is covered in the section on Nutrition: where energy comes from - what it has to do. We have so much energy - it's not an endless supply. If we tie a large proportion of that energy up digesting and sorting out overload and sorting out emergencies and problems, there is less for us to function with everywhere else. If we have diverted large chunks of our energy away doing other things, consciously or sub-consciously - we run the risk of not having enough energy, feeling tired all the time.

The reason to give a strong focus towards nutrition is that the more you look at health and fitness - the clearer it becomes. It has been the acknowledged basis of health since Hippocrates, 400 BC - and it is inescapable. It is the obvious explanation of so many aspects of good health and bad health.

The better the suitability of food, the better the body will function. Our requirements are for foods that give us energy, foods that help build and repair our structure, and foods that help to protect us.

[1] metabolic actions/metabolism – the sum total of all the bio-chemical processes that keep the cells alive, all the structural and functional activity of all the organs and systems. A complex inter-twining set of chemical processes by which life is made possible for a living organism, ie: what is going on inside us, all the time. The continual breaking down and joining up of simple components to provide what is needed.

I think most people do want to look after themselves but have just been led to believe or come to the conclusion that it is difficult, or expensive, or both.

It's lamentable really that our time is so limited with doctors and other health professionals. Perhaps the health of the nation would improve if people just had more time to talk about things and learn about things - but there are very few places, people and opportunities for us to find out more unless you have the time and ability and moreso the inclination to do good level research - it takes a lot of time.

The human body is truly wonderful - and that is the message we need to pass on.

We need to be interested in our health and treat it as though it matters. In some respects I think we had responsibility taken away from us, over many years, for a variety of reasons and a lot has changed since then - particularly what we eat and how we live. We need to get back into the loop.

We have stretched the NHS well beyond groaning point and we have to take individual responsibility back. We have to change the attitude that we do what we want, get ill and then expect someone to sort it out or we can take something.

We have to manage lots of things. We have to manage time, we have to manage priorities, we have to manage people, we have to manage budgets - and we have to manage our health.

And we have to remember that we are infectious - not just colds and flu - but wellness is catching. Yawning is catching, laughing is catching, being well is catching. It's your hormones.

We can directly affect - enhance, or suppress - our immune systems. Being well looks after our immune system - and our immune system is our best defence against everything.

The important thing is to know we have choices - and what those choices are.

Health and Wellbeing - Why it's important

- ✓ feel better
- ✓ have more energy
- ✓ have less aches and pains
- ✓ sleep better
- ✓ improved circulation and fitness
- ✓ look better
- ✓ improved self-esteem and confidence
- ✓ increased or enhanced ability - physically and mentally
- ✓ being well and healthy will have distinct benefits, in and outside work
- ✓ body working better - brain and mind working better
- ✓ manage better
- ✓ better communication
- ✓ improved leadership skills

We feel better

We feel better because when the body is well, it performs better.

All day, everyday and through the night, an extraordinary number of functions are being performed by the body. We are absorbing things, moving things round, throwing things out, we are breathing, we are repairing and renewing bones, muscles and tissue – all the time, we are secreting things that make other things happen – things that carry thoughts and information through and around our body.

Whether we are lifting our right foot or reading a book, we are relying, all the time on highly sophisticated chemical and electrical reactions. They report the messages to us that we need, whether we are cold or hot or hungry, what we think, whether we are happy, whether we need to be fearful, whether we recognize something we see. The result of all these functions is how we feel.

They are all the result of long sequences of chemical processes – some of which may take place in split seconds and they are all part of the continuous domino effect that runs our bodies.

They require our various organs and systems to operate and work well. If they aren't operating so well – whatever we are trying to do – lift our right foot, send messages to and from the brain, pump oxygen, pump blood, fight infection – will be affected, whether consciously or sub-consciously. On a sub-conscious level things just won't be happening so well and for some time we may not know. This is why it is possible to have conditions for some time before finding out there is something wrong and diagnosis. On a conscious level the most common things we may experience will be:

pain
laboured, difficult movement or thought
tiredness, or
colds.

There are many others, but those are the common and increasingly common ones - which most of us will have experienced at some time.

Just think how many people would like to go through a working week without pain, tiredness or a cold.

So, if we are well, everyday functions are performed properly and without pain – and we are nice, happy people.

How we feel in happy mode is also run by the same chemistry and biology that is taking place in our body all the time – the same chemistry and biology as lifts your right foot, repairs and renews tissues and pumps blood – it's your hormones.

Feeling good at a football game – winning the World Cup, being out on a walk, seeing something that really takes your breath away, the most wonderful hug and kiss you can imagine . . . the goose bumps, the all over tingling . . . it's your hormones.

The hormones we release at these times are amongst the most wonderful drugs you'll find – and they are free and accessible on demand – we just have to keep them in working order and know what to do.

Oxytocin, for example – shoots up when you are being hugged – the hormone which originally produced the nurturing behaviour in mammals – and this is why they are so strong, so powerful. They not only affect the nurturing mother and the nurtured babies – but they actually directly affect the dad, or other members of a group or witnesses – even if not physically involved in the nurturing. Just standing watching, seeing that picture, seeing that scene, can affect others too. These things are infectious. Having a hug can make us feel good – and watching a romantic film can affect us the same way too.

Everything we do is affected by the messengers that keep our body functioning. The production or synthesis of these hormones depends on the availability of their constituent nutrients – they are made of amino acids which we get from what we eat – and the work they do and their journeys depend on the health of blood plasma, our interstitial fluid and all the organs of the body that work together. They are very busy components of the human body; they instigate, regulate and manage all the reactions that go on in our body all the time.

And having these hormones and pathways in good working order directly affects our immune system – it relies on these messengers and pathways to be able to respond, to do what it has to do, to keep us well.

> Healthy hormones and systems and pathways – good immune system;
> poorly hormones and pathways – struggling immune system.

Being well looks after our immune system – our own, in-built, rapid-response team.

Have more energy

The energy is being produced well, is being used efficiently and because it is being produced well and used efficiently we will have enough for what we need.

Many people who feel tired may have their bodies operating on very restricted energy levels to begin with, from poor fuel/food and poor fuel processing. Even if we think we eat adequate (or too much) food, if it isn't the right sort of food, it won't have the right nutrients, vitamins and minerals that we need – so our body is still under-nourished. Plus the body is trying to do much more than it should do because we've cluttered it up and diverted energy to cope with non-nutritious substances, excess and invaders and it has to compensate where organs and systems are under-par. We may have over-burdened the body, as well as obstructing the means it has to carry out its processing. All day, everyday – our bodies are working non-stop specifically for our survival. We can make that easy for them, we can meet them halfway – or, as is easy to do and seems to be becoming more common, we can make that process more difficult – and lose the benefit of all that valuable energy. The thing to remember is that whatever we do to them, our bodies will keep on trying to function, they will keep on trying to survive. That's why we do get away with an awful lot – our bodies will try and cope with everything and a lot of the time they do remarkably well. Despite a significant amount of neglect or abuse our bodies are trying to look after us – but again, this can also camouflage the fact that there are things we shouldn't do. Because we are getting away with things – we aren't stopping to appreciate what is going on and make changes. If we eat good things and live a user-friendly lifestyle and take exercise and tune-up the organs and functions of the body, our energy levels respond – we have available energy. It isn't compromised by having to deal with too many, extra, imposed demands – which we may have been making without even knowing it. And this is extra energy physically and mentally. Energy is a key component in feeling good.

Have less aches and pains

Less backaches, headaches and migraines and joint pains; this is explained in the sections on nutrition, digestion, toxins and elimination. Good diet provides good nutrients and doesn't leave disproportionate amounts of debris and gunk behind. Poor diet and processed foods are a challenge to digestion, they don't have as much goodness, they take a lot out of the system, it takes a lot of energy to deal with them and many of them will leave a gluey, mucousy gunk and often toxins as well. The body has to remove toxins from the blood stream and the internal environment and the safest place to store unwanted toxins can be in fat and muscle tissue. This can make fat tissue harder to lose and causes aches, pain and inflammation in muscle tissue. Exercise will keep the cardio-vascular system and circulation strong to carry toxins away. Sufficient water will also help the cells of organs, muscles and tissues to work well and aid elimination – avoiding dehydration can significantly reduce pains, typically headaches. Fitness will keep the muscles strong to support limbs and joints and avoid aches and pain.

Sleep better

You allow your body the time and conditions it needs to rest and repair and health and fitness allow that body clock to work as it should. There is a dedicated section on Sleep.

Have improved circulation and fitness

Everything is working better. Cells and tissues are nourished and hydrated. You have more energy. Eating a good diet looks after your blood and your veins and your heart, improving circulation and mobility. Good foods help maintain the right acid/alkali levels for your blood and don't thicken the blood, adversely affecting blood pressure, clotting and valves. Healthy blood is less likely to leave fatty or calcium deposits in the veins and arteries. Good circulation helps fitness and fitness helps good circulation.

Look better

Being well and healthy shows in your skin, eyes, hair, teeth, nails, posture, fitness and energy – you can see this and so do other people – and it's all to do with the body and the organs and the systems and the cells having the required nutrients.

Improved self-esteem and confidence

You are feeling and looking better – benefiting physically, mentally and emotionally. The nutrients in our food also support our mood and emotional health. Lack or imbalance of vitamins and minerals can directly affect how we feel.

Increased or enhanced ability – physically and mentally

Improved cardio-vascular function, the heart, the blood supply and respiration.

We depend on that blood and oxygen supply through the body and the right food and exercise looks after our blood vessels and enables that transport and distribution network. The right combinations of proteins, carbohydrates, fats and oils - the ones we hear so much about, the essential fatty acids, omegas 3, 6 and 9 – maintain the health of the cells and the cell membranes allowing absorption and secretion, vital to how we perform. The correct nutrients support the production and activity of the hormones that enable us to perform well and influence our moods and ability.

Being well and healthy will have distinct benefits, in and outside work

Operating better has a direct effect on relationships with other people - relationships with work colleagues and personal and social colleagues, friends and partners. We are feeling and looking better - giving off a noticeable, bright, feel-good factor. We'll be one of those people people want to be with, take notice of. In a work situation it definitely helps command respect, up and down hierarchy. People who look after themselves are often respected, popular friends, respected bosses and respected team members, respected partners, parents and children.

Body working better – brain and mind working better

They aren't separate systems, they are intricately connected. They are dependent on each other. Our brain is like a muscle - it needs nutrition, exercise and relaxation - it needs looking after. We are supporting our physical, mental and emotional health and performance. Developing good energy levels and good sleep patterns, increasing our ability to cope and have less distractions, will affect our focus, concentration, mental ability and memory. All these systems work on a chemical, electrical and cellular level - managed by health and nutrition.

Manage better

Managing our health, our body, our life is part of our management skills - it is part of how we manage generally. We manage time, we manage people, we manage money and we manage our health. Managing is taking responsibility - responsibility for how we are, what we do. If we feel better, have more energy, have improved circulation and fitness, enhanced physical and mental ability, we will manage better and manage the people and things we are responsible for better.

Better communication

The better we are functioning the less impaired we are likely to be by tiredness, pain, difficulty in concentration - all the things that can affect how we come over to other people. We are often not concentrating properly on other people, even when we think we are - if at some level we may be distracted by a headache, backache, heartburn, tiredness or stress. We may not be paying the right attention or giving the right consideration to listening and speaking. Communication skills depend on listening and interpreting information and we can directly improve our health and ability to do that. We are nourishing our brain and all the hundreds of different neurological pathways which process information.

Improved leadership skills

So if you feel better, have more energy, sleep better, have improved circulation and fitness, look better, relate with people better, manage better, command more respect, communicate better - think was this will do for leadership skills. Leadership skills are communication, management, thinking, commanding respect, setting an example.

Work Life Body is about being as well as you can - if you want to.

One of the Doctors I particularly admire who speaks on health and nutrition, is Dr Paul Clayton and a quote from some of his work is:

> *'Underpinning all my research and advice is this simple fact. Given the right nutrition and lifestyle, our bodies have amazing powers of self-healing and regeneration.*
>
> *'They have to - because almost every cell and tissue in your body breaks down and is replaced on a regular basis. Bone is re-absorbed into the body and then renewed, cartilage in joints experiences wear and tear but is renewed, membranes of nerve and other cells are broken down and replaced.'*

Dr Paul Clayton graduated summa cum laude in Medical Pharmacology from Edinburgh University, prior to obtaining his PhD. He is Fellow and former President of the Forum on Food & Health of the Royal Society of Medicine, FRSA, and a former Senior Scientific Advisor to the UK government's Committee on the Safety of Medicine. He has worked with leading doctors and clinical scientists at centres of clinical expertise in the UK and abroad, and trained the pharmacists in Britain's largest chemist chain in preventative nutrition. Dr Clayton frequently presents at and chairs international conferences on nutrition and health. He is a Visiting Fellow at Oxford Brookes University, and chair of the scientific advisory boards of BiotheraPharma (USA) and Itogha (Norway). He is also Technical Director of the Szent-Gyorgyi Instititute of Clinical Pharmaconutrition (Hungary).

What is health?

There are lots of definitions of health:

the absence of disease
the absence of any symptoms or pain
being in optimum condition
being completely well
feeling full of vitality and energy
being able to take on all moderate physical tasks without discomfort
good appetite
going to sleep and waking easily
good humour and moods
ease in thought and action.

Most people would like to be completely well, many would be prepared to settle for a lot less as they may not think health is achievable. Others may be living with a disability that causes pain. For everyone there is an optimum state of health and in many cases it could be better than it currently is.

As an example of everyday health, remember the idea of a working week without headaches, migraines, backpain, tiredness, lack of energy, concentration and memory problems, colds or flu. For some people that would be normal – many other people have come to accept their headaches or backpain or tiredness or recurring colds as normal.

The 'normal' weekly stats of painkillers and anti-inflammatories taken is frightening.

Understanding more about how the body works and how different things will have different effects on our health, allows us to have greater choice in how healthy we want to be.

Some factors we have some control over and some we do not.

Eating well, taking exercise, good posture, good social skills and social framework and a good psychological outlook will all contribute enormously to good health – and we really need a combination of all of these, as they all work together. Any one of these factors will positively improve our health – but by combining all of them or as many of them as we can – the benefits are even greater. This sort of good health is feeling good, looking good, having enough or more than enough energy and mental ability.

Equally, if one of those aspects of health declines – it can easily come to affect our overall health.

On a physical level lack of exercise, pollution, poor diet, poor posture, dysfunctional breathing, stressful lifestyle, rushed meals, lack of sleep, smoking, excess alcohol, poor housing conditions, chemicals in the home and the natural environment, all compromise our body's ability to regulate itself. We do have control over many of these factors and this is where we can make the most difference.

On a mental level, lack of stimulus, lack of social framework, personal or work-related stress, divorce, bereavement and depression, can all adversely affect health. Many of these we cannot help occurring but we can adopt healthy ways of dealing with them – and we can try and keep ourselves in the best shape to be able to deal with them. Managing emotions and mental health is a helpful and practical way of overcoming some side-effects and preventing these developing into longer-term and more serious conditions.

We can also inherit a predisposition to ill health. Inherited weaknesses from our parents and grandparents and beyond can influence how well we are. We cannot change our parents or our genes but we can look after ourselves so that latent or potential problems have less opportunity to manifest themselves.

All of these factors affect the immune system throughout the body and metabolism at cell level, influencing our ability to regulate and repair.

There are more than 45 known nutrients that are essential to health and it can be possible to be deficient in many at once so it is easy to see the effect this can have on overall health.

The immune system

The immune system does not just fight bacteria and viruses, it plays a huge role in both clearing rubbish from the tissues and helping tissues and organs repair themselves. It is one of the most complex systems in the human body. Cell metabolism provides the energy necessary for this to happen and mostly takes place in small power stations in each cell[1]. If these are damaged or do not have enough nutrients, there is not sufficient energy to power the immune system. Ensuring sufficient nutrients and looking after our bodies will play a major part in good health.

If alerted the immune system can produce a million anti-bodies a minute to identify and overcome an attack from invaders (antigens). A strong immune system is the difference between a cold being 24 hours or 1 week+, a one-off occasional occurrence or a recurring nuisance; or a minor, short-term, stomach bug and serious food poisoning.

Exercise, state of mind and what we eat, all affect our immune system. They are all part of the body's information and messaging system that runs the show. Over-exercise and arduous training can deplete the immune system and endurance athletes and explorers have to monitor and compensate for this. Positive mental and physical exercise, especially those focusing and harnessing the mind and body – can increase the T-cells of the immune system by around 40%.[2]

Main points of entry into the body are the GI (gastro-intestinal) tract where things come in from the outside via food and drink; the lungs where things come in from the outside via the air we breathe and the skin where we absorb things from the external environment or can become injured.

Healthy, strong, mucous membranes of the GI and respiratory tracts and healthy skin are front lines of defence.

All the time we have some immune cells roaming the body. When an invader is identified more immune cells are produced in the bone marrow and the thymus and posted out to the lymph nodes, the tonsils, the appendix, the spleen and patches in the GI tract. That's why lymph nodes in the neck, armpits and groin can become inflamed during infection. Lymph doesn't have a pump in the body, it makes its way round the body relying on our physical activity, it is moved by the movement of the muscles – so

[1] mitochondria

[2] eg: t'ai chi, yoga and Pilates and many more and you can create your own version at home – smooth, positive movement and focus.

inactivity significantly reduces the ability of our lymphatic system and lymphatic drainage.

The immune system is completely dependent on the adequate intake of vitamins and minerals. The nutrients in our food are used to create our immune system armies: T-cells, T-helpers, T-suppressors, macrophages and NK (Natural Killer) cells. It is dependent on food for: vitamins C, E, A, B1, B2, B6, B12, folic acid, zinc, magnesium, selenium, manganese and copper – to name a few! These ingredients need to be in balance, excesses can stop the system working properly. Beware of self-diagnosis – it's quite a complicated business. All we have to do is eat a great variety of great food. If we do think there are problems, for any reason, seek professional, qualified advice.

Bacteria also have a key role in our immune system – on the inside as well as the outside. Our good bacteria, probiotics, produce lactic acid and hydrogen peroxide which are natural anti-biotics. They stop bad bacteria growing and make it difficult for them to survive. They are important in overpowering bad bacteria and they boost the immune system.

Development of disease depends on 3 factors:
genetic predisposition, environmental influences and a trigger.

Genetic predisposition is now well studied and becoming increasingly understood. This includes inherited illnesses and problems that run in families.

Environmental factors are the nutritional status of the individual, the amount of exposure to the bacteria/virus/fungus/toxin (antigen) and the state of regulatory capacity of the patient, the immune system. Environmental toxins are also possible threats, such as, heavy metals, asbestos, various chemicals and solvents.

Triggers for immune dysfunction could be periods of prolonged stress, viral diseases, or an extra chemical load.

The immune cells the body produces for fighting infection are generally white blood cells, including lymphocytes, leucocytes, monocytes and macrophages. These cells are concentrated primarily in immune locations like lymph nodes, the spleen, thymus, tonsils, the gut and appendix but are present throughout the body.

Anything that is not part of the healthy body has to be dealt with and eliminated or a disease may develop. This includes by-products of our metabolism and digestive processes, some of which are quite toxic, an example of which is ammonia produced from the breakdown of proteins. It also includes cells that have been damaged and are even cancerous, these are destroyed by lymphocyte type cells called Natural Killer cells. Every day even the healthiest person can produce cancerous cells and not develop cancer whilst the immune system can produce NK cells and get rid of the cancer cells. The liver, which has the job of detoxifying poisons, is also part of this system.

The immune system operates on a state of alert and depends on challenges to keep it primed and in working order. Whereas we need to keep ourselves clean and avoid serious contamination, over-sanitized lifestyles and sterile environments can reduce our immune system's ability to function - we need a few bugs so that we remember what to do.

We can also view the immune system as a caretaker, keeping everything clean and organized and in working order and noticing when parts need repairing. Many repair processes take place at night and are affected by our hormones. If these hormones are out of balance we may not sleep well at night and the repair processes are compromised. Sleep plays a big part in immunity. This is why we need to sleep or rest when we are ill to give the body the chance to recover properly. We will generally recover more quickly from illnesses if we do rest and the immune system will come through stronger to fight another day. If you do work through an illness, still try to take as much rest as you can and give your immune system the rest it needs as soon as you can. Incomplete recovery, especially on a repeated basis, if you run your immune system down, may eventually lead to a lot more time off which isn't good for you or your work. There's two parts to recovery, being better yourself and giving the system chance to top up. Feeling OK doesn't necessarily mean you've recuperated - so try and gauge yourself whether you should be going full tilt or reigning back. Being well and adequate recovery will usually mean you work better and have less time off.

Many bacteria and viruses we face are much the same as they were for our ancestors from an immune perspective but our immune systems have faced a significant challenge from the new lifestyles, man-made toxins and chemicals it is presented with now. We have invented thousands of new chemicals and put them into the air and onto our food. This puts extra pressure on the immune system and in some cases it can become overloaded or disrupted as some of the toxins will block or interfere with immune reactions. The immune system is constantly evolving and finding ways of coping but the scale of the changes over the last 100-200 years would be a challenge for any system.

The immune system needs to be supported by giving it all the nutrients it needs and by cutting down exposure to as many toxic chemicals as possible. We can help with this by being selective about the food we eat and the chemicals we use around the home and on the skin in our cosmetics, soaps, shampoos and bathroom kit.

The ideal diet for the immune system is, strangely enough, the ideal diet for everything else; sufficient protein - but not too much which would suppress the system; and good EFAs (essential fatty acids) boost the immune system. Saturated or hydrogenated fats suppress it and clog up the lymphatic vessels.

Well-balanced, good, natural foods:
seeds, nuts, fruit, veg, pulses, wholegrains, fish, garlic.

Try and eat as great a variety as possible, especially seasonal produce - and including some raw items if you can. Cook other items as lightly as possible to retain vitamins and minerals and some crunch.

Our immune system is our defence and protector in maintaining good health. It needs looking after to do its job properly.

Anatomy and Physiology

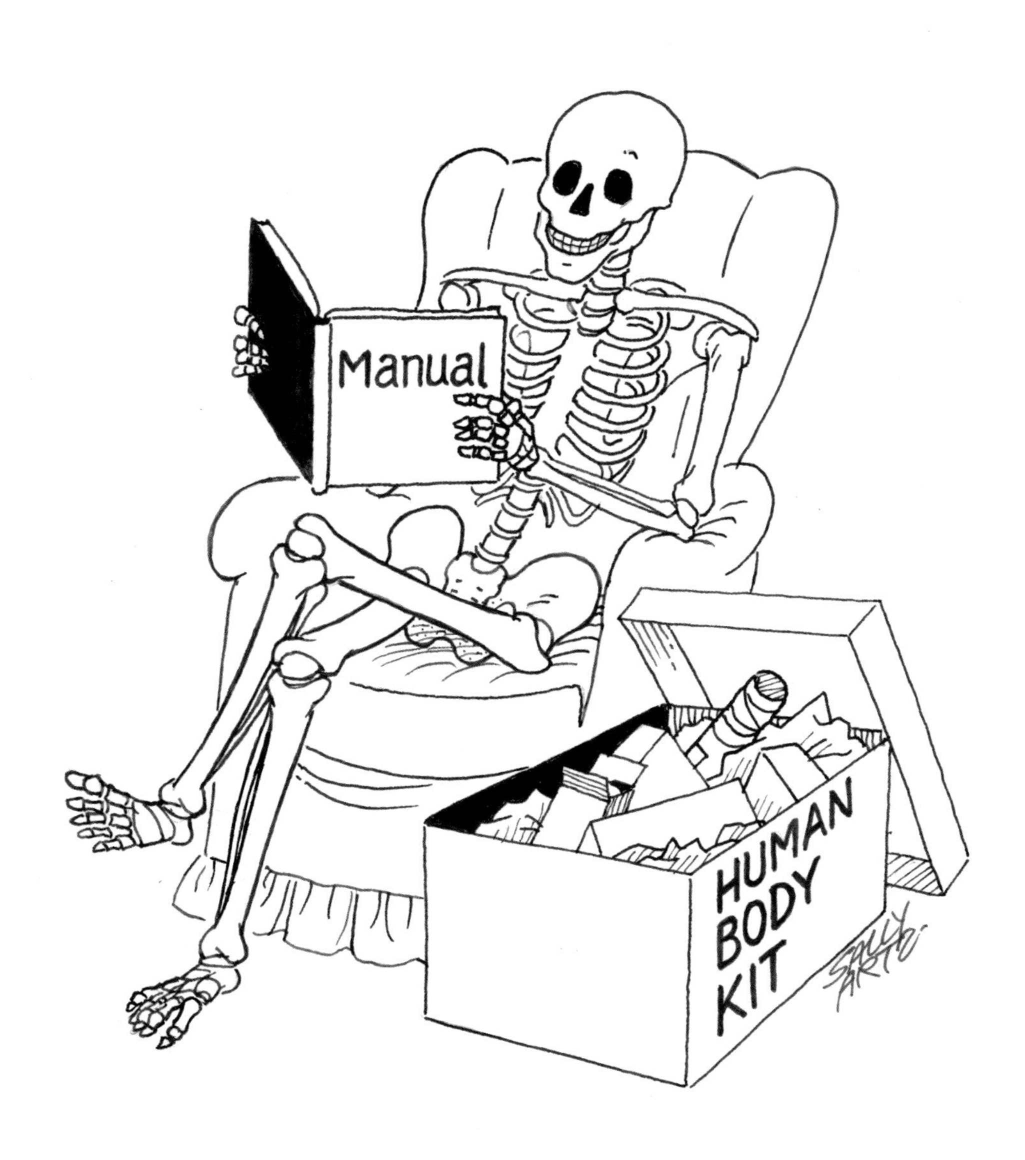
Manual
HUMAN
BODY
KIT

The Brain

The brain is our 'control centre'.
It is where our mind is and it is where control over the body comes from.

The brain is made up of a mass of nerve cells that control the body in two ways. The Central Nervous System (CNS) allows us to make muscular movements and to process visual information and the Autonomic Nervous System (ANS) which is primarily concerned with maintaining a stable internal environment. All the descriptions you have heard of the brain are probably the best we can do – a lovely dollop of spaghetti and a firework show – the spaces being as important as the substantial tissue.

The brain governs functions that are not otherwise under our control, such as breathing, digestion, temperature regulation, heart rate, etc – plus motor functions, consciousness, language, thought-processing, emotions and memory. It is constantly processing millions and millions of messages, so that we and our bodies know what to do.

It is one of the largest organs in an adult, consisting of around 100 billion neurons (brain cells) and 900 billion glia (packing material, means 'glue'), 900 billion is 9 times

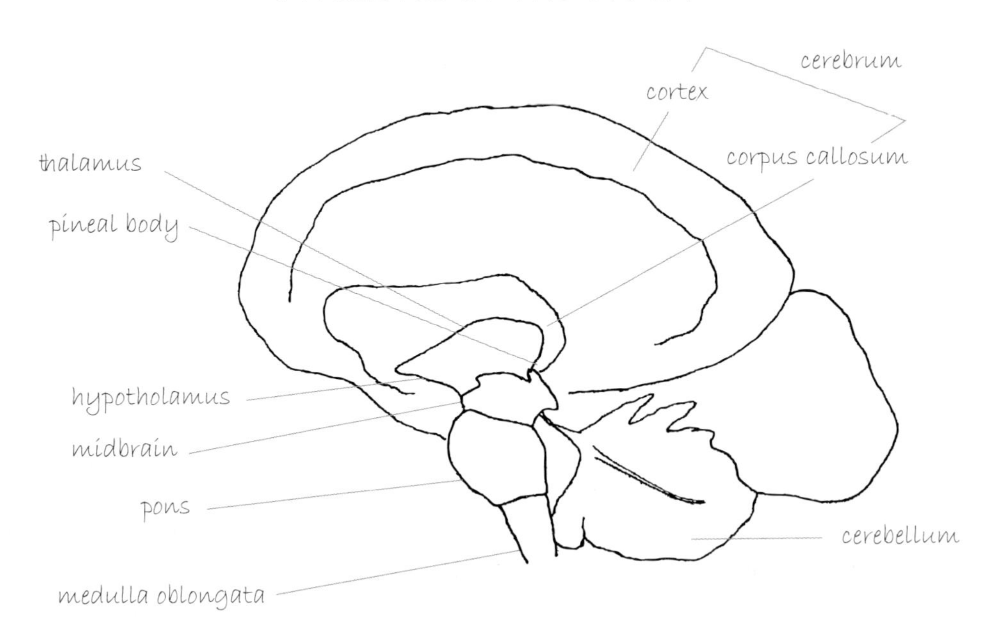

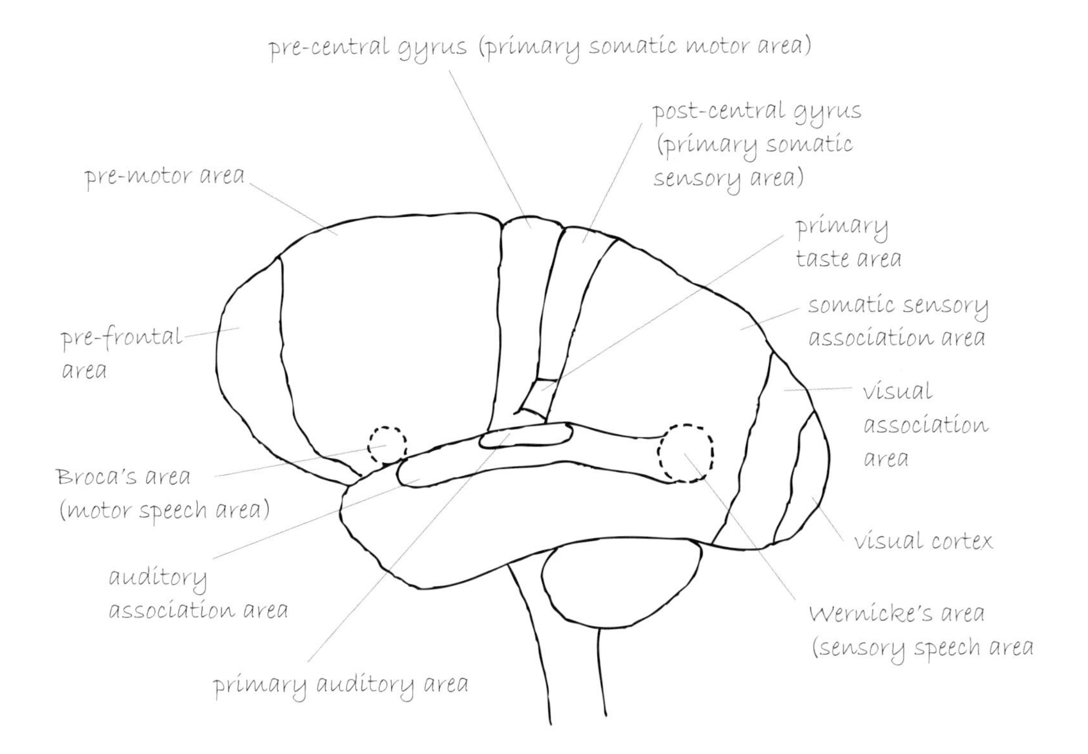

the number of stars in the galaxy. The brain weighs approx 1.4kg (3lbs). It grows very rapidly for the first 9 years and then more slowly until full size at approximately 18 years.

The other major substance in the brain is fat. Every nerve cell is coated with a layer of fat (called the myelin sheath). Nerve cells conduct electrical messages like electric cables. The nerves, like the cables, have to be insulated or electrical impulses would jump or short from one nerve to another causing random patterns of firing – and chaos. The insulation on nerve cells is fat – but not just any fat – it is composed of essential fatty acids – such as the ones found in nuts, seeds and fish. This is why we often hear of the importance of Omega 3 oils and oily fish in connection with brain food and brain health.

The brain is about 85% water and is very sensitive to dehydration. Alcohol, for instance, acts as a diuretic – meaning it results in you losing more liquid than you've taken in. A hangover is largely due to lack of water in the brain and the best cure for a hangover is to drink lots of water – as close to the consumption of the alcohol as possible. Hours later, after sleeping for example, won't be as successful because the brain cells have been dehydrated all that time and rehydrating them will take longer to be effective. Other dehydrators are tea and coffee. Anyone suffering from regular or daily headaches may be able to put that right, or find significant improvements, simply by drinking more water, and/or less coffee or tea.

The brain uses 30% of all energy produced in the body. In order to use that energy, it needs nutrients – vitamins and minerals, making it one of the highest users of nutrients of any of the organs of the body. So, when there is a shortage of nutrients in the diet the result may be headaches, lack of concentration, memory lapses, irritability, depression and behavioural problems.

The brain is held suspended in cerebrospinal fluid, around the brain, spinal cord and within the cavities and canals of the spinal cord and the brain. The brain is such an essential organ it is very heavily protected by the skull, tough muscular tissue and the fluid surrounding the brain. If exposed to too high trauma or impact, as we know, damage can be severe as demonstrated in accidents and injuries, such as road accidents, sports accidents and injuries from violence.

Possible causes of brain damage also include pre-natal infections, mechanical trauma to the head during or after birth, nerve-damaging poisons and reduced oxygen supply. Damage to brain tissue can cause cerebral palsy, spastic paralysis, hemiplegia, paraplegia, triplegia and quadriplegia. A common example of the destruction of neurons in the motor area of the brain is a CVA (cerebrovascular accident) or stroke – a haemorrhage from or cessation of blood flow through the blood vessels in the brain, this disrupts the oxygen supply and stops the functioning of the neurons, sometimes causing the death of the neurons.

The list of brain associated conditions is unpleasantly long: Dementia – including Alzheimer's Disease, Parkinson's Disease, Huntington Disease, epilepsy, stroke, paralysis, cerebral palsy, encephalitis, meningitis and more.

The brain is literally fantastic and still continues to flaberghast the most revered scientists, researchers and doctors. It is way beyond our real understanding – with far more performance, power and ability than any computer. It is the most complicated, intricate and delicate structure we can possibly imagine.

So, the brain is our control centre, in charge of many functions. A dollop of spaghetti and a firework show of nerves, neurons, glia and fluid. Highly developed. Uses 30% of the energy of the body and composed 85% of water. It requires vital nutrients like all the other organs, tissues and systems of the body.

A NEURON (brain cell)

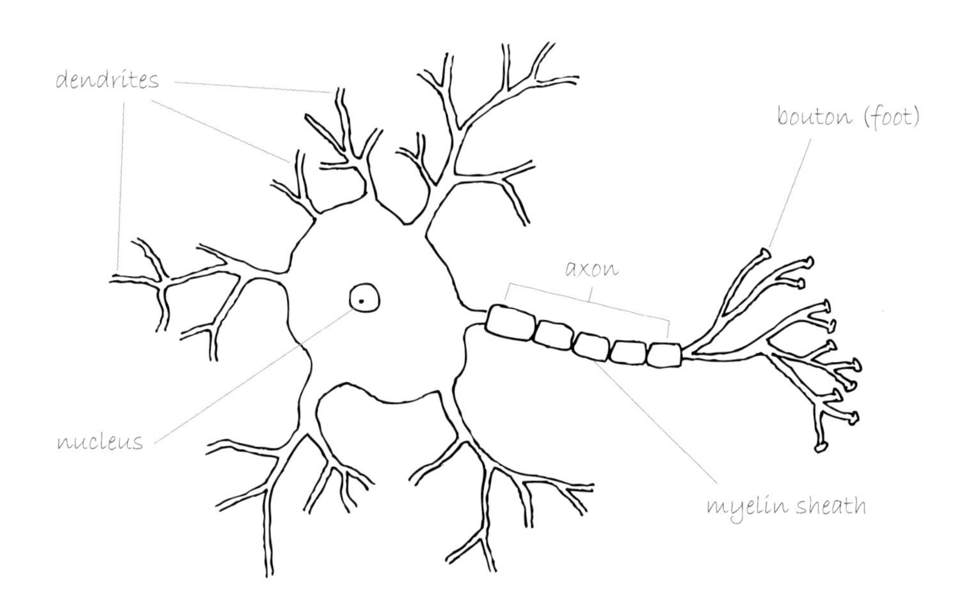

A SYNAPSE

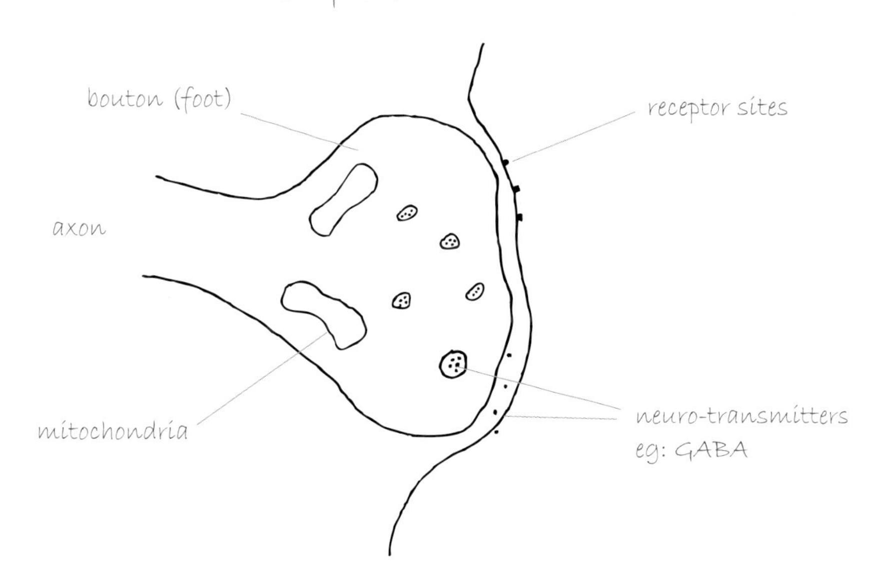

The complexity of the world's entire telephone systems is equivalent to a part of your brain the size of a garden pea. John Townsend

University of Toronto – Department of Nutritional Sciences
Nutrition and Brain Function / Behaviour
Research in this area examines the susceptibility of brain to fluctuations in nutrient intake, with changes in both brain metabolic processes and behaviour as outcome measures. Studies encompass various stages of lifespan, ranging from paediatrics to geriatrics and involve diverse outcomes including cognitive function, mood disorders, appetite regulation and susceptibility to neurodegenerative disorders.

According to Professor Mark Rosenweig:
the myth that brain power declines with age has been exploded.

- If the brain is stimulated NO MATTER AT WHAT AGE new protuberances will grow on each brain cell's tentacles and increase the total number of possible connections.

- Some of the world's most creative men have been exceptionally prolific at advanced ages; Gaugin, Michelangelo, Haydn, Picasso.

- We generate new brain connections more rapidly than the average loss of brain cells. Even if we lose 10,000 brain cells a day from birth, the total number lost at age 80 would be less than 3%.

THE BRAIN IS A WONDERFUL ORGAN.
IT STARTS WORKING THE MOMENT YOU GET UP
IN THE MORNING AND DOESN'T STOP UNTIL
YOU GET INTO THE OFFICE.

Robert Frost

BRAINS – LEFT AND RIGHT

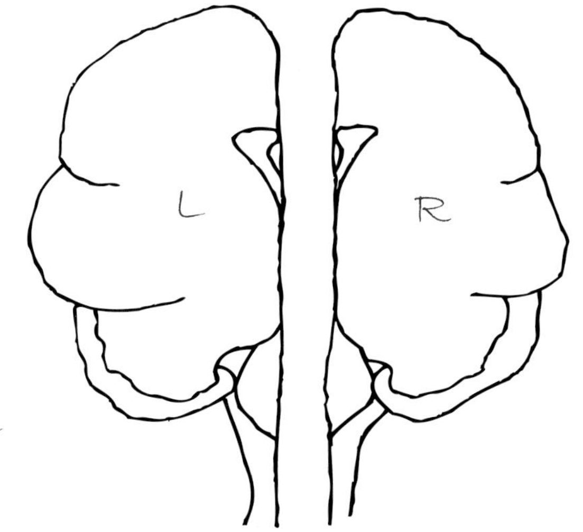

Speech
Calculations
Intellectual analysis
Reading
Writing
Naming
Ordering
Sequencing
Complex motor sequences
Critique
Evaluation
Logic

Artistic activity
Musical ability / rhythm
Emotions
Recognition
Comprehension
Perception of abstract patterns
Spatial abilities
Facial expressions
Holistic ability
Intuition
Creativity
Images
Colour

STRUCTURE OF MAMMALIAN HEART

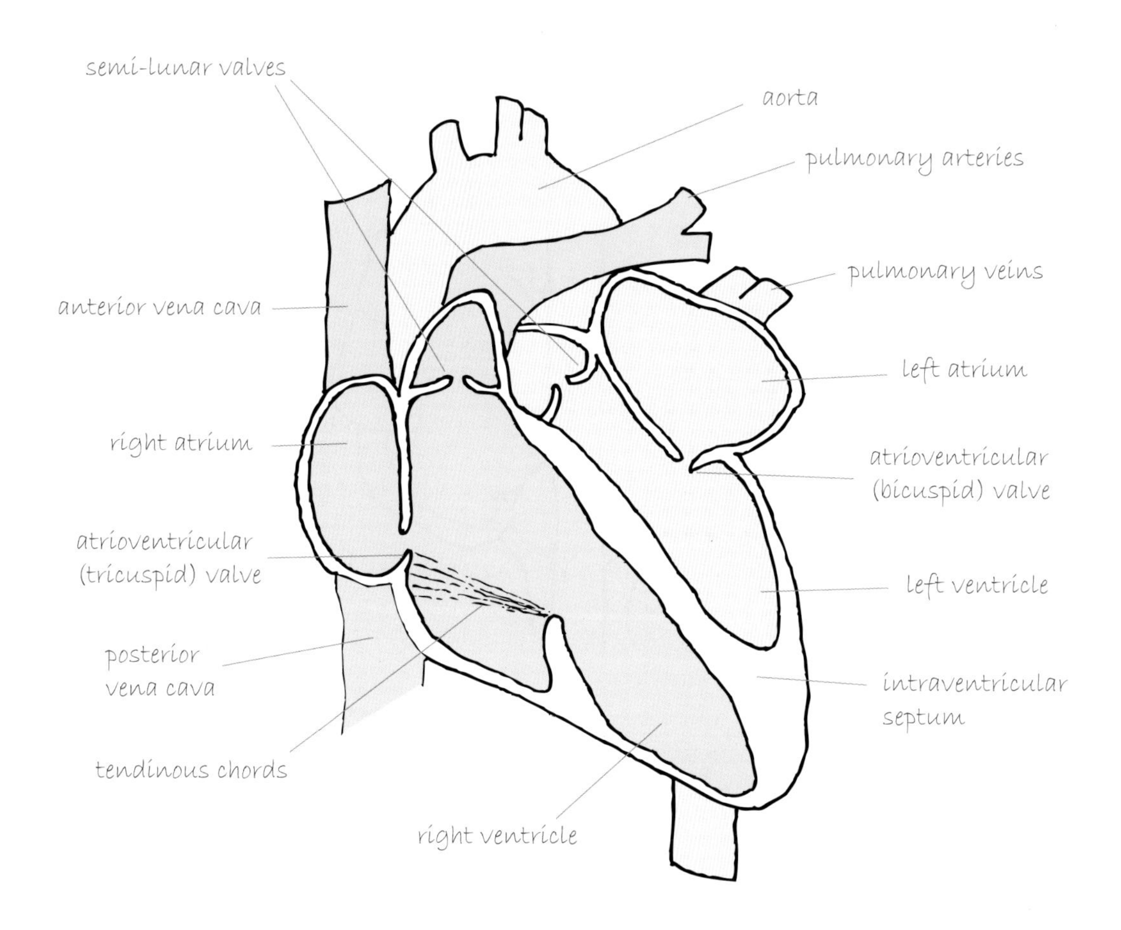

The Heart

The heart is effectively a pump which moves blood around the body. It is almost all muscle tissue and is the strongest muscle in the body. The heart beats very regularly more than 115,000 times a day. It needs a good supply of oxygen and glucose to provide the necessary energy for it to work well. Small amounts of micronutrients such as magnesium and zinc are also vital for a healthy heart.

The structure of the heart consists of:

- the pericardium – the fibrous sac around the heart
- the heart wall – the epicardium, the outer layer, which is muscle
  – the myocardium, the middle, substantial layer of wall, which is muscle
  – the endocardium, the inner layer, of delicate scale-like tissue
- 4 chambers – 2 atria, the superior (upper) chambers receiving blood from veins
  – 2 ventricles, the lower chambers, passing blood to the arteries
- valves – atrioventricular valves, allowing blood flow from the atria to the ventricles
  – semilunar valves, preventing backflow from aorta to ventricles
- the heart skeleton – a fibrous structure of rings supporting valves and cardiac muscle.

The **pericardium** protects and cushions the heart, it is made of tough, white, fibrous tissue, lined with smooth, moist membrane.

The wall of the heart is made of the specific layers.

The **epicardium**, the outer layer of the heart wall.

The **myocardium** is a layer of specially constructed and arranged cardiac muscle cells, composed of endless branching cells, joined into a continuous mass, held together by rings or discs. Each join, or disc, includes gaps and the join is held, or made, electrically – combining the expansive muscle tissue into a single, functioning mass. The cells pass desired actions around the whole wall of the heart, eg: contractions – and because the whole wall of the heart can operate as one, as a single, encompassing wrapping, it can apply great force to the cavities, vessels and blood within the heart itself (like your hand around a squeeze ball).

The **endocardium** is the inside layer. It is a very fine, delicate layer of tissue, made of scale like cells which form continuous sheets of tissue that contain no blood vessels. The endocardium coats projections of the myocardial wall, some of which create the major valves involved in regulating blood flow through the heart.

The Chambers of the Heart

The heart has 2 sides, separated by a muscular **septum**. The right side passes de-oxygenated blood to the lungs. The left side passes oxygenated blood to the rest of the body.

Both sides have 2 chambers. The upper chamber on each side is the **atrium**, they receive/collect blood from the veins. The lower chamber on each side is the **ventricle**, they force blood into the arteries.

The atria and ventricles on each side of the heart are separated by valves (atrioventricular valves). These work by allowing in-flowing blood through in the correct/desired direction, because the blood flow itself pushes the flaps flat against the walls of the blood vessel (see below).

Blood Flow

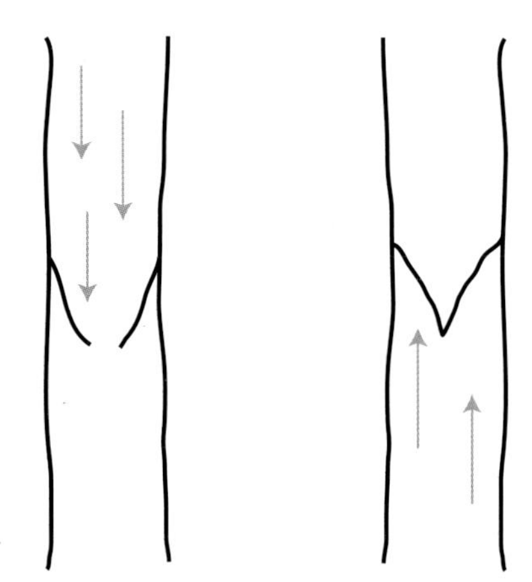

When the ventricle contracts - with the normal rhythmic beating/pumping of the heart - the blood could flow back from the ventricle to the aorta but because it is going against the direction of the flaps of the valves, it causes the flaps to fill and close, until the next pump back in the normal circulation direction causes them to open again.

In the lining of the pulmonary artery and aorta there are also semilunar valves - small, protruding flaps. Mechanically they work in the same way as the atrioventricular valves, allowing blood flow in one direction - from the ventricles to the aorta and pulmonary artery and preventing it in the other direction – from the aorta and pulmonary artery into the ventricles.

The **skeleton of the heart** is made up of fibrous twists of tissue – a bit like skeins of fine, strong yarn – which twist round and hold and support the different areas of the heart, especially the valves, it also provides an electrical barrier between the wall of the atria and the wall of the ventricles.

So, the heart is a pump which moves blood around the body. It is almost all muscle tissue and is the strongest muscle in the body. It has 4 chambers and various valves. The heart beats very regularly more than 115,000 times a day or 70 times a minute. It requires vital nutrients, like all the other organs, systems and tissues of the body.

Additional note:

In the cardiac field of work, cardiologist Dr Dean Ornish has shown that support programmes offering a combination of healthy diet, exercise, stress reduction and emotional support reversed coronary artery disease. The emotional support and emotional expression were as effective as the other physiological interventions.

MAMMALIAN BLOOD CIRCULATORY SYSTEM

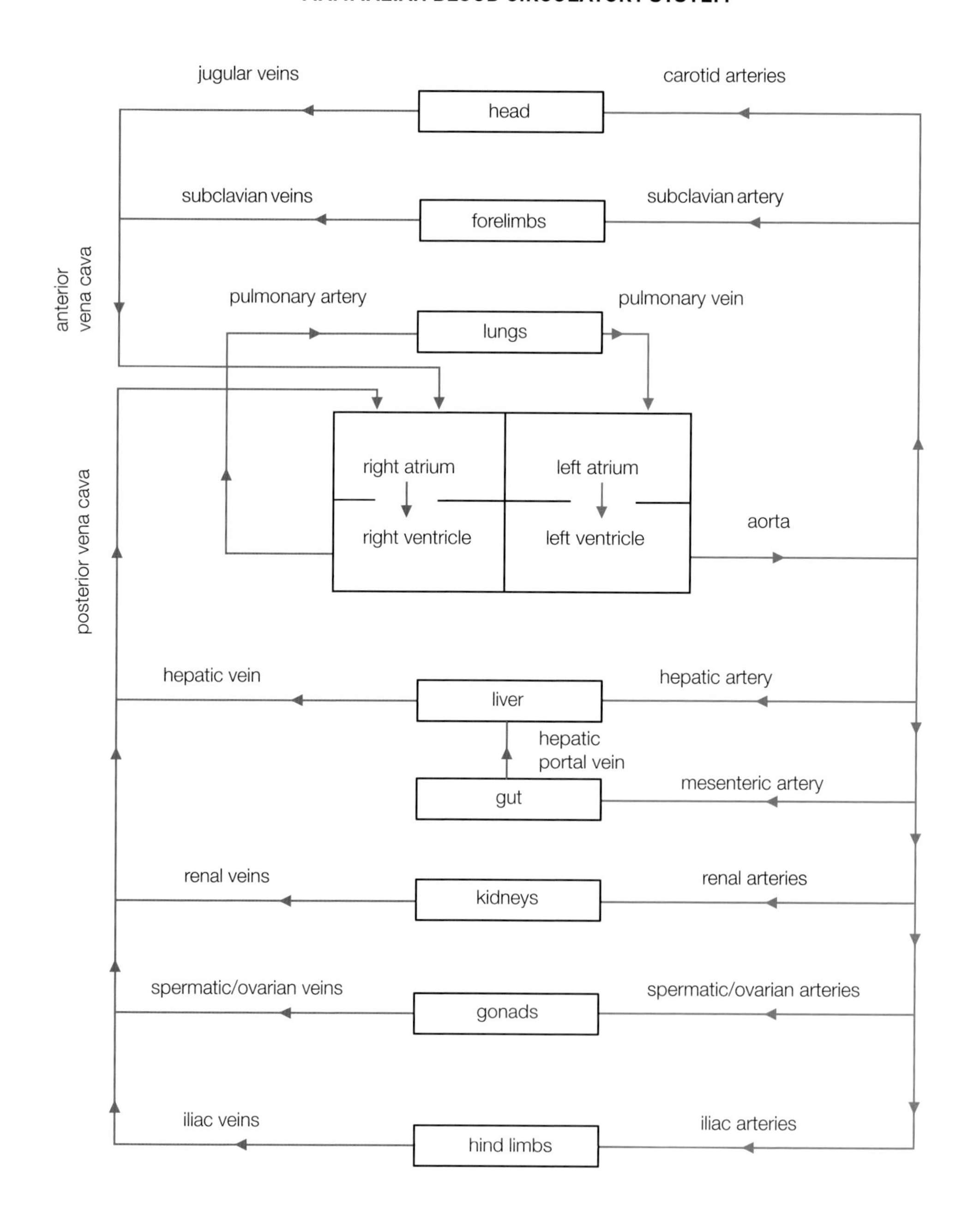

The Lungs

We have two lungs that fill most of the chest cavity and surround the heart. The wind pipe or trachea leads down from the mouth and nose, branches into two 'bronchi' and into the two lungs.

The bronchi then divide again and separate further and further into an extensive network of tiny, tiny delicate airways and then into tiny air sacs called alveoli. The fine network of respiratory airways is surrounded by very fine networks of tiny blood vessels called capillaries and it is where these very fine vessels lie against each other that oxygen can pass from the airways into the blood to be used throughout the body – and carbon dioxide from the blood can pass back into the airways to be carried away and exhaled.

Oxygen is needed by the body to 'burn' glucose to produce energy just like a fire needs to have air to burn. The by-product of the burning process is carbon dioxide which is a waste gas and must be eliminated, so it is released from the blood into the lungs and breathed out.

In normal circumstances air is drawn into the lungs by the downward movement of the diaphragm which swells the abdomen. Air is released and pushed out of the lungs when the abdominal muscles contract making the chest cavity smaller. When we are stressed, by nervous or psychological pressure or by physical exertion, air is drawn into the lungs by movement of the chest cavity, which produces shallow breathing. This is less efficient in the long term and leads to lack of oxygen in the cells of the body. Trained singers, actors, narrators and public speakers who need good breath control are taught to breathe from lower in the abdomen.

The airways are very fine and delicate and easily affected by contaminants or excess mucous or moisture.

The nostrils and mouth are adapted to filter and warm the air we breathe in before it reaches our bronchi and lungs. The voicebox (larynx) is at the top of the trachea.

'Normal' breathing is approximately 15 complete respiratory cycles per minute.

Our breathing can be influenced by:

- physical activity
- speech and singing
- emotional activity – crying, laughing, fear
- drugs – eg: sedatives, alcohol
- sleep.

So, the lungs permit the distribution of air and the elimination of respiratory gases. They require vital nutrients like all the other organs, tissues and systems of the body.

Additional note:

40 or so years ago the text books used to say that if you could unravel the lungs and spread them out, they would cover the area of a tennis court, it may even have been two tennis courts. The books don't seem to say this any longer - but it is a very useful way to think of how extensive and fine the network of tiny airways is.

The Liver

The liver is the largest organ, or gland, of the body.
It weighs approx 3-4 lbs, that is 1.5 kg.
It has two main lobes separated by a ligament.
The right lobe is the very large lobe, it is approximately five sixths of the overall liver, and the left lobe is one sixth.

Vessels, tissues and cells of the liver are called hepatic; 'hepat' means liver.

The liver is one of the most complex organs of the body and has the only tissue that can regenerate. Where surgery is necessary, if half the liver was removed, the remaining half can re-grow in 6 months – (if it is well, not if it's not).

The liver is just below the diaphragm on the right side but towards the centre of the body.

The right lobe consists of:

- the right lobe proper
- the caudate lobe
- the quadrate lobe.

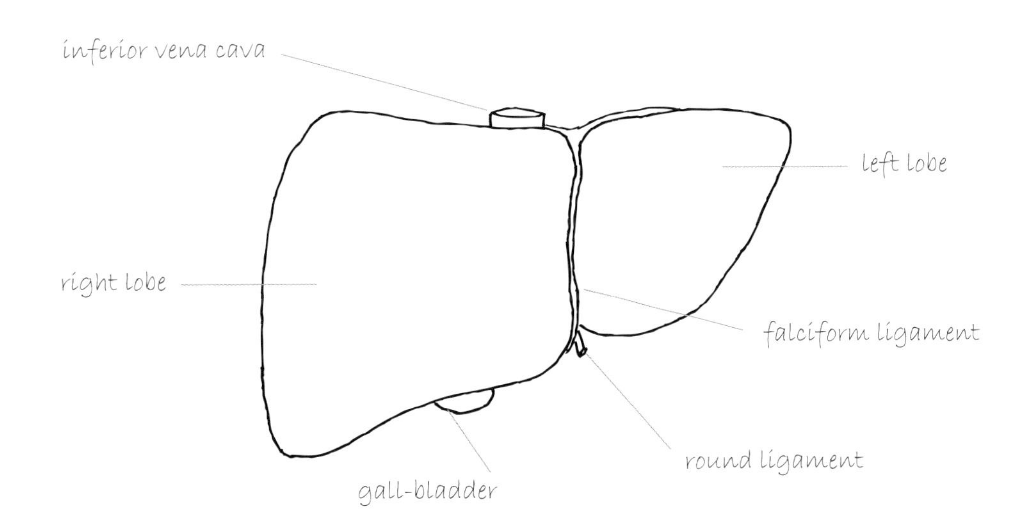

Each lobe is made up of lobules. The lobules are tiny shapes (hexagonal or pentagonal prisms) about 2mm high x 1mm in diameter. A small vein (hepatic vein) runs through each lobule and the vein is surrounded by cells (hepatic cells).

From each lobule there are:

- branches of hepatic artery
- branches of portal vein - interlobular veins
- branches of hepatic duct - interlobular bile ducts.

From those - branches of interlobular veins run between the hepatic cells to the central vein.

Blood enters the lobule from the hepatic artery and portal vein. The arterial blood oxygenates the hepatic cells. The blood from the portal vein goes to the liver to be quality-checked, for cleansing, detoxification and filtering. In the branches of veins running between hepatic cells (sinusoids) there are phagocytic cells that can remove bacteria, old red cells and other particles.

THE LIVER - inferior view (from the back)

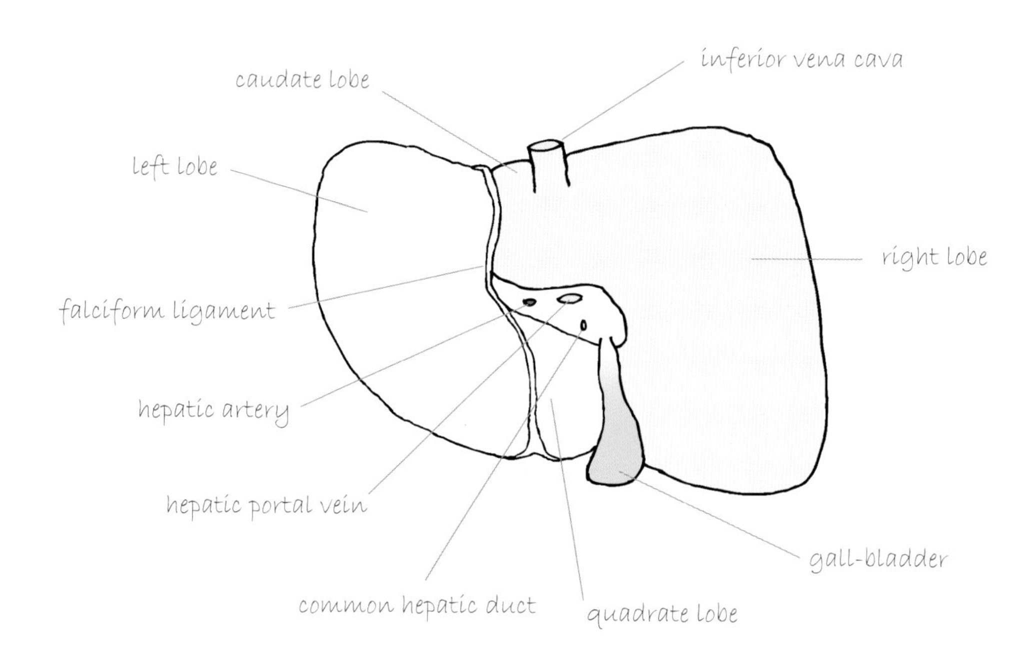

Vitamins, minerals and nutrients to be stored or metabolized[1] (used or chemically changed in order to be used) by the liver, enter the hepatic cells. The body uses nutrients in 2 main ways; as an energy source and as building blocks for making more complex chemical compounds. Before they can be used they have to be assimilated, ie: changed/prepared.

Toxins from the blood are also taken into the hepatic cells and detoxified.

The blood flow continues to the vein at the centre of each lobule which leads to the main hepatic vein and into the vena cava.

Bile formed by the hepatic cells goes via vessels in the spaces around the cells[2] to the bile ducts.

The smaller network of bile ducts runs to two larger ducts - the right and left hepatic ducts - which then combine into one hepatic duct.

The hepatic duct from the liver and the cystic duct from the gall-bladder also merge and form the common bile duct which opens into the duodenum, 2-4 inches below the pyloric opening from the stomach.

The liver has many, many functions:

- to detoxify various substances
- to secrete bile (about 1 pint a day)
- to take part in metabolism of proteins, carbohydrates and fats
- to store substances, eg: iron, copper, vitamins A, B12, D, E, K, riboflavine, niacin, pyriodoxine, folic acid
- to produce plasma proteins and host blood cell production during foetal development
- to break down erythrocytes and defend against microbes
- to inactivate hormones, including insulin, glucagon, cortisol, aldosterone, thyroid and sex hormones
- to synthesize vitamin A from carotene, the provitamin in carrots and greens
- to produce heat: the liver uses a lot of energy and has a high metabolic rate, so produces a lot of heat - it is the main heat-producing organ of the body.

[1] metabolic actions/metabolism – the sum total of all the bio-chemical processes that keep the cells alive, all the structural and functional activity of all the organs and systems. A complex inter-twining set of chemical processes by which life is made possible for a living organism, ie: what is going on inside us, all the time. The continual breaking down and joining up of simple components to provide what is needed.

[2] canaliculi

To look at some of those functions more closely:

1 The liver is involved in carbohydrate metabolism by storing glucose which is an important energy source in the form of glycogen. The rate at which the liver releases glucose from glycogen stores helps to control blood sugar.
2 The liver is involved in protein metabolism by producing many blood proteins, including blood proteins needed for blood coagulation. It also breaks down small protein molecules called amino acids. This process releases ammonia as a by-product and ammonia is toxic so the liver turns it into urea to be excreted.
3 The liver is involved in fat metabolism by synthesizing cholesterol and triglycerides. The average diet may contain about 200-800mg of cholesterol but the liver regularly manufactures 2,000mg per day. (Cholesterol is essential throughout the body, for innumerable functions; healthy cell membranes including brain cells, synthesizing and modulating hormones, the nervous system, transport of substances between cells, reproduction and foetal development).
4 The liver forms bile and secretes bile pigments into the gall-bladder. These help with the digestion and absorption of fat.
5 When drugs have done their job, they need to be broken down and eliminated and this is something else done by the liver. It also detoxifies other poisons and breaks down steroid hormones. Poisoning of the liver is common because anything absorbed from the stomach is carried first to the liver, which therefore gets a higher concentration than other organs and is often damaged in the process of neutralising the poisons to protect the rest of the body. The most common poison is alcohol, though many drugs and industrial chemicals also damage the liver.
6 The liver has an immune function. It contains phagocytic cells which act as a sieve for bacteria, bacterial components and other antigens (irritants), to eliminate them.

So, the liver is the largest organ or gland of the body. Weighs approximately 3-4lbs, or 1.5kg. It is one of the most complicated organs with a wide range of functions, all closely interlinked with other systems in the body. It detoxifies, it is significantly involved in the digestion of all the food groups, it stores vitamins and minerals, it plays a crucial role in the immune system and it is our major source of heat – as well as many other things. It requires vital nutrients, like all the other organs, tissues and systems of the body.

Additional notes:

To look at 3 major functions:
1 Detoxification
2 Bile secretion
3 Metabolism

1 **Detoxification.** Poisonous substances enter the blood from the intestines or skin. They are carried by the blood stream to the liver. In their existing make-up they are foreign/unfamiliar and unacceptable/threatening to the body. In the liver, chemical reactions undo the existing make-up of the toxin and separate the components and then if necessary re-combine them with other components to make compounds which are acceptable/will not harm the body, eg: metals from chemicals, vaccinations, drugs, dental fillings. The metals will be removed from the molecules in the blood and if they can't be eliminated, they will be stored/hidden in fat or muscle tissue.

2 **Bile secretion.** Bile is formed from bile salts, bile pigments and cholesterol. The salts aid absorption of fats and are then absorbed themselves towards the end of the small intestine (the ileum). 80% of bile salts are recycled back to the liver to be used again in bile. Old or sub-standard erythrocytes (red blood cells) are destroyed in the spleen and released in haemoglobein. The haem part is converted into bilirubin and taken in the blood back to the liver. The bile salts filter out the bilirubin and excrete it into the bile. Bile is secreted via the right and left hepatic ducts, into the common hepatic duct, into the cystic duct from the gall-bladder, into the common bile duct. The bile produced in the liver is stored in the gall-bladder at between 5 and 10 times concentrated strength and the gall-bladder ejects the concentrated bile into the duodenum as part of the digestive process.

3 **Metabolism of Carbohydrates, Proteins and Fats.** Metabolism is a combination of two processes; catabolism and anabolism.

Catabolism is the breaking down of nutrients, usually by oxidation and so releasing energy.
Anabolism is the joining up of simple components and requires energy.

By breaking down and simplifying the nutrient components, or building them up to our own customized specification, the liver delivers the amino acids, sugars and fatty acids in a form the body likes and wants, that it can use and that isn't harmful.

The Kidneys

We have 2 kidneys, one each side of the middle of the back. They are like large, pinky-coloured, red kidney beans. An average kidney measures approximately 11 cm x 7 cm x 3 cm (4.3 in x 2.7 in x 1.2 in). The left kidney is often slightly larger than the right. The top of the kidney is just slightly higher than the 12th rib (the bottom rib at the back - we only have 10 at the front). A heavy cushion of fat usually encases each kidney and holds it in position with connective tissue anchoring them in place. The right kidney is often a little lower than the left - because of the position of the liver.

The kidneys receive 25% of cardiac output (the blood from the heart) at any one time, their primary role is filtering blood. The kidneys are guardians of the internal environment deciding what to keep and what to throw away in order to maintain fluid levels. They re-work the body fluids 15 times a day. When the body breaks down proteins, first into amino acids and then into smaller molecules, ammonia is produced as a by-product. This chemical is very dangerous and quickly detoxified in the liver into urea - this needs to be eliminated from the blood, so is excreted with water from the kidneys in the form of urine. Urine passes from a tube from each kidney to the bladder where it can be expelled from the body.

Excess protein in the diet does overwork the kidney, sometimes dangerously and is a very real caution in relation to high-protein-based diets.

The kidneys are also involved in the regulation of water levels in the body and elimination of water and salts (eg: sodium and potassium) dissolved in the blood, called electrolytes. This process helps to maintain a constant blood pH. Metabolic waste products and toxic substances are eliminated and nutritionally useful substances are kept.

The chief functions of the kidneys are to process blood, excrete urine and maintain fluid/electrolyte balance. They do this by varying the amount of water and electrolytes leaving the blood and passing into the urine. Many blood constituents cannot be held within normal (safe) ranges of concentration if the kidneys fail; typically sodium, potassium, chloride and nitrogenous waste - especially urea.

Kidney failure means homeostatic failure - ie: if not resolved, death.

The kidneys also influence the rate of secretion of various hormones.

The basic functional part of the kidney is the nephron.

The kidneys are very intricate organs performing a constant balancing act, processing blood constituents and passing them on via routes of elimination or absorbing them through the walls of the tubules back to the blood. They are involved in very fine adjustments and filtration in order to keep us well.

The medical term relating to things to do with the kidney is renal, eg: renal artery, renal function, renal failure.

So, the kidneys are smallish organs, either side of the middle of the back – constantly processing and filtering the blood, producing urine for elimination and reabsorbing useful elements. They require vital nutrients, like all the other organs, tissues and systems of the body.

Additional notes:

Hypertension can be caused by reduced blood flow through the kidneys from hardening and narrowing of the blood vessels. When this occurs a part of the kidney produces renin, an enzyme that changes one of the blood plasma proteins to produce angiotensis which acts as an agent restricting the blood vessels further and increasing blood pressure.

Dialysis acts as an artificial kidney – if an individual's own kidneys aren't functioning correctly. Blood is taken via the radial artery in the arm and passed through a tube which has a semi-permeable membrane which separates large particles from smaller particles. The tube is snaked through a bath, or tank, of dialysis solution containing various concentrations of electrolytes and other chemicals. The pores in the membrane are small, so the small urea particles are passed out and taken away and the blood retains the larger blood cells which are passed on to re-enter the patient via a wrist or leg vein. The solution in the dialysis tank has to be constantly replenished with freshly mixed solution to keep levels of waste low.

A patient with complete kidney failure will need 2 or 3 complete dialysis treatments a week.

Gout is a condition characterized by excessive levels of uric acid in the blood. The body produces uric acid from the metabolism of purine, ingested matter from digestion present especially in glandular meats or produced within our own body. Blood uric acid levels can become elevated because of increased dietary intake, excessive production in the body or defective excretion by the kidneys. Because uric acid is not as soluble as many waste products the body has to find somewhere 'safe' to put it and it tends to be deposited in the joints and tissues of the body to try and keep it out of the blood. Deposits of uric acid in the kidneys produce kidney stones.

Single kidney

Many people are born with a single kidney. It is more common in males and the left kidney is the one more often absent. The ureter (the tube that takes urine from the kidney to the bladder) on the affected side is usually abnormal or absent. In other cases, from somebody with two kidneys, one kidney may need to be surgically removed, leaving a single remaining kidney. Removal of the kidney (a 'nephrectomy') may be required as a result of an anatomic abnormality such as obstruction, or because of a tumour, or from a severe traumatic injury after an accident. Conversely, a kidney can be donated to someone who has kidney damage or kidney failure.

A single normal kidney will often grow faster and get larger than a normally paired kidney. For this reason, the single kidney is larger and heavier than normal and so is more vulnerable to injury. It is important to be aware of the increased risk of injury with certain heavy contact sports and participation in various physical activities. There is evidence to suggest that people with one kidney should avoid sports that involve higher risks of heavy contact or collision (boxing, football, rugby, hockey). The consequences of losing a single kidney would clearly be very serious.

Most people with a single normal kidney have few or no problems, particularly in the first few years. Some longer-term problems have been recognized and most doctors believe that people with a single kidney, particularly from birth or during early childhood, should be followed up more closely than people with two normal kidneys. Children who have had a kidney surgically removed may have some slightly increased chance of developing abnormal amounts of protein in the urine and some abnormality in kidney function in early adult life. Similar abnormalities have been found in individuals born with a single kidney. In addition, there is a greater chance of developing a slightly higher blood pressure than normal. The decrease in kidney function is usually mild, and life span is normal. In general, special diets are not needed by individuals who have one healthy kidney. The advice is the same as for others; a healthy well-balanced diet, low salt intake and to aim to drink 6 to 8 glasses of water a day/a minimum of 2 litres.

The Spleen

The spleen is another fairly large organ, as an average much the same size as your fist - it varies in size from individual to individual and at different times. It swells during times of infection in the body and reduces in size in old age. The spleen is directly below the diaphragm above the left kidney and descending colon. Its fibrous, spongey texture is full of blood and lymphoid tissue. After birth, blood cells are formed in the bone marrow but they are stored in the spleen which acts as a reservoir in emergencies. The spleen does a form of quality control on them and old red blood cells and platelets are broken down and destroyed. The spleen also produces antibodies for the immune system. Day to day we aren't very aware of our spleen and only notice if we get 'stitch'.

The 4 main roles of the spleen are defence, the process of blood cell formation, the destruction of worn-out and imperfect red blood cells and platelets and as a blood reservoir.

Defence: as blood passes through the spleen special white blood cells of the immune system - macrophages - remove and destroy micro-organisms identified as invaders.

Blood cell formation (haematopoiesis): before birth, red blood cells are formed in the spleen, liver and thymus - after birth they are formed in the bone marrow - but some of the special immune system white blood cells - monocytes and lymphocytes - complete their development in the spleen. (The spleen can also still produce red blood cells in cases of severe haemolytic anaemia - anaemia resulting from the destruction of red blood cells from toxic agents or inherited blood disorders).

Red blood cell and platelet destruction: as blood passes through the spleen, worn-out and imperfect red blood cells and platelets are removed and destroyed - again, by macrophages. The haemoglobin molecules from the destroyed cells are broken down and the iron (haem) and globin are salvaged and returned to the bloodstream and stored in the bone marrow and liver.

Blood reservoir: Blood is continually moving slowly through the spleen and at any time it would hold a considerable amount of blood - a normal volume being approximately 350ml. It isn't an extra supply of spare blood but it can act as a reservoir if needed. The volume of blood in the spleen could decrease from 350ml to 200ml in less than a minute, giving a sort of DIY transfusion, typically in the event of blood loss by accident or haemorrhage.

So, the spleen is a largeish, spongey organ – continually processing blood, supporting the immune system, removing micro-organisms, tidying up the tired cells and recycling the iron. Blood moves slowly through the spleen so at any time it may act as a reservoir if needed. It requires vital nutrients, like all the other organs, systems and tissues of the body.

Additional note:

Although the spleen's functions make it a most useful organ, Dr Charles Austin Doan undertook the first splenectomy in 1933 - on a 4 year old girl. It was a very radical operation for the time. The little girl recovered and so proved that it is not a vital organ, we can live without a spleen but would need long term anti-biotic medication following the removal. Spleen removal is now usually only undertaken if someone's condition is considered otherwise life-threatening. Risk of infection is greater after a splenectomy, particularly for pneumonia, scepticaemia and malaria.

Sometimes the spleen filters too much of the blood causing bruising, bleeding and anaemia. Sometimes it causes pain if it swells up. Sometimes it splits after an injury and bleeds very seriously. This is the most common reason for a spleen needing to be removed.

The Skin

The skin is the largest and thinnest organ and provides a protective layer between the internal environment of the body and the external world.

The skin of an average-sized adult would be approximately $1.6m^2$ - $1.9m^2$.

The thickness of the skin varies from less than 0.05cm in places, to more than 0.3cm, eg: there is thicker skin on parts of the hands and feet and very fine delicate skin on the eyelids.

In biological terms the skin is referred to as integument - so the integumentary system is the skin, hair and nails - our covering.

The skin is a cutaneous membrane (Latin: cutis - of the skin) of 2 main layers, the epidermis and the dermis. The outer layer is the epidermis and the inner layer is the dermis. Those two layers are also made up of their own sub-layers; 5 layers to the epidermis and 2 to the dermis.

Beneath the dermis is a loose sub-cutaneous layer, rich in fat, with collagen and fibrous gel. The fat content varies according to the nutrition of the person.

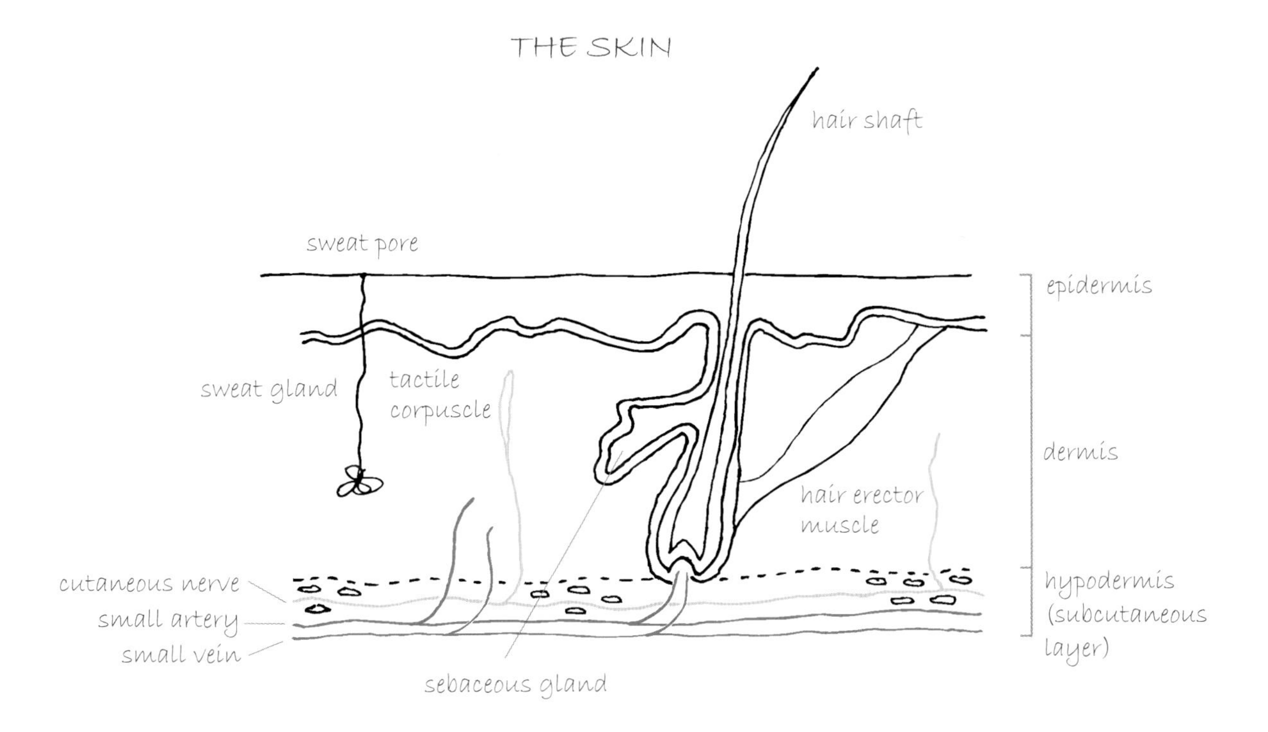

The epidermis is continually shedding and renewing itself from within. It is made up of 5 layers:

Layer 1 (stratum corneum) - made up of cells from inner layers moving to the outside. As the cells reach the surface they die and are continually being shed. The cells contain keratin which makes this layer strong and able to withstand considerable wear and tear. Keratin also makes the skin water-repellent, stopping unwanted fluids entering the body and limiting water loss from the body. This layer is an important barrier for us against micro-organisms, bacteria, chemicals and pollutants. If the barrier is damaged, contaminants can pass through.

Layer 2 (stratum lucidum) - these cells are filled with a soft jelly (eleidin) which will eventually become keratin. This layer is only present in areas of thicker skin, eg: palms and soles.

Layer 3 (stratum granulosum) - where keratin begins to form. Again, this layer is not present in thin areas of skin.

Layer 4 (stratum spinosum) - which is rich in RNA (ribonucleic acid) to start the synthesis required to produce keratin.

Layer 5 (stratum basale) - where skin cells multiply to transfer out to the other layers.

One of the most important functions of the skin is its ability to create and repair itself - especially following disease or injury. We have to make new skin cells at the same rate we lose them (or we'd fall apart). Even at rest, we are producing millions and millions of new cells to replace the old ones. This constant cycle of production and renewal relies on our body being able to provide all the elements and nutrients we need to create and maintain healthy cells - the correct proteins and fats and water and the healthy environment for that to happen. The normal cycle of the production of cells to being shed, is 35 days. This may happen faster if the skin was subject to increased abrasion, which, if prolonged, would shorten the production cycle so that cells were to reach the outside layer early, which results in a thicker, tougher external layer, eg: calluses.

The dermis is the mechanical strength of the skin. It has a specialized network of nerves and nerve endings, processing pain, pressure, touch and temperature. The dermis acts as a reservoir for water and electrolytes. This is also where we have hair follicles, sweat and sebaceous glands, many blood vessels and muscle fibres.

The dermis has 2 layers:

Layer 1 (papillary layer) - a layer of loose connective tissue and a fine network of collagen and elastic fibres. It is this layer that has the ridges of our skin which we see in the epidermis and which gives us our fingerprints and enables us to grip things and walk on slippery surfaces.

Layer 2 (reticular layer) - a more dense network of collagen and elastic fibres. Collagen for strength, elastic fibres to be stretchy and supple. This layer is where we have small bundles of muscles holding hair follicles and attachments to some muscles, eg: facial muscles. If we experience fear or cold, these are the muscles that contract making our skin hair stand up and giving us what we call 'goose bumps' or 'goose pimples'.

Between the bottom layer of the epidermis and the top layer of the dermis - is the dermal-epidermal junction of fibrous filaments and gel which hold the 2 layers together.

The dermis does not continually shed and regenerate, like the epidermis. It does maintain itself but rapid regeneration only occurs in special circumstances, eg: healing of wounds. A deep incision, like the site of an operation, triggers the cells in the dermis[1] to reproduce quickly and form an unusually dense mass of new connective tissue fibres, which may or may not become normal tissue, depending on severity. If it does not transform to normal tissue this will remain as scar tissue.

If the elastic fibres are stretched too much - eg: the abdomen during pregnancy or obesity - the fibres weaken and tear which is how we get stretch marks. They are pink whilst they are tears and as they heal and lose that colour, they become white.

Skin colour is determined by the quantity of melanin in our epidermis. We all have similar numbers of melanocytes throughout the base layer of the epidermis - but the variation in skin colour is determined by how much melanin they produce - light and dark. Production of melanin is influenced by heredity/genes, exposure to sunlight and age. Carotene also influences the yellow tones of skin colour.

[1] fibroblasts

Functions of the Skin

Protection
Sensation
Growth and movement
Synthesis of chemicals, eg: melanin, keratin
Synthesis of hormones, eg: vitamin D
Excretion
Temperature regulation
Immunity

Protection – the stratified cells of the epidermis provide a good, strong barrier protecting inner tissue from threats from micro-organisms, chemical hazards, physical trauma, the unwanted entry of some fluids and water loss from the body, plus melanin providing basic protection against ultra-violet rays.

The epidermis is covered in a thin surface film consisting of residues from sweat and sebaceous glands and excess, cast-off cells. This chemical composition consists of: amino acids, sterols, phospholipids, fatty acids, triglycerides and waxes from sebum[1], water, ammonia, lactic acid, urea and uric acid from sweat.

Sensation – the skin is a sophisticated sensory organ due to millions of different somatic (cell) receptors throughout the entire body surface. The receptors detect stimuli – pressure, touch, temperature, pain and vibration so that the body can respond.

Permitting growth and movement – as the body moves the skin must be supple and elastic. It grows as we grow and stretches and recoils to permit change in body shape and position without tearing or breaking.

Synthesis of chemicals and hormones – some substances and chemicals are absorbed through the skin: vitamins A, D, E and K, oestrogens, other sex hormones, cortisol hormones, some drugs, nicotine, nitroglycerine. The skin produces melanin and keratin.

Excretion – through the skin, by managing the volume and chemical content of sweat, the body can manage the total fluid volume and waste products, such as uric acid, ammonia and urea. The role of excretion via the skin can be significantly increased in certain diseases or pathological conditions. We shed approximately 1lb/450g of waste products daily through the skin. The skin also breathes, taking in oxygen and exhaling carbon monoxide formed in muscles and tissues.

[1] secretion from the sebaceous glands – see page 50

Temperature regulation – maintaining stability of body temperature is critical to survival because healthy survival depends on bio-chemical reactions which depend on enzymes functioning which require/can only work within prescribed temperatures. The body must balance the amount of heat it produces with the amount it loses. If the body temperature rises too high, the skin plays a critical role in heat loss by evaporation, radiation, conduction and convection. If the body temperature falls too low the sensory cells of the skin detect the fall and pass the information to the brain to act.
Immunity – there are specialized cells in the skin which attach to and destroy pathogenic micro-organisms, and Langerhans cells and T-cells which trigger reactions to diseases, playing an important role in immunity.

Appendages of the Skin

Hair growth begins when cells of the epidermis spread down into the dermis, forming a small tube – the follicle. Blood capillaries around the follicle nourish the matrix which forms the hairs and they push upwards in the follicle and become keratinized/strengthened as hair. As long as the matrix stays alive, the hair regenerates even if it is cut, plucked or otherwise removed. The root lies hidden in the follicle. The visible part of the hair, the surface, is the shaft; the inner core is the medulla. In the cells there is melanin, which again, determines the colour of the hair – brown or black. A unique type of melanin containing iron is responsible for red hair.

Straight hair has a round, cylindrical shaft. Wavy hair has a flat shaft, which is not so strong and is more susceptible to being broken and damaged. Two or more sebaceous glands secrete sebum into the hair follicle to lubricate the hair and keep it from becoming dry, brittle and easily damaged. Hair alternates between periods of growth and rest. On average head hair grows just under 12mm (½in) a month or about 11cm (5in) a year. Body hair grows more slowly.

Head hairs reportedly live between 2 and 6 years, then die and are shed. New hairs replace those lost – unless baldness occurs. The known causes of baldness are the coincidence/combination of inherited genes for baldness and the presence of testosterone.

Hair growth is not stimulated by frequent cutting or shaving.

Nails are heavily keratinized epidermal cells. The visible part of the nail is the nail body, the rest of the nail – the root – is in the cuticle. Under the nail is the nail bed. Like hair, nails grow from cells in the skin just under the top layer (stratum corneum). On average nails grow 0.5mm a week but finger nails grow faster than toe nails and both grow faster in the summer than the winter.

Sweat Glands

Some sweat glands (eccrine sweat glands) are tiny, very numerous and distributed throughout the body. They function over the whole lifespan to produce a transparent, watery liquid – perspiration or sweat – rich in salts, ammonia, uric acid, urea and other wastes. A single square inch of skin contains about 3,000 sweat glands. These glands are seated in the sub-cutaneous level with ducts through the dermis and epidermis to the surface of the skin.

The other type of sweat glands (apocrine sweat glands) are deep within the sub-cutaneous layer of the skin, in the armpit, near the breast and the pigmented skin around the anus. They are larger than the eccrine sweat glands. They are connected with hair follicles. Apocrine glands enlarge and begin to function at puberty and produce a more viscous and coloured secretion. Odour often associated with sweat from these glands is not caused by the secretion itself – it is caused by contamination and decomposition of the secretion by skin bacteria – this is directly affected by what we eat, how much and how well our body is functioning and eliminating waste products and hydration.

Sebaceous Glands

Sebaceous glands in the dermis secrete oil for the hair and skin. Wherever hairs grow from the skin there are sebaceous glands, at least two per hair. The oil, or sebum, keeps the hair and skin soft and supple – it is nature's own protective skin cream. It is rich in triglycerides, waxes, fatty acids and cholesterol that have an anti-fungal effect and contribute to reducing fungal activity on the skin surface. Sebum secretion increases during adolescence stimulated by increased blood levels of sex hormones. The sebum can accumulate and enlarge some of the ducts forming white pimples. With oxidation the sebum darkens, forming a blackhead. Acne can also occur during adolescence as a result of over-active secretion of sebum clogging sebaceous glands with sloughed skin cells and becoming contaminated with bacteria which can cause secondary infections within or beneath the epidermis, in the hair follicle or sweat pore. Again, this can be greatly affected by what you eat and how well the body is functioning.

It is quite possible that even our daily, morning bathroom routine, the first few minutes of our day, can expose us to in excess of 200 chemicals – before we've started to eat anything or go outside. The skin is a permeable membrane and will absorb a proportion of all these things. To that we can add, gardening chemicals, cleaning and household chemicals, chemicals in and on foodstuffs, air pollution – the list is a very long one. The skin can often be an early indicator of health and toxicity - affected by dryness, rashes, lumps and bumps. Many diseases are detected by skin changes.

The skin needs the body to be able to supply adequate amounts of hormones, enzymes, proteins, fats and other nutrients, water and energy for the production and renewal of skin cells. This is a non-stop process.

So, the skin is a very large, thin organ – a water-repellent barrier between our internal body and the outside world – involved in protection, sensation, growth and movement, synthesis of chemicals and hormones, excretion, temperature regulation and immunity and home to our hair, nails, sweat glands and sebaceous glands – constantly reproducing and replacing itself. It requires vital nutrients, like all the other organs, tissues and systems of the body.

Additional note:

Skin Care

The multi-million pound skin care industry is vast and extremely high profile. There are many products to help us look after our skin. The skin's best ways of looking after itself come from within. Good diet, water and healthy lifestyle will support, protect and nourish the skin. Including crushed flax seeds in the diet helps maintain moisture in the skin and so does drinking flax seed oil! Including lecithin in your diet helps emulsify lipids and fats which help support skin moisture levels and suppleness. Smoking, alcohol and many drugs will age and dehydrate the skin.

One dot of olive oil or sesame seed oil rubbed around the hands and wrists can be as good as some of the most expensive creams, lotions and potions (also scalp, shins and feet). You hardly need any.

Protection has to include sun screens. Too much sun and tanning also ages and dehydrates the skin and burning can be painful and dangerous. There is lots of information available to help find and use a good, effective sun screen.

The Gastro-intestinal Tract

ORGANS OF THE DIGESTIVE SYSTEM

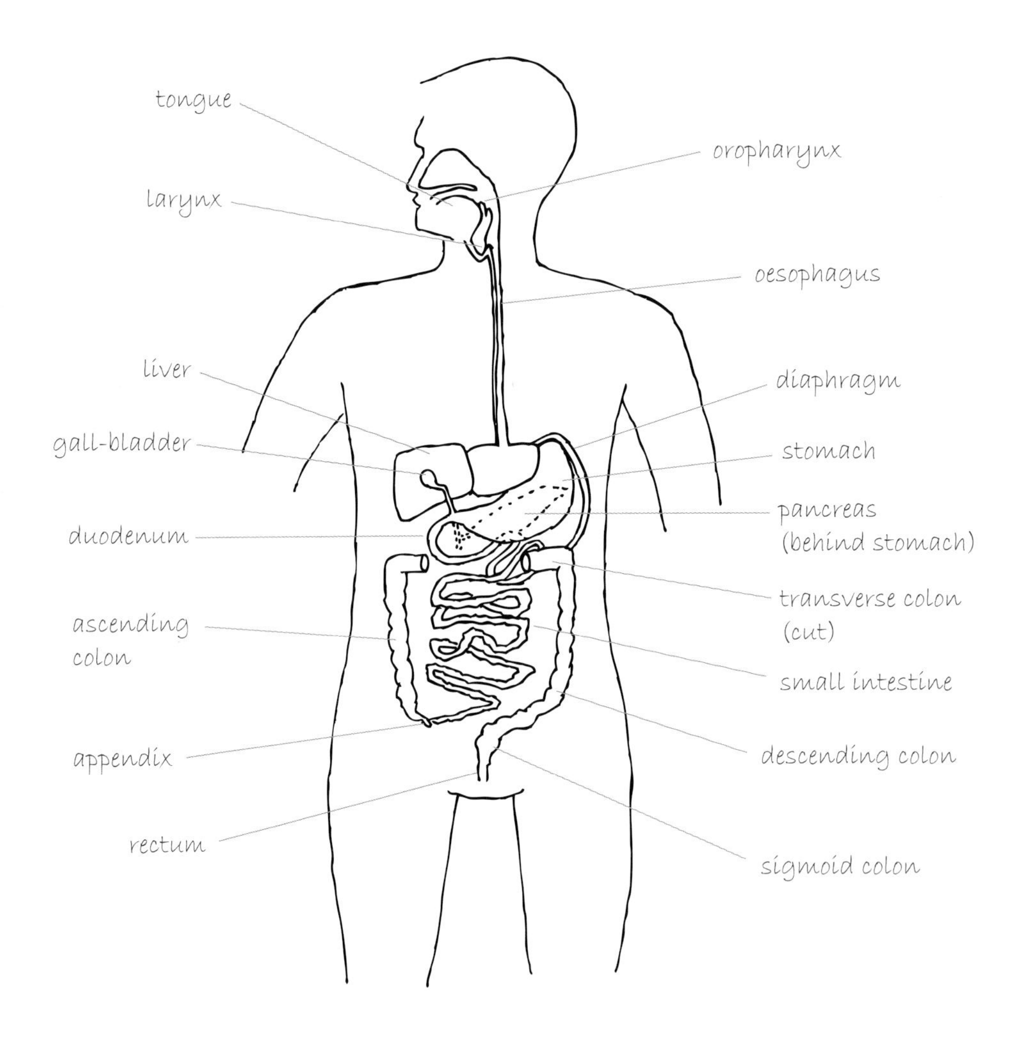

Digestion - the big picture

The primary function of the digestive system is to maintain a constant level of nutrient concentration in the internal environment.

- This is done by breaking up complex nutrients into simpler nutrients so that they can be absorbed. The digestive system also provides the means of absorption.
- Digestion provides a means of survival for the entire body and requires the function of many other systems.
- As well as beginning the digestive process in the mouth, the teeth and tongue also work with the nervous system and the respiratory system in producing spoken language.
- In the stomach, acid assists the immune system by destroying potentially harmful bacteria.
- To transport nutrients through the body/gastro-intestinal tract, the digestive system needs the secretion of digestive juices and enzymes and the regulation of muscles and the nervous and endocrine systems.
- The oxygen needed in these processes needs the respiration and circulation systems.
- The body's framework - the skeletal and integumentary systems - are required to support and protect the digestive organs and the gastro-intestinal tract.
- The skeletal muscles have to function for ingestion, chewing, swallowing, peristalsis and elimination.

This is the part digestion plays in homeostasis - the constant state of balance in the internal environment. Maintenance of temperature, blood pressure, oxygen, carbon dioxide, water and electrolyte concentrations and pH concentrations, despite external events and changes.

The digestive system cannot operate alone - nor can any system or organ. The body is an integrated system, not a collection of independent components.

SUMMARY OF DIGESTION

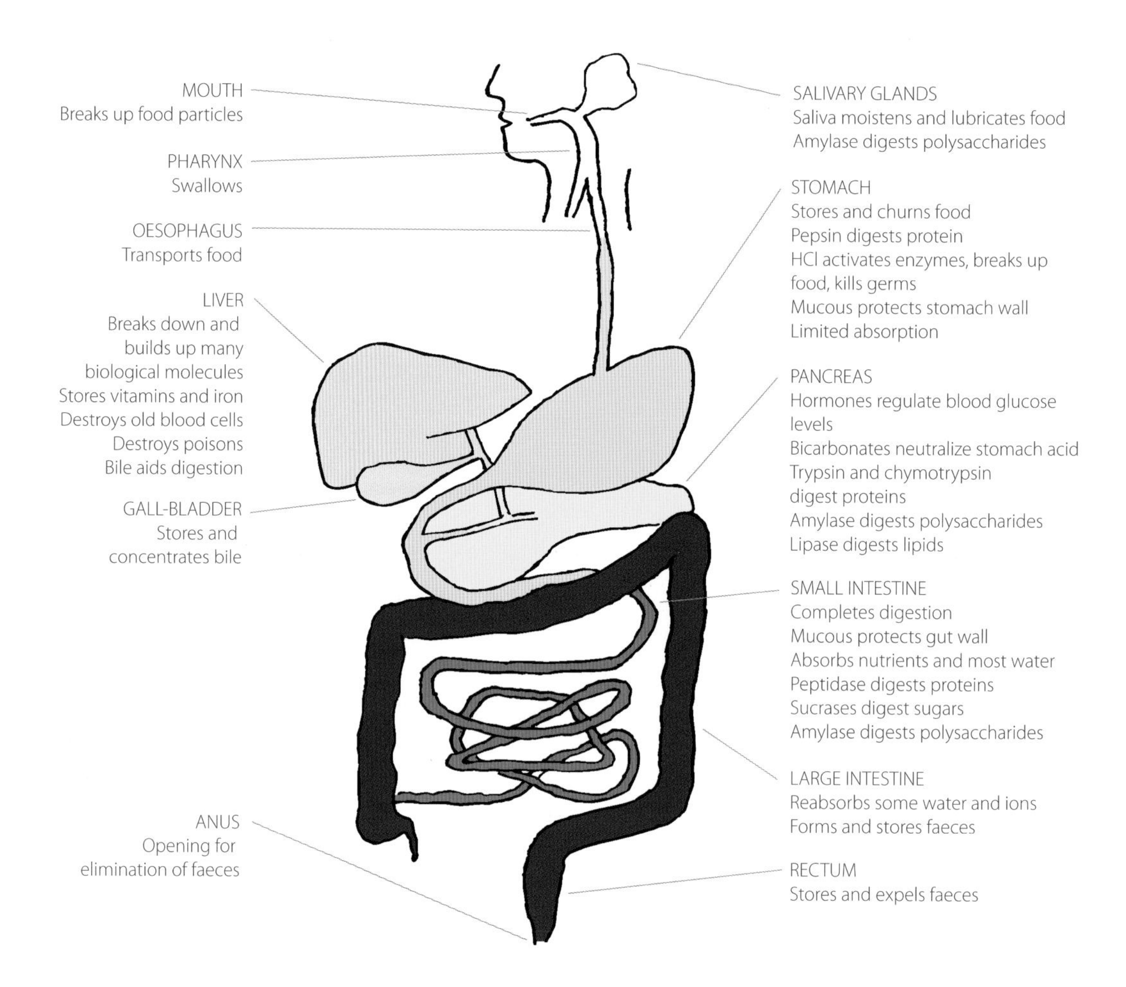

The Mouth and Gullet

The gastro-intestinal tract (GI tract) is basically a corridor through the body, open at both ends. It is how we can pass things into and out of our body without them being passed into the 'internal environment' – the blood, organs and tissues – of our body. The food enters from one end and the waste products leave from the other end and we absorb what we want to use, somewhere in between. Most of our food is in a form that our body cells can't use and the digestion process has to transform it to smaller and simpler forms. The digestion process is both mechanical and chemical. The mechanical process consists of biting, chewing, mashing and mixing whilst the chemical process consists of production of juices containing enzymes to break the food down into simpler, smaller molecules so that it can be absorbed into the body. At the end of this process the unusable parts and waste are eliminated from the body.

The Mouth

Digestion starts even before we start to eat – when we smell, see and then taste food. Stimulation of these senses produces saliva in the mouth from the saliva glands under the tongue and at the sides of the mouth. When we are hungry, the sight and smell and anticipation of food starts the digestion process. Saliva contains enzymes called amylase, which start the breakdown of large molecules into smaller ones.

In order for food to be absorbed the particles must be very small. Chewing food well starts the breakdown process and this continues through the gastro-intestinal tract, as most molecules are too large to go through cell walls and they have to be broken down into smaller molecules. Amylase can only breakdown carbohydrates.

When we start to eat, our teeth chew up the food before swallowing, partly to break down the lumps of food but also to expose as much of the food as possible to amylase. The longer we chew the more the food is broken down and exposed to the enzymes and the easier it is to swallow and later to be absorbed. It is better to chew food really well to prepare it for digestion. This is true of all food, our body likes us to chew food well in the mouth – our stomach doesn't have teeth. Our mouth is very well equipped for this, it has teeth, it has a large tongue to mash and churn and pummel the large food particles around and lots of sets of muscles in the cheeks and jaw. Breaking our food down as much as possible in the mouth is a huge help to the digestive system and what our body was designed to do. (It is also a very helpful stage in weight loss.) It is much harder work to break down large food pieces in the stomach and intestines and can cause

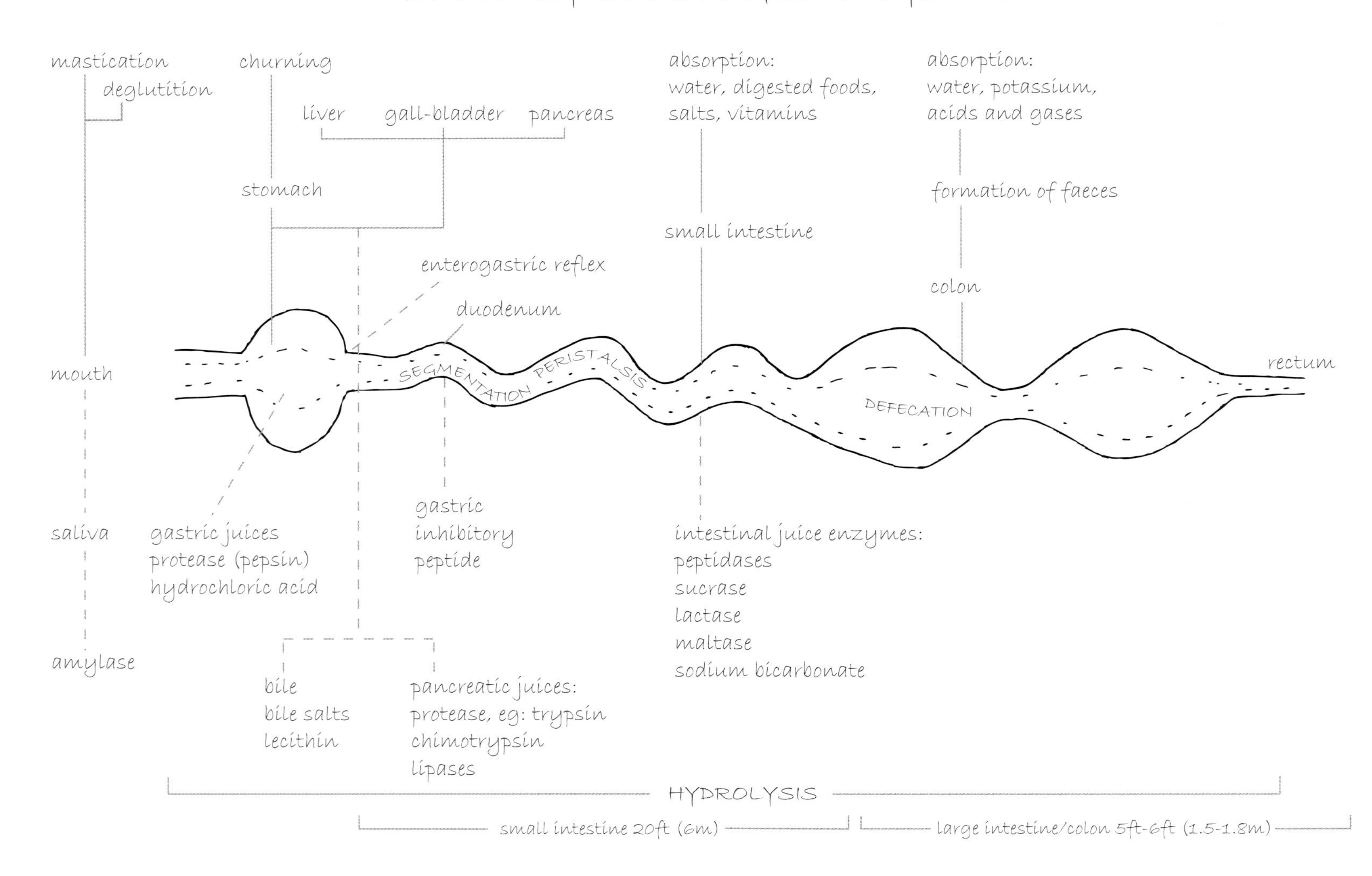
A JOURNEY THROUGH THE GASTRO-INTESTINAL TRACT /
ALIMENTARY CANAL / DIGESTIVE SYSTEM
mastication
deglutition
churning
liver
gall-bladder
pancreas
absorption:
water, digested foods,
salts, vitamins
absorption:
water, potassium,
acids and gases
stomach
formation of faeces
small intestine
enterogastric reflex
colon
duodenum
mouth
SEGMENTATION
PERISTALSIS
DEFECATION
rectum
saliva
gastric juices
protease (pepsin)
hydrochloric acid
gastric
inhibitory
peptide
intestinal juice enzymes:
peptidases
sucrase
lactase
maltase
sodium bicarbonate
amylase
bile
bile salts
lecithin
pancreatic juices:
protease, eg: trypsin
chimotrypsin
lipases
HYDROLYSIS
small intestine 20ft (6m)
large intestine/colon 5ft-6ft (1.5-1.8m)

complications. Not chewing enough or swallowing large pieces of food will obstruct digestion and the extra work will steal energy from our body – not to mention heartburn, hiccoughs, wind, toxicity, slow transit time and festering, putrefying, undigested matter.

The Gullet

Food is swallowed down the oesophagus or gullet and into the stomach for the next stage in the digestive process. The exit at the back of the mouth carries the air we breathe to our lungs and swallowed food to the gastro-intestinal tract. Then these two pathways fork and separate. As we swallow, a flap of skin called the epiglottis, covers the opening to the windpipe (trachea) which leads to the lungs and prevents food from going into the windpipe and lungs, which would cause choking, ie: 'going down the wrong way'. If this happens, it usually makes us cough to expel the food, so that we don't choke.

Food travels down the oesophagus by peristaltic movement. This happens by the rings of muscles around our throat rhythmically pushing the food down.

At the top of the stomach is a one-way valve called a sphincter. When the stomach is working vigorously to mash food up, the valve closes to stop food, acid and digestive enzymes coming back up. Occasionally if the valve doesn't shut properly some of the stomach contents can come back up into the oesophagus, which we call gastric reflux. This most commonly happens if we have eaten too much and the stomach is too full, or if we are eating in a slumped over position so that our chest is compressed. The acid in the regurgitated food can burn the delicate tissue of the oesophagus which is uncomfortable and may be painful. Correct posture is important for good digestion.

So, in the mouth our food is broken down from large pieces to smaller pieces, by mechanical and chemical actions. The gullet takes the food from the mouth to the stomach.

The Stomach

Although people often call the belly, the stomach - this isn't strictly speaking true. The stomach is quite high up in the abdominal cavity just under the rib cage. It is where our food goes to next, after being swallowed.

In the stomach the food continues to be jostled around and turned and stirred by muscular action - a muscular action that mashes the food particles, rather like a squashing action. The job here is still to break food particles down from larger particles to ever smaller ones. Digestive juices and an enzyme[1] called pepsin are secreted in the stomach - which mix with the food particles which eventually become a thick, milky consistency, called chyme. Every 20 seconds the stomach releases a small amount of chyme into the duodenum to control the flow - this is controlled by hormone and nerve mechanisms.

The presence of fats and nutrients in the chyme released from the stomach into the duodenum, the first part of the small intestines, triggers the release of more digestive hormones into the blood[2]. The hormones are instructions to reduce the activity of the gastric muscle in the stomach wall to slow the peristaltic wave. The nervous control is from receptors which sense the presence of acid and the distention within the gastro-intestinal tract. This also checks the rate of passage, giving the digestion process chance to work on the food and regulate the amounts passing from the larger volume stomach to the smaller volume duodenum. Further digestive juices[3] are also secreted in the intestines when chyme is present which assist the stimulus for peristalsis.

So whilst the stomach is working on food the instructions were to slow down whilst the stomach does what is has to do - and on leaving the stomach the instructions are for the peristaltic muscles to get going again.

In the stomach the gastric juices have to increase the acidity (lower the pH). This is done by secretion of hydrochloric acid. The hydrochloric acid has 2 functions. It enables the proteins to be digested more easily because the enzymes at work here work better in an acidic environment - and it also provides an acid bath which acts as a barrier to any stray bacteria or viruses that have been taken in with the food.

[1] Proenzyme pepsinogen is converted to pepsin by hydrochloric acid from parietal cells in gastric glands. The parietal cells also secrete intrinsic factor which protects molecules of B12 from stomach acids and stays attached to B12 to the lower small intestines where it can be absorbed.

[2] gastric inhibitory peptide – GIP

[3] Cholecystokinin-pancreozymin – CCK

The stomach is a very acid environment indeed for digestion, the sort of acidity that would burn our skin - mainly involved with the digestion of protein.

Mucous is also produced in the stomach, to cover the entire surface of the stomach to protect itself from the acid.

The stomach serves as a reservoir, storing food until it can be moved along; secretes gastric, digestive juices; churns food breaking it down into smaller pieces; carries out a limited amount of absorption, some water, some alcohol and short chain fats; and helps protect the body by destroying pathogenic bacteria.

Another secretion, called intrinsic factor, is also released here which protects molecules of vitamin B12 from being destroyed by stomach acids and stays attached to B12 until it reaches the lower small intestines where it is absorbed. (Vitamin B12 is needed to make use of proteins, help the blood carry oxygen, essential for energy, needed for synthesis of DNA, essential for nerves and essential for production of new blood cells.)

It takes between 2-6 hours for the stomach to empty after a meal. Hormones and nerves control this so the duodenum is not overloaded.

So, the stomach accepts food from the gullet, squashes and mashes it and turns it into chyme – and releases it into the duodenum – the next stage along the way. It's a very acid environment for the digestion of proteins.

The Pancreas

The juices from the pancreas also enter the digestive process before the food leaves the stomach. As well as digestive juices, the pancreas produces sodium bicarbonate and insulin. The sodium bicarbonate is alkaline to neutralize the acidity produced in the stomach and maintain homeostasis and insulin.

The pancreas is a long, thin, dual-purpose organ, just under the diaphragm and mostly to the centre and left.

Our food doesn't pass into the pancreas, the pancreas sits on the sidelines and secretes juices to work on the food in the stomach and duodenum, on the way to the small intestines. It is a digestive gland which is part of the system, like the salivary glands in the mouth but not somewhere that the food actually goes. In German it is called the abdominal salivary gland.

The pancreas primarily produces pancreatic juice, a mixture of different digestive enzymes, which continue to breakdown larger food particles into smaller molecules that can be absorbed when they reach the small intestines. The enzymes breakdown proteins, carbohydrates and fats.

The pancreas also produces hormones, insulin and glucagon that help control blood sugar. So this organ is very directly related to obesity and diabetes. Both hormones are secreted directly into the blood.

Insulin helps the take-up of glucose from the blood to the cells for storage and use as energy.

Glucagon hormone promotes the release of glucose from tissue cells - mainly the liver but also the muscles - into the blood where it can be used as energy.

So basically, the pancreas sits on the sidelines, the food does not enter it – it secretes digestive juices which help the breakdown of all foods, proteins, carbohydrates and fats. It also secretes insulin and glucagon which help to control blood sugar.

Additional notes:

All glands in the body are either exocrine or endocrine and the pancreas is, very unusually, both.

Exocrine glands secrete the hormones (and/or ligands[1]) they produce, to the body, via ducts, eg: salivary glands, intestinal glands, sweat glands, sebaceous (skin oil) glands. Endocrine glands are ductless glands, they secrete the hormones (and/or ligands) they produce directly into the blood or interstitial fluid (fluid in the microscopic spaces between the cells, extracellular fluid, including lymph), eg: the pituitary gland, thyroid gland, adrenal glands.

Producing hormones to work on blood sugar – is what is called an endocrine role[2] – because the juices are released directly into the blood.

Producing digestive juices to work in the stomach and duodenum – is what is called an exocrine[3] role – because the juices are released into glands and ducts, then on into the GI tract.

[1] Ligand(s) – an ion, molecule or group of molecules that binds to another chemical to form a larger complex.

[2] Endocrine – secreting into blood or tissue fluid rather than into a duct; opposite of exocrine.

[3] Exocrine – secreting into a duct, as in glands that secrete their products via ducts onto a surface or into a cavity; opposite of endocrine.

The Liver and Gall-bladder

The liver is one of our most complicated organs and has lots of roles in digestion.

The liver:

- makes the bile for use in digestion - approx 1 pint/day
- receives ingested vitamins and minerals
- receives and sorts ingested food particles and transforms them for use or storage
- metabolizes and converts fats, proteins and carbohydrates
- absorbs dissolved toxins from the blood
- receives blood via the portal vein for inspection and processing

amongst other things.

The gall-bladder sits on the underside of the liver attached by connective tissue. It is a little sack approx 7-10 cms (3-4 ins) long and 3 cms (just under 1½ ins) wide.

Early in the digestion process, the liver makes bile. The bile ducts from the liver merge with the duct from the gall-bladder which opens into the duodenum - the first part of the small intestines.

Bile is a mixture of substances and once produced in the liver it is stored and concentrated in the gall-bladder.

The lecithin and bile salts in the bile break down large droplets of fat, making them more easily digestible.

Bile also contains some sodium bicarbonate which, like the sodium bicarbonate produced in the pancreas, helps to neutralize the acidic chyme from the stomach.

The liver also excretes cholesterol in bile where this has been picked up in the body and taken to the liver for disposal.

At the end of digestion the liver receives all the broken down, ingested food particles, sorts them and transforms them into new substances needed for our bodies or stores them for later use.

All the blood vessels serving the gastro-intestinal tract lead to the portal vein in the liver and so this is the first port of call for digested foods. Many food molecules need to undergo more transformation to make them usable by the body and this is carried out in the liver. The liver is involved in the digestion of all the food groups; carbohydrate, fats and protein.

The liver takes **carbohydrate** molecules in the form of glucose and either releases them back into the blood to be used for energy immediately or links them together in long chains for storage – this is called glycogen. This glycogen is stored in the liver until it is needed, eg: when blood sugar levels drop or when we exercise.

Fat molecules arriving at the liver are reformed, degraded or stored. The liver is able to convert between fats, proteins and carbohydrates depending on shortfalls of any of these groups. It is able to make cholesterol which is essential for forming hormones like cortisol, for nerve insulation and for cell walls.

Protein foods, now in the form of amino acids arrive at the liver where they may take one of several routes.

1 The liver may simply export the amino acids into the blood stream where they make their way to other cells and tissues to be built into new proteins such as collagen in bone and muscle protein (myosin) in muscles.

2 The liver may combine the amino acids to form the proteins it needs itself, or it exports these new proteins into the blood for use by other cells.

3 The liver makes blood proteins (fibrinogen, albumin, and globulin) which are essential for the functions carried out in and by blood.

4 Excess amino acids are broken down into molecules of ammonia and molecules of keto acid. The ammonia is very toxic and is converted by liver cells to urea to go on to be excreted in urine. The keto acid molecules are converted to glucose or glycogen, or to fats – all of which can be used to supply energy

About 4g of bile salts and 1.5g of bile pigments are secreted every day in the bile. After they have done their job of helping fat digestion most of the bile salts are reabsorbed by the intestines and delivered back to the liver so they can work again. The liver also secretes sodium chloride and sodium bicarbonate with the bile. This fluid passes out of the liver down the bile duct into the gall-bladder where it is stored until it is needed. While in the gall-bladder, sodium, chloride and water are actively reabsorbed so the bile becomes more concentrated.

Once digestion has started with food being chewed in the mouth, nerve impulses and a hormone[1] cause the gall-bladder to contract so that bile is released and pushed down

[1] cholecystokinin (CCK)

the bile duct into the duodenum to the food being digested. It acts on fatty substances to break them down, emulsify them and aid absorption.

So, the liver makes and secretes bile to break down fats in digestion, it sorts out ingested foods for use or storage, it stores vitamins and minerals, stores glycogen and makes blood proteins.

Additional notes:

Besides these digestive-related functions the liver also has all its other roles (see Anatomy and Physiology section, page 35).

Gall stones

Gall stones are solid clumps of material, mainly cholesterol, which form when the concentration in the bile is too high. Instead of remaining fluid, little crystals occur forming small 'stones'. The stones can become larger with time. When a fatty meal is eaten and the gall-bladder is stimulated to contract, the stones are pushed down into the narrow bile duct where they can become stuck. This leads to severe pain and sometimes to fever. Until the gall stones can be removed by an operation, fatty foods have to be avoided to try and prevent contraction of the gall-bladder. Gall stones can be avoided by drinking plenty of water so that body fluids do not become too concentrated and by not overloading the liver. Stones are more likely if the gall-bladder doesn't empty regularly and high cholesterol bile stays in the gall-bladder for long periods of time. (A similar process happens in the kidney with the formation of kidney stones.)

The Small Intestine

In the small intestine the food particles receive further processing. They are jostled by the muscular actions of peristalsis and segmentation. This mixes the incoming chyme with digestive juices from the pancreas, liver and intestine wall. They are liquefied, joining with water to dilute down into simpler compounds[1] and worked on by many further enzymes[2]. Many enzymes in the various digestive juices are active during the liquefying process. In the small intestines the presence of two of the digestive enzymes[3], regulate the speed with which the food passes so that the larger or more complex molecules can be slowed down to maximize the time the digestive functions can work on them. The digestive juices continue to work on all the food groups, carbohydrates, fats and protein.

It is in the 20-ish feet of the small intestines that almost all the ultimate absorption takes place, about 90%. The tiny particles of food pass into the intricate folds of the lining of the intestines where they are taken up by the tiny blood vessels - capillaries. The large surface area provides the sites for the molecules to pass from the external environment, the GI tract, to the internal environment, the rest of the body. An average transit time from the beginning to the end of the small intestines, from the stomach to the large intestines, for a typical, healthy person would be approximately 5 hours.

We take food from the outside, external environment, into our body to provide nutrients in the internal environment. Food needs to be able to get to the cells and to be in the right state. The contents of the gastro-intestinal tract are in a channel running through the body and only when they are absorbed through the gut wall do they enter the internal environment and are available to the blood, tissues, organs and cells of the body.

It is important to have a healthy population of good bacteria in the small and large intestines, to assist in the breakdown of food particles and to allow the scavenger cells to do away with the bad bacteria.

So, the small intestines carry the food from the stomach to the large intestines. They are approximately 20 feet long – and this is where the food we have eaten becomes absorbed and passes from the tube or corridor that is the gastro-intestinal tract – into the internal environment of our body and all its cells, tissues and organs.

[1] hydrolysis – chemical process in which a compound is split by addition of HI and OH portions of a water molecule

[2] including peptidases for amino acids, and sucrase, lactase and maltase for carbohydrates

[3] GIP and CCK

The Large Intestine

The large intestine is about 1.5-1.8m (5-6ft) long and on average, approximately 6cms (2½ins) diameter, decreasing towards the lower end. What we eat reaches the large intestine about 8-10hrs after being eaten.

The residue of food from the small intestine enters the large intestine passing through a valve that stops it flowing backwards[1]. The appendix is very close to this valve. It is like a little finger off the intestine, about 8-10cms (3-4ins) long and contrary to some references it does have a function in the body. The appendix acts as a holding bay for good bacteria and is also where they can multiply. We can get by without an appendix but it is very useful to have one. The bacteria of the large intestine help prevent disease and assist in digestion and the absorption of essential nutrients, they play a major role in nutrition and digestion. Overall there should be around 1.5 kg of symbiotic, friendly bacteria living in the gut. It is the numerous by-products of these bacteria which differ according to what we eat, that can be very toxic and odorous! especially if we aren't eating a good, varied diet. The by-products of good food aren't too unpleasant; the by-products of not so good food, are not so good.

When food residues enter the large intestine they are acted upon by bacteria and some of the enzymes still present. The food residues move slowly through the large intestine allowing bacteria to digest the unused cellulose and other fibres. As the colon content moves towards the rectum, the mass of solids, of food origin, gradually diminishes and the debris from the bacteria's activity gradually increases. Nearly one third of the stool's solid mass is of bacterial origin.

The colon content is moved along by peristalsis. When we eat, presence of food in the stomach stimulates peristalsis, pushing previously eaten foods and waste along further on and towards the exit (rectum).

The time taken for a meal to get through the gut from mouth to exit, or transit time, should be about 18 hours. (2 hrs stomach, 5-6 hrs small intestine, so it may be about another 8+hrs in the large intestine). You can see what your transit time is by eating either sweetcorn or beetroot or linseeds and seeing when they reappear. If you do this, you will need to avoid whichever food it is you choose to use for about a week beforehand for this to work accurately. This transit time is influenced by the amount of fibre and water in the diet. Lots of fibre enables food residues to travel through the gut in a faster time as it stimulates the peristaltic contractions of the gut wall muscles. A transit time of

[1] ileocecal valve

slower than 18 hours may benefit from eating more fibre foods such as vegetables and wholegrain cereals and higher water content foods and drinking more water.

A slow transit time means that food wastes are in the colon for a long time, gently composting and festering, which is where windy gases may be produced – and beginning to produce toxic breakdown products that can damage the delicate lining of the colon if they are around for too long. Slow movement through the colon can lead to constipation and the risk of diseases of the colon (eg: diverticulosis and colitits).

When the food residue enters the large intestine it is very liquid. One of the main functions of the large intestine is to absorb water and minerals which help with the body's fluid balance, so the stool becomes drier as it gets towards elimination. As we secrete more than 8 litres of digestive juices, much of which is water, this would be a lot of water to lose, not to mention a lot of trips to the loo. Most of this water is recycled back into the blood.

Two minerals whose balance is essential to the wellbeing of every cell are sodium and potassium. The bowel is able to absorb these minerals from the waste parcels in the colon, along with some vitamins. Drugs can also be absorbed from the large intestine.

If the bowel is healthy and we are eating a good diet with plenty of vegetable fibre and water, we should have a bowel movement after each meal but at least once a day (perhaps two being the norm). If the bowel opens less often than once a day, then the body is constipated and this can impact on many functions and organs of the body and increase risk of bowel disease. Efficient working of the bowel is one of the single best ways to health.

Ignoring times you should go to the loo and eating low fibre food both contribute significantly to constipation. Laxatives used for constipation either increase the amount of water in faeces or contain irritants that stimulate the colon wall. Becoming dependant on laxatives eventually destroys normal bowel function. Excess use of laxatives, nervous stress, infection and high toxins in the bowel, can all produce watery faeces – diarrhoea.

It cannot be stressed enough that a healthy bowel and efficient elimination are two critical ways to avoid many acute and chronic conditions, from skin irritations to tiredness, colds and cancer. We know we eliminate through our skin, our nose and our mouth as well – but the primary routes of elimination are through our gut and urinary system – and it is vital to keep them functioning well. What we put in has a very significant effect on how they work and how well they can manage.

As well as considering what we eat and our nutrition, any other ways in which we manage any symptoms which may be affecting us should be done with professional, qualified advisers. It's important not to worry or leap to unilateral decisions on anything we are not sure of or change medications. The important thing is to find out more and see if any there are any changes that will help.

So, food residues enter the large intestine where gut bacteria act on the food residues, water is reabsorbed and vitamins and minerals are absorbed into the blood stream. Movement is slow to allow time for the bacteria to do their work and for absorption to take place. The residues of food and bacterial activity are expelled.

Additional notes:

Gut Bacteria

The type of bacteria that turns milk into yogurt is called lactobacillus acidophilus and is just one of many of the strains present. Other important types are Bifidobacteria, Lactobacillus bulgaricus, Lactobacillus casei. You may see these names on many 'probiotic' products available. These bacteria feed on our leftovers but in return produce vitamins, help to eliminate unhealthy bacteria and are in effect part of our immune system.

Some of the major beneficial functions of lactobacilli:

1. Some strains act to destroy hostile invading bacteria by producing natural anti-biotic substances.

2. They reduce the level of cholesterol, lessening one of the factors of cardio-vascular disease.

3. They help to produce important B vitamins.

4. They help prevent cancer by detoxifying or preventing the formation of chemicals which are carcinogenic.

5. They are able to control proliferation of hostile yeasts such as candida albicans.

6. Through their production of lactic acid they preserve and enhance the digestibility of foods which are fermented with them, such as soy products (tofu, miso), sauerkraut, pickles, etc.

7. They enhance and allow digestion of lactose.

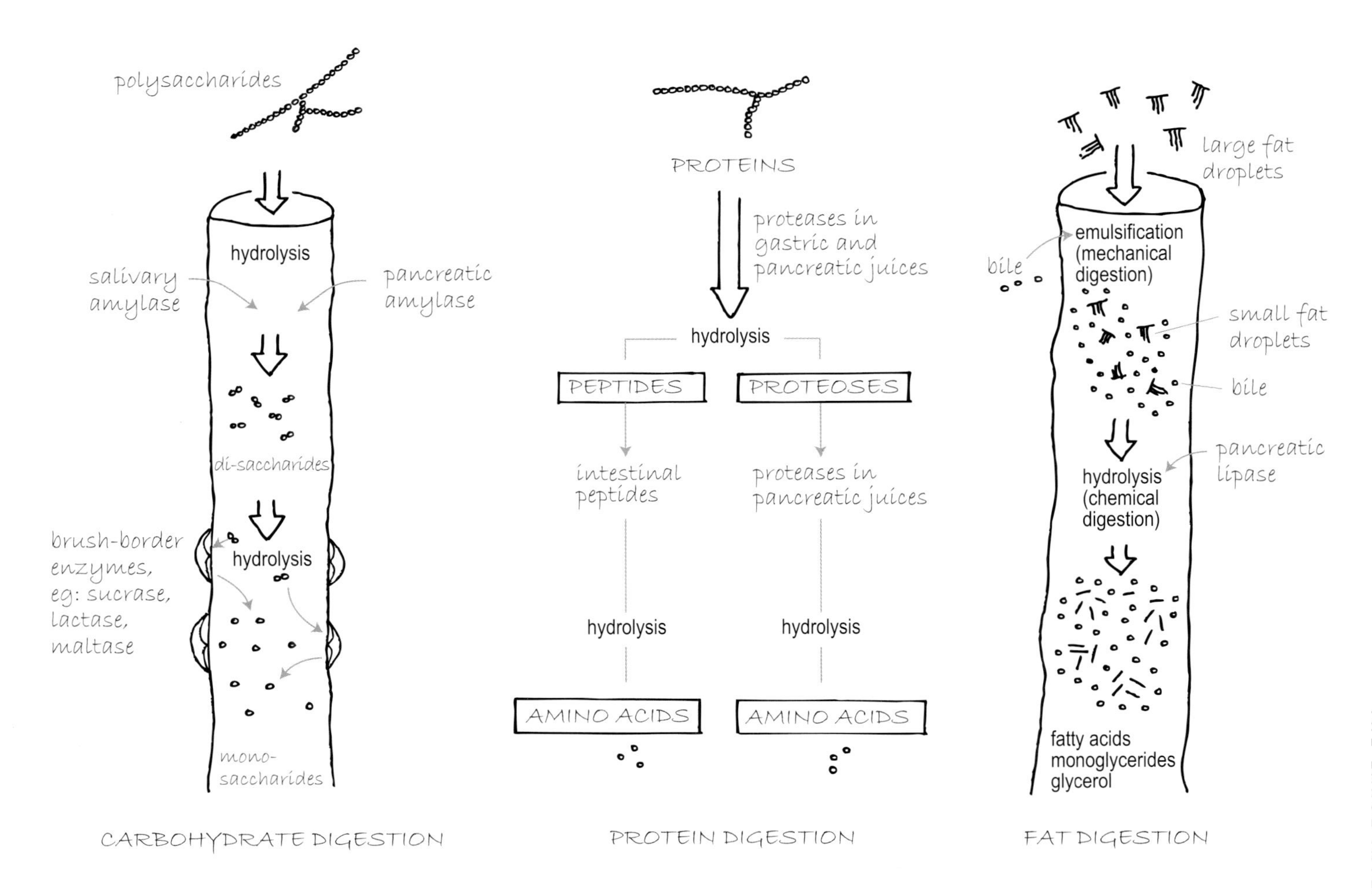
polysaccharides
hydrolysis
salivary amylase
pancreatic amylase
di-saccharides
hydrolysis
brush-border enzymes, eg: sucrase, lactase, maltase
mono-saccharides
CARBOHYDRATE DIGESTION
PROTEINS
proteases in gastric and pancreatic juices
hydrolysis
PEPTIDES
PROTEOSES
intestinal peptides
proteases in pancreatic juices
hydrolysis
hydrolysis
AMINO ACIDS
AMINO ACIDS
PROTEIN DIGESTION
large fat droplets
bile
emulsification (mechanical digestion)
small fat droplets
bile
pancreatic lipase
hydrolysis (chemical digestion)
fatty acids monoglycerides glycerol
FAT DIGESTION

A sandwich's route through the gastro-intestinal tract

The simple, basic fate of a tuna sandwich.

The bread would be the main carbohydrate and so source of energy.

Bread: white and processed

- poor carbohydrates, low nutrition
  broken down in mouth and intestines into single sugars
  gives some energy but poor in relation to the work required in digestion
  slow transit time and creates sticky mucous.

Bread: brown and processed – much the same

Bread: good, wholemeal, brown

- more nutrients
  better energy payback
  fibre helps bowel, faster transit time, wheat flour will create some mucous.

The tuna would be the main protein.

Tuna:

- good protein, worked on by the acid in the stomach
  broken down through the gut and absorbed
  provides helpful building blocks and nutrients.

Mayonnaise: sugar, fats, eggs, additives, preservatives

- sugar – processed sugar, adds to toxic load, no nutritional value, uses more resources than it can provide, upsets blood sugars
- fats – poor quality, depending on the oil – processed to energy or surplus stored
  butter – broken down, mainly as it passes liver and pancreas and absorbed as fatty acid, not a lot of benefit because it is saturated fat, provides some energy but mostly surplus
- eggs – some protein, depending on the type of egg plus some more fat and more carbohydrate.

Salt, in bread, mayo and possibly the tuna and any additives
- adds to sodium level and will cause some dehydration.

If sweetcorn:
- good energy from plant sugars (and some more calories)
  some fibre, helps transit time.

If lettuce:
- light coloured, watery lettuce, eg: iceberg
  some fibre and water - not much in the way of nutrients
- Cos/Romaine hearts - fibre, water, vitamins and minerals
- green leafy, organic lettuce - fibre, water, vitamins, minerals.

SNACK 1

If you eat:
- a chocolate bar
- packet of crisps
- and a fizzy drink

you can generally expect:
- low nutrients
- poor quality carbohydrates – low energy contribution
- no fibre
- excess sugar and fat, disrupting blood sugar levels and affecting tiredness/energy
- slow transit time
- poor contribution to immune system, body repair or health.

Ditto – if you eat:
- pizza, burgers, pot noodles, many processed meals or snacks.

SNACK 2

If you eat
- a piece of fruit
- some nuts and seeds
- and drink water

you can generally expect:
- good nutrients
- good fibre
- body-friendly fats and sugars
- good energy payback
- good contributions to immune system, body repair and health.

Ditto – if you eat:
- rice, pulses, vegetables, wholegrains, good home-made meals or snacks.

The Cell

Every part of us is made of cells, the organs, the fluid, the bones, tissues and muscles are all made of cells – the cell is the essential basic unit of us, of life and all living things. There are around 100 trillion cells in the human body. Almost every one is microscopic, ranging from 7.5 micrometers to 150 micrometers (the average full stop on a printed page is approximately 100 micrometers).

The health of our cells is the true picture of our health. We need our cells to be healthy for us to be healthy. The health of our organs and tissues, is the health of the cells they are made of.

Each cell has a membrane, has a gel-like middle called cytoplasm and has a nucleus[1]. Each cell also has its own special team – a team of special components called organelles[2], which do all the things a cell has to do. They produce energy, produce protein, tackle invaders, ship out waste and many, many things. Cells are busy doing lots of things, all the time.

We start life as one cell formed from the joining of the sperm and the egg of reproduction and the genes from the sperm and the egg hold the code for our growth and development and who we are. Our original cell, at conception, contains a copy of our DNA and as that cell divides and multiplies, there is a complete copy of the DNA – our genetic code – in each resulting cell. The genes hold the instructions for the cell to multiply and develop and become our limbs and organs. At the beginning of life the original cell divides into two and those two divide and so on and the initial tiny cluster of cells is unprogrammed and can become any type of cell – these are the embryonic stem cells. The genes present in each cell hold the instructions for which type of cells they become and what they will do and we develop from a single cell, to cells with

[1] The nucleus of each cell contains the genetic material, in 23 pairs of chromosomes, made of DNA. (Chromosomes are strands of amino acids, which are derived from protein). These are the instructions which tell the cell what to do.

[2] Some of the Organelles:
the mitochondria is the energy centre providing the energy for the activity of the cell by converting sugar/glucose;
the lysosomes attack invaders and package up waste to be eliminated;
ribosomes make proteins;
the endoplasmic reticulum controls the production of protein;
the golgi apparatus parcels up the proteins to send them off to where they are needed.

defined roles, forming skin, spine, brain and all the parts of the body. We have over 200 different types of cell in our bodies. Tissue is a collection of cells organized together for a specific purpose - and our organs are collections of those tissues organized together. Cells divide and multiply from embryo stage to create us - and in adulthood they divide and multiply as part of the continual process of replacing cells which are wearing out and dying.

All the time things are passing in and out of our cells, through the cell membrane. Nutrients, oxygen, water and dissolved chemicals pass into the cell - and the products made by the cell, eg: proteins, hormones, repair and renewal material and waste substances are passed out. The cell membrane has gateways, like pores, that let these substances pass through - but the substances have to be recognized and fit with the keys in the cell membrane to allow entry or exit. There are different gateways and coded entry and exit systems for all the different things that have to pass in and out. The cell membrane has to be healthy and work properly to allow this to happen. It is made of a double-sided, flexible, fatty layer that protects the cell from invading infections, bacteria and viruses and monitors what is passed in and out. How well the cell can work and the cell membrane can perform relies on the presence of the nutrients, oils (lipids) and fatty acids it needs and the conditions and environment provided. We provide that environment by how we live and what we eat.

Once allocated to their various tissues and organs, all the cells are programmed and have a job to do - something to produce or change and this depends on the tissue and organ that the cell is part of. Adult stem cells can multiply to reproduce and replace old cells within particular parts of the body, eg: liver, blood, skin. Our new, red blood cells are made by stem cells inside our bone marrow, the soft white tissue inside some of our bones.

The functions of all the individual cells are chemical processes, forming and transforming the various substances received and passed on. Millions of our cells are dying and being replaced, all the time. We are in a constant balance of cells dying and being replaced. Skin and bone and blood cells are continually lost and replaced - but brain, heart and cartilage cells are not and have to be looked after to last a lifetime. Different types of cell have different ways of multiplying, creating new cells - but typically they split into two and each new cell has its copy of the genetic code and its instructions.

Our blood, lymph and nervous systems are made up of cells and the cells and cell membranes are our communication and transport system, within and between organs and throughout the body

If we don't provide the nutrients for our cells to function well - we are making it difficult for them to carry out all the essential functions they are programmed for. If we put the supply of nutrients, oxygen, water and chemicals out of balance we affect what they can do and the environment within our body.

Our DNA and our cells do what they do without us having to think consciously about it. We don't have to think about what they need and what they are doing. So long as we provide what is necessary and don't subject them to conditions they can't cope with – they know what to do. Normally we wouldn't have to measure and regulate things for our cells, we just provide a grand selection of everything they need and they sort it all out. We do need to safeguard that general arrangement for them – and prevent imbalances that could overwhelm the system. Nutrition, what we eat, is the supermarket for our cells.

Our cells are busy working together to keep us well but if we become unwell it is because something is going wrong in some of the cells, the cells not being able to work properly, being damaged – scientists research infections and disease by looking at cells. Cell damage can be caused by infections, genetics, injury or lifestyle – what we eat or what we do.

Life is changing all the time and some changes are taking place very quickly and very intensely, subjecting our cells and our chemistry to significant change and imbalance. The body is a wonderfully adaptive and evolutionary thing – but some of these changes can become stresses and strains if we can't adapt quickly enough – and some people may be able to adapt more quickly than others. We all have different thresholds for coping with deficiencies or overloads. Nutritional deficiencies can cause problems and drugs, alcohol and other excesses or infection can cause problems.

If we take hydration / **dehydration** as an example:

A typical characteristic of modern lifestyle is rushing and a faster pace of life and a greater exposure to chemicals in modern products. These sorts of conditions can easily cause dehydration. Once upon a time our most regular drink would have been water, because it was virtually all there was to choose from – but now there is a vast range of drinks, in bottles, tins, packets and sachets – so it is possible to quench our thirst or enjoy a drink whilst not actually taking in that much water. Even for those not involved in a fast pace of life, there may be a higher sodium, chemical or pollutant load in food, drink and environment which can cause dehydration. Our bodies are 80% water – a high level to keep topped up – and water is continually being used in all the bodily functions and processes.

Extra demand, long sustained demand or stress, ie: extra things for the body to do/extra processing, mobilizes extra nutrients which uses more water. This results in the cell becoming less hydrated, which can have two effects; a mucous forming in the cell because the fluid is less liquid and the cell trying to hang onto what water there is. It

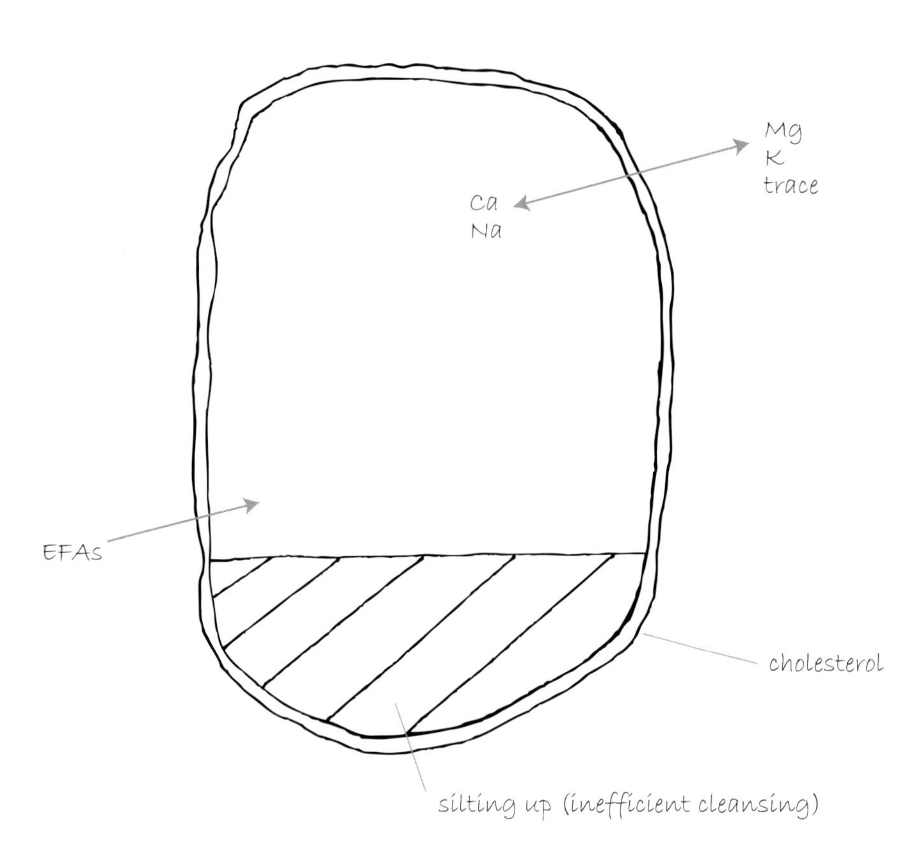

Elimination

the main route is:

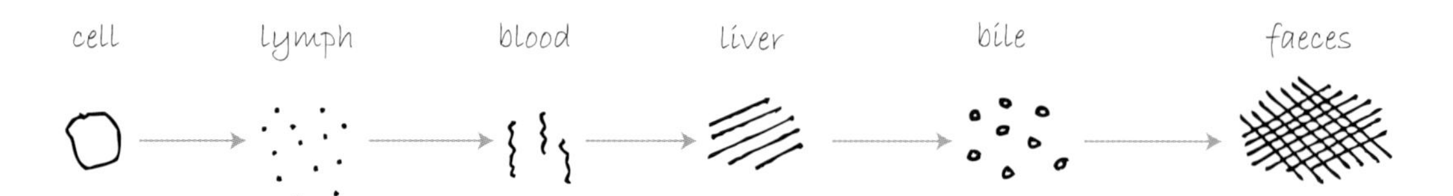

If there is any overflow, because any of the routes of elimination are not working efficiently, or if the load is too great, the overflow goes to the kidneys, lungs, skin, nose, eyes and ears. In females excess elimination may also be passed in menstrual fluid/tissue.

senses a lack of water and acts to protect itself. To do this the cell forms an extra layer, a coating, to prevent water loss and keep hydration in – and this coating is cholesterol. In this state the cell may not be cleansing as it ideally would, things are not being passed in and out of the cell via the cell membrane as easily. The mucous formed inside the cell may be holding some waste products – toxins – that it should be passing out. Although these are natural short term reactions, they aren't good sustained over a prolonged period of time. All the time the cell needs to be taking in what it needs and eliminating waste. This can also explain why people may be under-nourished and deficient in vitamins and minerals, even though they are eating well – if the nutrients cannot be absorbed sufficiently or are not being processed into a form that the body can use them. When cell cleansing and the processing that should be taking place is not taking place, or is compromised, toxins formed can build up. The cells in the liver can sometimes take the greatest impact because it is one of the most active organs, with so much to do. The liver de-saturates essential fatty acids, produces hormones, stores vitamins, converts fats into energy and detoxifies, as well as much more – so stressed cells and strong imbalances can have a large knock-on effect. When the cell has an increased coating, the daily/overnight mineral exchange is also not taking place, or not taking place properly – magnesium and potassium and trace elements passing into the cell and calcium and sodium being passed out. These work in partnership so they all need to be present, in balance, to work properly. This is also called the electrolyte exchange and is covered in the next section (page 81).

To restore the balance, we would need to turn off the stress alert, whatever that may be: rigorous exercise, poor/unbalanced diet, work, vaccines, infections, etc, or trauma – for example an operation or injury, big emotional or anxiety event. Turning off the stress alert means rectifying or reducing what is causing it, removing the stress – which we may or may not be able to do, plus drink more water and optimize elimination (see page 78). Even when we cannot easily turn off the stress alert – by being aware of what is happening, we can drink more water, address the dehydration and adjust the diet to help elimination. By eating things of a high water content and easily digestible foods, we will be increasing the intake of water and reducing the water needed in digestion, reducing the stress on the system. (There is a separate section on Stress, including the role of nutrition, page 158). Restoring the environment the cell likes will enable it to resume normal metabolism.

Histamine also affects the water in the body. Dehydration makes histamine levels go up and rehydration helps levels of histamine go down. High histamine creates inflammation, amongst other things, hence anti-histamines.

Aldesterone, produced by the adrenals, is one of the general regulators of water in the body.

Cells carry out the vital activities of all living things: movement, respiration, sensation, growth, reproduction, excretion and nutrition.

Examples of cells:

muscle cells are squashy and stretchy to contract and release

gland cells make hormones to lubricate your skin and hair

osteoblasts produce bone proteins to maintain the skeleton

macrophages kill viruses and bacteria

cardiac cells contract for your heart to pump blood

nerve cells (neurons) are very long and thin and carry electrical messages for the entire body to and from the brain.

There is an excellent web site on the cell - www.centreofthecell.org - by Queen Mary University of London and Barts and The London School of Medicine and Dentistry.

Electrolytes

Electrolytes is the descriptive name for a large group of compounds that break up in solution to form changed particles. They are a chemical substance which, when dissolved in water or melted, separate into electrically charged particles (ions), capable of conducting an electric current. They include sodium (Na), potassium (K), calcium (Ca), magnesium (Mg), chloride (Cl), bicarbonate, phosphate and sulphate – all of which occur in the food which we eat and drink. The electrolytes are involved in metabolic activities and are essential to the normal function of all cells. The concentration of sodium and potassium either side of the cell membrane produces the effect of the fluids and electrolytes being drawn from one side to the other and this provides the means by which electrochemical impulses are transmitted in nerve and muscle fibres. The concentration of all the various electrolytes in body fluids is maintained within a narrow range. This is dependent on adequate intake of water, the presence of electrolytes and the mechanisms within the body that regulate absorption, distribution and excretion of water and the particles dissolved in it.

Again, this is something we do not normally have to be consciously aware of. Our body and our cells just get on with electrolyte balance. The most common time for us to think of it, or talk about it, is in connection with exercise and nowadays in relation to sports drinks. Because we lose more water from our body when we exercise, some electrolytes will be lost in that water. Most of the time the body can put that right and rebalance things. If it is particularly hot or we are doing particularly strenuous exercise, it is important to replace the fluid lost. Usually just replacing the water, will enable things to sort themselves out. If the exercise is prolonged or strenuous, then we may also need to replace electrolytes, usually sodium, and perhaps energy. Most commercial sports drinks fall into 3 categories, isotonic, hypotonic and hypertonic.

An isotonic drink would have a moderate concentration of sugar/energy, to replace fluid and provide fuel/energy during exercise, eg: 200ml of orange squash per litre and a pinch of salt.

A hypotonic drink would have a lower concentration of sugar/energy, to provide a more rapid fluid replacement without providing much energy, during or after exercise, eg: 100ml of orange squash per litre and a pinch of salt.

A hypertonic drink would have a higher concentration of energy/sugar, to replenish energy/glycogen, after exercise, this would not help rehydration during exercise, eg: 400ml of orange squash per litre and a pinch of salt.

For sessions of moderate exercise, for up to an hour, water is usually all we need. If the exercise is more intense, or for longer periods, or in hot conditions, the addition of carbohydrate and electrolytes may be more helpful - judged on provision of fuel/energy and fluid replacement.

As well as exercise, other conditions that can affect fluid loss from the body and electrolyte balance are diarrhoea and vomiting. Again, the body can often rebalance these losses itself but in frail people or infants or even poorly pets, trained medical staff may administer electrolytes to help restore the balance. The effects of fluid loss from the body can range from impaired performance, lack of muscular strength, exhaustion, hallucinations and circulatory collapse.

The effects of an electrolyte imbalance are not isolated to a particular organ or system. In general, however, imbalances in calcium concentrations affect the bones, kidney and gastro-intestinal tract. Calcium also influences the permeability of cell membranes and thereby regulates neuro-muscular activity. Sodium affects the osmosis of blood and therefore influences blood volume and pressure and the retention or loss of interstitial fluid. Potassium affects muscular activities, notably those of the heart, intestines and respiratory tract, and also affects neural stimulation of the skeletal muscles.

That gives a general summary but there are some additional notes for a little more detail.

Additional notes:

Electrolytes are categorized into 4 main groups: acids, bases, buffers and salts.

Acids - by definition an acid is any substance that will release a hydrogen ion when in solution. It is the concentration of hydrogen ions that accounts for the chemical properties of acids. Hydrochloric acid is an important acid in the body, produced in the stomach to aid digestion.

Bases - are alkaline compounds. When in solution they combine with hydrogen ions. Bicarbonate is an important ion in the body and plays a critical role in the transportation of respiratory gases and in the elimination of waste products.

Buffers - minimize changes of certain ions in our body fluids. They act as a reservoir for hydrogen ions and they donate or remove hydrogen ions from the solutions in the body fluids to maintain a constant pH. The normal pH range of blood and other body fluids is very narrow - between 7.36 and 7.41. Maintaining pH within this range is critical.

Salts - a salt is any compound that results from the chemical interaction of an acid and a base. Like acids and bases, salts are electrolyte compounds that change in solution. If the water is removed they will crystalize and form salts. When an acid and a base react in solution the positive ion of the base and the negative ion of the acid will join to form a salt and additional water. Salts are common in many body fluids and tissues, such as bone. The proper amount of such mineral salt electrolytes as potassium, calcium, and sodium are required for the proper functioning of nerves and for contraction of muscle tissue.

Sodium chloride, calcium chloride, magnesium chloride, sodium bicarbonate, potassium chloride, sodium sulphate, calcium carbonate and calcium phosphate are examples of several salts which contribute important electrolytes required for numerous body functions.

Homeostasis

Homeostasis is the constant state of balance in the internal environment, inside the body – the maintenance of temperature, blood pressure, oxygen, carbon dioxide, water and electrolyte concentrations and pH (acidity) concentrations, despite external events and changes.

The word comes from the Greek meaning stable, or steady. The person acknowledged as having discovered this concept in relation to human biology was the French physiologist, Claude Bernard in 1865 and Walter Cannon an American physiologist adopted the word in this connection in 1930. (Walter Cannon is also the physiologist who, in the 1920s first explained the understanding of the 'flight or fight' response).

Homeostasis is maintained by control systems which detect changes in the internal environment and respond to/rebalance/correct the change. These are commonly referred to as either positive or negative feedback mechanisms. Negative feedback systems work by a situation being detected and then a response to counteract it. Most of our control mechanisms are negative feedback.

A control system has 3 basic components: detector, control centre, effector.

The detector detects the change; the control centre decides the acceptable limits of the change and when to instigate an adjustment and instruct the effector; the effector produces the required change; the detector detects the change.

The example most often used to demonstrate this is temperature change, which flatteringly likens us to a central heating system (see diagram page 85). In the body, fall in temperature is detected by special temperature-sensitive nerve endings, the detectors. They send information to groups of cells in the hypothalamus, in the brain, which in this instance is the control centre. The output from the hypothalamus (hormones) activates effectors to raise body temperature: these may be muscles to cause shivering, narrowing of blood vessels in skin to reduce blood flow to and from heat loss surfaces, and instructions for behavioural change – putting on clothes, curling up, seeking a warmer place, lighting a fire, putting the heating on, closing the window, etc.

When body temperature returns to within acceptable range, the temperature-sensitive nerve endings stop stimulating the cells of the control centre and they stop producing the hormones that instruct the effectors.

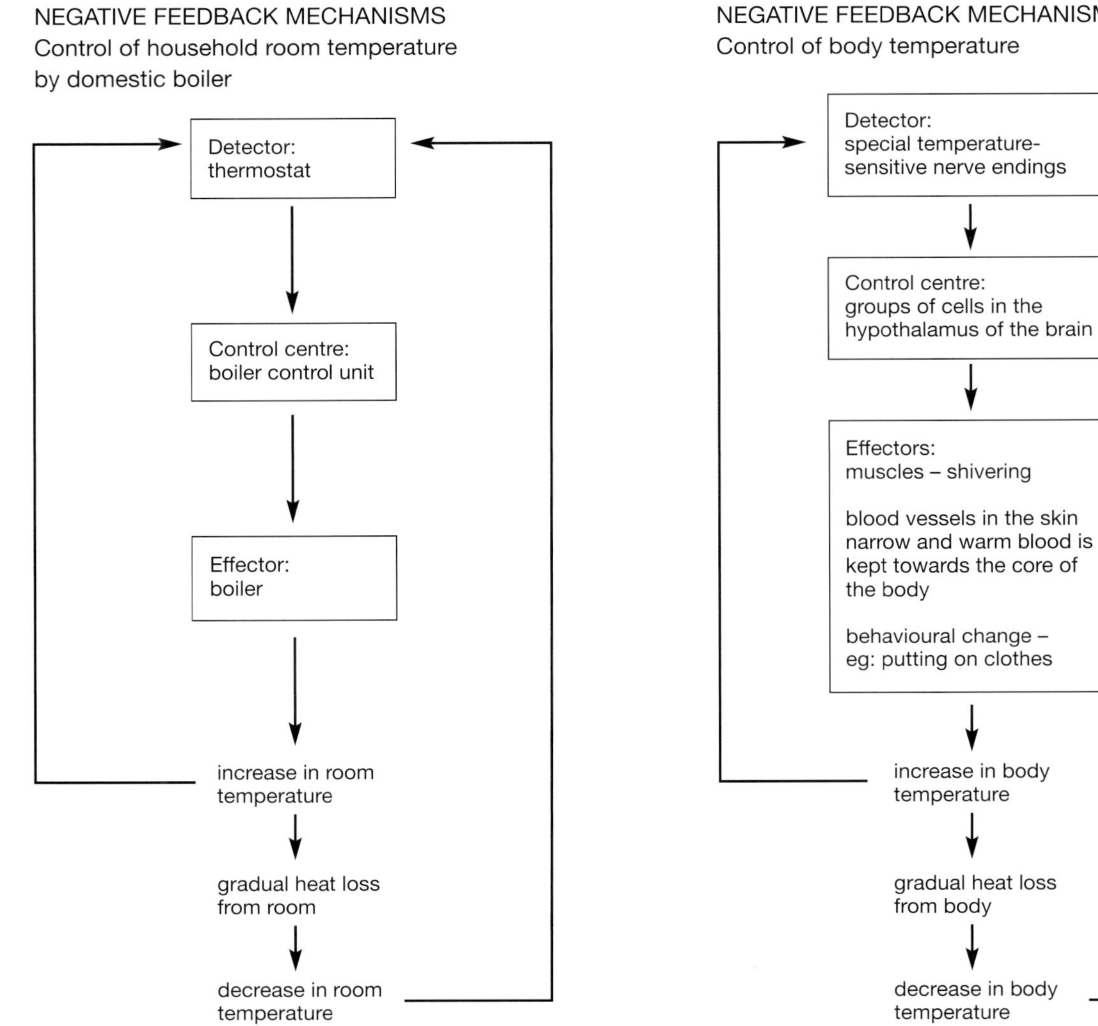
NEGATIVE FEEDBACK MECHANISMS
Control of household room temperature by domestic boiler
Detector: thermostat
Control centre: boiler control unit
Effector: boiler
increase in room temperature
gradual heat loss from room
decrease in room temperature
NEGATIVE FEEDBACK MECHANISMS
Control of body temperature
Detector: special temperature-sensitive nerve endings
Control centre: groups of cells in the hypothalamus of the brain
Effectors: muscles – shivering
blood vessels in the skin narrow and warm blood is kept towards the core of the body
behavioural change – eg: putting on clothes
increase in body temperature
gradual heat loss from body
decrease in body temperature

A feedback system includes:

hormones - chemical messengers
nerves - electrical messengers
receptors - specialized nerves or endocrine glands
control unit - manager, usually/often the brain
effectors - organs, muscles, glands.

Positive feedback mechanisms occur much less in the body because they can be harmful or dangerous. They could be fatal if they didn't stop/went out of control. Positive feedback mechanisms work by detecting a situation and then instead of counteracting it, emphasizing or increasing it. This happens in blood platelet production and clotting to heal an injury, causing a fever, or building contractions at childbirth. All these things are helpful to deal with the immediate situation but could cause real problems out of control.

Like metabolism, maintaining homeostasis is what we are doing all the time. This is why we use 1,000-2,000 calories a day, even before we think we are doing anything - because our bodies are busy doing things all the time. All the time our internal environment may be becoming too acidic and being balanced, having high or low blood pressure and being balanced, becoming too hot or cold and being balanced, running out of oxygen and breathing, running out of water and absorbing some more. These things have to be maintained within safe, healthy limits and it's a non-stop job and involves all the different systems and parts of the body, working together - and this is why what we do and how we look after our body can make such a difference.

Many illnesses and conditions are caused by homeostatic imbalance and as we get older some of the detectors and control systems will become less effective. Any time there is too much of something harmful and we can't correct it, or not enough of something essential and we can't correct it, that is homeostatic imbalance. Ideally our control mechanisms deal with this but if the mechanisms don't work properly, that is when medical intervention may be used or illnesses occur.

NOTHING CREATED BY MAN
COMPARES TO THE DESIGN
OF THE HUMAN BODY.

Patrick Holford

Nutrition

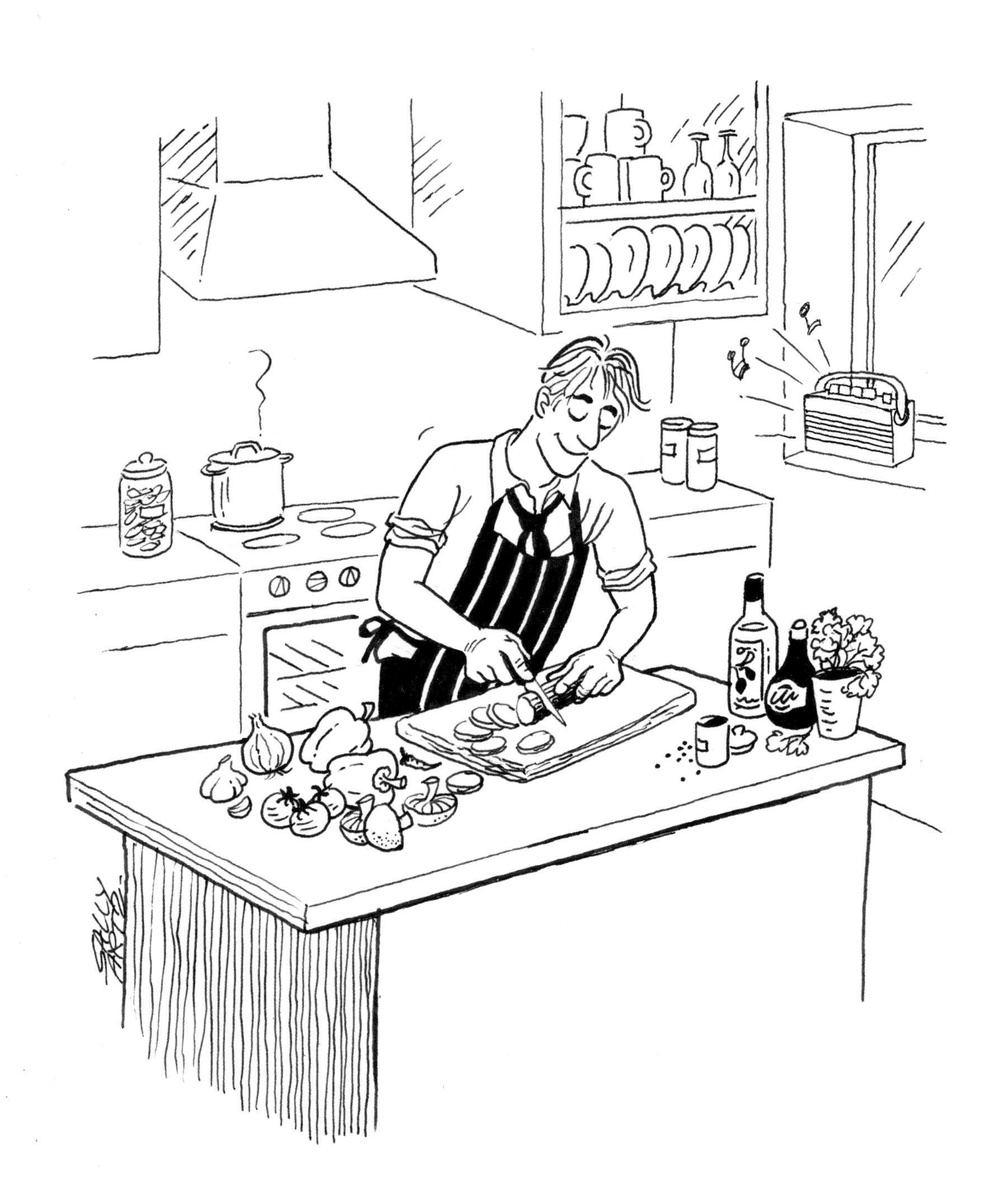

Nutrition

from Latin: nutrire – nourish

- the supplying or receiving of nourishment, food
- nutrient: substance serving as or providing nourishment
- nutritious: nourishing, efficient as food
- nutritive: serving as nutritious food, concerned in nutrition, nutritious article of food
- nutriment: nourishing food

nurse, from Latin: nutricia, nutricius, nutrire

nutrition /nu·tri·tion/ (noo-trish´un) the taking in and metabolism of nutrients (food and other nourishing material) by an organism so that life is maintained and growth can take place. nutri´tional

Nutrition, the food we eat as fuel to keep our bodies alive and well. The better the suitability of the food, the better the body will function. Our requirements are for foods that give us energy, foods that help build and repair our structure and foods that help to protect us. Nutrition is the food we eat, it's not an alternative therapy.

The body needs nutrients to grow cells, repair wear and tear, protect against infection and to function properly.

Nothing created by man compares to the exceptional design of the human body.

- 2.5m red blood cells made every second in the bone marrow to keep body cells supplied with oxygen

- the heart beats approximately 115,000 a day, pumping blood through over 20 miles of blood vessels

- 10 litres of digestive juices are produced and secreted every day to break down food and assist absorption through the gastro-intestinal wall

- the gastro-intestinal wall is 30 feet long with the surface area of a football pitch and effectively replaces itself every 4 days

- the immune system replaces its entire army every week

- the external skin surface replaces itself every month

- most of the body is renewed every 7 years.

Your body is working very hard - all the time - even when we think we're not doing anything. We're breathing and the lungs inflating and deflating and the heart beating and the blood circulating, the muscles and skin holding and altering our position, continual renewal and repair, cleansing and elimination - all the metabolic actions, the sum total of all the bio-chemical processes that keep the cells alive, all the structural and functional activity of all the organs and systems and all the constant messaging.

Energy produced from food powers all these continual, sub-conscious, vital processes - leaving plenty leftover to keep us warm and allow us to move and undertake physical activity as well. We are very aware of the energy needed to walk, carry heavy shopping or suitcases, or run – either for pleasure or an emergency. It is easy to forget all the rest of the energy we are using all the time. This is why what we eat is so important. Our body is composed entirely of molecules derived from food, macronutrients and micronutrients, all taken in and digested, and health and integrity depend on what we eat. We will burn somewhere around 1,000 to 2,000 calories a day just staying alive, before undertaking conscious exercise and activities.

Nutrition is not a set of rules. It is entirely up to all of us, what and how we eat – and the most important thing is to enjoy good food. Nutrition has been first and second nature to us for years and years and years. Animals and humans do have an innate, valuable, cumulative wisdom of food sources and requirements. Those instincts have been disrupted and very strongly influenced by recent trends and developments of the last 50-100 years. There are exceptional, potential health benefits for everyone in thinking about food and what is good for us. Nutrition isn't new, it isn't a fad but it did become overlooked for many people, for various reasons. Knowing more about food and more about our own design and how we work is simply reminding us of the basic wisdom we have always had.

Our nutritional status depends on 4 factors:

- quality of our food
- quantity of food
- how efficient our digestion, absorption and utilisation are
- our bio-chemical and genetic make-up.

Nutrition isn't only for sports people, athletes and celebrities – it does the same for them as it does for all of us. It affects: mental performance, emotional balance, physical performance and resilience to illness. The right food gives us the best chances of feeling well, performing well and having a good, strong immune system.

The quality of the food we eat has direct influences on our nutritional status. Good food grown in good soils supplies good carbohydrates, proteins and fats, rich in vitamins and minerals. If food is grown in depleted soil, the food will be depleted in nutrients and we will eat and absorb significantly reduced nutrients, vitamins and minerals. Food quality is affected by how food is grown, how it is harvested, how it is stored, how it is processed and then what we do with the food in preparation and cooking. At each stage nutrients can be depleted and lost. Also, at each stage unhelpful or even unhealthy substances can be added to it.

In Britain there is rarely a problem of too little food, often a problem of too much food and as a consequence, malnutrition is endemic. Malnutrition doesn't only affect people who don't have enough to eat. People who eat a lot will still have malnutrition if what they are eating isn't providing the nutrients they need or they are unable to absorb them. In developing countries, there is often not enough food and in these places we see cases of malnutrition from under nutrition. Too much food can lead to as many health problems as not enough. Where we have more food than we need, food choices are what make the important difference.

Our ability to be able to absorb nutrients is as important as what we eat. Modern lifestyles and personal habits often interfere with digestive processes – so that even if we are eating good food, we may not be getting the benefit of that goodness and being able to use it. If we eat too much sweet food, we will upset the balance of the bacteria in the gut, which will interfere with the absorption of nutrients. If all the right nutrients aren't available, that can interfere with absorption because many nutrients work in combination with others. If we eat too much gluey, gunky food (wheat, meat, dairy), this can build up on the inside of the gut wall which will interfere with the absorption of nutrients, especially if we aren't eating enough fibre. If there are too many toxins in the gut, they will reduce the absorption of nutrients. If we don't chew our food well and/or if we eat too fast, this will interfere with digestion, the secretion of digestive juices and reduce absorption and can increase toxicity. Toxicity is simply the load of toxins on the body, the things that are a threat to the body and internal environment, that have to be neutralized and/or eliminated. If the amount of toxins taken in or produced is too high, the body has a lot of extra work to do and if it can't neutralize or eliminate those toxins quickly enough, we will be affected by aches, inflammation or reactions of some kind, as well as tiredness. There are lots of foods that are easy on the body, easy on digestion and create a very low toxic load.

We are all individuals, with different genetic make-ups and different needs. We are likely to have 300 different strains of bacteria, unique to us as an individual. There is no 'right diet' for everyone. What we need depends on age, growth, sex, illness, pregnancy, breast feeding, psychological and/or emotional stress, activity level, genetics and other considerations such as toxic overload and drugs. Once, our taste buds and cravings would lead us to the nourishment we needed at that time, which is how many animals still live – we would instinctively know what was good for us – but we have generally overridden and confused those instincts by modern, artificial flavours and foods and habits. Now we have to re-educate our brains to make decisions about our nutritional needs. We have to do it consciously as opposed to sub-consciously – and we don't come with a maintenance manual.

Our bodies just want us to eat a good mixture of good food (and it would quite like us not to eat too much of the others!).

As well as the major food groups; proteins, fats, carbohydrates and water, there are about 45 different vitamins, minerals, amino acids and essential fatty acids required by our bodies to be healthy. In addition there are other essential ingredients including air (oxygen), warmth, shelter, sunlight and companionship. A deficiency of any essential nutrient will produce anything from mild, almost imperceptible, ill-health to terminal conditions and death. It is rare to have isolated deficiencies but quite common to have multiple deficiencies, especially in people who are unwell. A typical modern diet tends to consist of dietary excesses and shortages which have very big effects on the body's metabolism and health.

We often only stop to think about what the body needs when something goes wrong - but we are designed the other way round - we are designed to maintain a state of health as our best resistance to illness.

So what we eat goes on to become the cells of our limbs and organs, our systems, our blood and all the fluids, enzymes and hormones that we are made of. Some foods are very easy for our bodies to breakdown and use and give us energy. Other foods clutter up the system and slow it down. They need a lot of work done on them to become useful, they don't provide good nutrients in the right combinations and they create a lot of waste. The wrong foods take a lot of extra work to digest and process which will make us tired or have less energy than we would have had - and at the end of all the extra work and processing, the energy gained will be very poor in comparison (which I have already referred to as a bad pay-back arrangement). If they are sweet and fatty foods, or contain a lot of toxins, there is not only the waste that makes its way out of the body - there is the waste that is left behind.

Natural, whole foods are always recommended because that makes life really easy for our body and our digestive system. The goodness is absorbed, they don't over-tax the system, they give back good nutrition and energy, they don't leave debris and gluey gunk around in the intestines. Processed foods are a challenge to the digestion, they don't have as much goodness and what there is won't be so easily absorbed, many of them do leave a gluey gunk behind and possibly toxins as well - which may be eliminated, or may be pushed away into fat and muscle tissue. The body has to get excess toxins safely away from the blood stream and in the internal environment, the safest place to store unwanted toxins is in fat and muscle tissue. This can make fat tissue harder to lose and causes aches, pain and inflammation in muscle tissue. It is also associated with the formation of cellulite.

Food groups

Carbohydrates, proteins and fats - the macronutrients
Vitamins and minerals - micronutrients.

Energy foods are generally carbohydrates such as grains, potatoes and fruit and also fatty foods such as oils and butter. These foods are broken down to form simple sugars such as glucose (as explained in the chapter on digestion).

Glucose enters a bio-chemical cascade[1] - which is what is taking place inside us all the time to provide the continual supply of energy - for everything.

Glucose combines with oxygen to produce energy molecules[2] that can be used immediately or stored. These energy molecules power most cell and body processes that are going on all the time, the building, the repair, the breathing, the continual chemical transactions, the digestion, the circulation, plus moving muscles and limbs, etc. (Fats also enter the cycle after some modification and produce energy).

There are 3 major food groups - carbohydrates, proteins and fats. Each group of foods has a different way of being digested and utilized in the body. We need a healthy combination of them all.

Carbohydrates

Carbohydrates are energy foods, including, potatoes, fruit, sugars and grains, eg: pasta, bread and rice. Some carbohydrates are digestible such as starch and some are not digestible because they contain fibre. Grains and potatoes contain starch and when we eat them, these foods are broken down by digestive enzymes to form simple sugars (eg: glucose). Glucose enters its bio-chemical cascade and produces energy.

Fibre may not be digested but it still has a very important role in digestion. Fibre can bind with water and increase the bulk of the waste parcels as they form in the colon which makes it easier to transit the system and decreases the time it takes to reach the exit. This is good because it does quite a good job of cleaning up the system and decreases the exposure of the delicate bowel walls to the waste products of digestion which are often toxic. Fibre includes cellulose and lignin which are found in plant cell walls. Vegetables and grains contain a good proportion of fibre.

[1] called the Krebs cycle/citric acid cycle

[2] ATP – adenosine triphosphate

Proteins

Protein foods help with building, repair and regulation and are generally found in eggs, nuts, seeds, beans, pulses, meat and fish. Grains such as rice have a protein portion as well as a carbohydrate portion. Protein foods also form muscle, bone, connective tissue, collagen and cartilage. Some proteins have a metabolic function, forming hormones like insulin, digestive enzymes and anti-bodies.

The smallest unit of protein is the amino acid. The largest chains of amino acids form the DNA in every cell. Other smaller chains link together to form hormones like insulin, or strands of muscle tissue. There are about 20 different amino acids that plants and animals build up in long chains, that we need. 12 we can produce ourselves (from other amino acids). 8 are termed essential because the body cannot make them, they have to come in in the diet – we have to make sure that we eat foods that provide those amino acids.

Fats

Foods containing fat are essential in our diets for the cell wall of every cell, to provide an energy store, to enable brain activity, to provide insulation and to be used to form biological substances essential for the normal working of the body – eg: hormones. Dietary fats include oils, butter, cheeses, meat, nuts and seeds. All fats are made up of small building blocks[1]. They consist of different fatty acids, depending on the food they came from. There are dozens of fatty acids in nature, which generally fall into two groups known as saturated fats and unsaturated fats. Saturated fats are the solid, hard fats; unsaturated fats are the softer, oily fats. We need both types of fat in our diets although in a typical western diet there is generally too much saturated fat and not enough unsaturated fat.

Fats can also enter the energy production cascade[2] after some modification. Fats are used in this way when there are no sugars available but they aren't as efficient in energy production as sugars.

The fats and oils debate is an area often surrounded by confusion. There are many sources of information and conflicting messages about whether to eat margarine or butter, which is the best oil to cook with and which are the healthier oils. The answers aren't necessarily simple and depend on various factors, generally to do with molecules – molecular bonds, hydrogen and oxygen – but easy solutions for us are quite simple. (This is covered later in the chapter, page 107.)

[1] of carbon, hydrogen and oxygen, triglycerides: 3 fatty acids and a molecule of glycerol

[2] Krebs cycle

Examples of unsaturated and saturated fats

Unsaturated	Saturated
almond	fats, especially hard fats
avocado	beef
dark green leaves	lamb/mutton
cashew nuts	pork
flax seeds	
hemp seeds	butter
mackerel	cocoa butter
olive	shea nut butter
peanut	
pecan	coconut oil
pumpkin seeds	palm oil
safflower oil	
salmon	the body converts excess sugar into
sesame seeds	saturated fats
sunflower oil	
soy bean	
trout	
walnut	
oils of wild seeds, eg: blackcurrant	

Micronutrients

We also need a good supply of other nutrients to work properly along with the carbohydrates, proteins and fats. Nutrients include vitamins and minerals. The metabolic actions of the body that are going on all the time[1], take place due to various reactions and these reactions are brought about by enzymes – enzymes are dependent on these vitamins and minerals. Without them our metabolism stops functioning properly and disease, various conditions and symptoms would result.

[1] metabolic actions/metabolism – the sum total of all the bio-chemical processes that keep the cells alive, all the structural and functional activity of all the organs and systems. A complex inter-twining set of chemical processes by which life is made possible for a living organism.
ie: what is going on inside us, all the time. The continual breaking down and joining up of simple components to provide what is needed.

Foods can help protect us from disease by supporting the immune system, eg: vitamins A, C and E and minerals like selenium and zinc. Proteins are needed to form the cells that fight bacteria and viruses – and nutrients such as vitamins and minerals are needed to help the enzymes and other systems to clear away waste products. Other vitamins and minerals play vital roles as the activating substance in numerous enzyme systems. Anti-oxidants also play a large role in protecting vulnerable molecules in the body (see page 109).

Vitamins

The word is derived from 'vital mineral'. A vitamin is a substance that the body needs to function properly and that it cannot produce itself so it must be present in the diet. Vitamins activate enzymes which in turn enable all the body processes. They are needed to balance hormones, produce energy, boost the immune system, make healthy skin and protect arteries; they are vital for the brain and nervous system and throughout the body. Vitamins A, C and E are anti-oxidants, they slow down the ageing process and protect the body from cancer, heart disease and pollution. B and C vitamins are vital for converting food into mental and physical energy. Vitamin D, from our food and made in the skin in the presence of sunlight, helps to control calcium balance. B and C vitamins are richest in fresh fruit and vegetables. Vitamin A comes in two forms: retinol, the animal form and beta-carotene, found in red, yellow and orange fruit and vegetables. Vitamin E is found in seeds and nuts and in seed and nut oils.

Vitamin C is one of the best known vitamins and was discovered when it was linked to a disease called scurvy. Sailors at sea in the age of sailing ships (1500-1700) often did not have access to fresh foods for months at a time. They often developed bleeding, swollen gums, a dry, scaly skin and bruising, often culminating in massive bleeding from which they could die. Even before they knew what the deficiency was, it was found that by eating citrus fruits the condition could be avoided – attributed to a British naval surgeon, James Lind, in 1753. British ships would dock at southern European ports to take on citrus fruits before going on longer voyages and because the sailors often ate limes they became known as 'limeys'. Citrus fruits are high in Vitamin C which prevents scurvy. Eating citrus fruits to protect against scurvy was finally adopted by the British Navy in the 1790s.

Vitamin C is needed for the maintenance of healthy connective tissue and bones, for the normal metabolism of cholesterol, for the production of cortisol by the adrenal gland, for the metabolism of various brain chemicals, for the synthesis of the hormone noradrenalin (which has powerful effects upon pulse rate and blood pressure), as a powerful anti-oxidant and it has anti-viral and anti-bacterial properties.

Other vitamins are vitamin A, vitamins B1, B2, B3, B5, B6 and B12, folic acid, biotin, choline, inositol, vitamin C, vitamin D, vitamin E and vitamin K. (See Vitamin Table for more information, page 100.)

Minerals

Like vitamins, minerals are essential for all the vital body functions.

Minerals come from rocks and find their way into plants via the soil. Plants need minerals to grow and we need the minerals present in the plants, though usually not in very large quantities.

Calcium, magnesium and phosphorous help in the formation of bones and teeth. Nerve signals, vital for brain and muscles, depend on calcium, magnesium, sodium and potassium. Oxygen is carried in the blood by an iron compound. Chromium helps control blood sugar levels. Zinc is essential for all body repair, renewal and development. Selenium and zinc help boost the immune system. Brain function depends on adequate magnesium, manganese, zinc and other essential minerals. These are just a few of thousands of examples.

Minerals are often divided up into 2 main groups, macro-minerals and trace elements.

The macro-minerals include calcium, phosphorus, magnesium, sodium, potassium and chlorine and are needed in quantities of several hundred milligrams per day. They are involved in structural functions, bones and cells, as well as metabolic ones.

The trace elements include iron, zinc, copper, manganese, iodine, chromium, selenium, molybdenum, cobalt and sulphur. They are required in very small quantities of a few milligrams a day or less and have subtle but vitally important effects on metabolism. (See Mineral Table for more information, page 101.)

We only need small quantities of vitamins and minerals but because they are only present in our foods in very small amounts, it is easy to become deficient in them. We may need large amounts of food to get the recommended levels. Most modern diets are relatively deficient in many of these nutrients which would be a contributory factor in susceptibility to illness.

A healthy diet will have a good combination of protein, carbohydrate, fats and nutrients of all types, in a good balance and in an easily digestible form. Dark green, leafy vegetables, root vegetables, fruit, beans, seeds and nuts, every day, will provide the variety and fibre we need.

Nutrition advice and food labels often refer to vitamins and minerals by RDA, or Recommended Daily Amounts/Recommended Daily Allowance/Recommended Dietary Allowance. There are greatly varying opinions on RDAs and some are set extremely low, hardly even constituting a bare minimum.

vitamin	sources	benefits / function	contra-agents
Vitamin A (beta carotene)	Orange/red coloured fruit, veg, fish, eggs, liver oil, dairy products, beef, liver	Healthy skin, eyes, immune system, mucous membranes, helps convalescing	Coffee, alcohol, excessive iron, vitamin D deficiency
Vitamin B1 (thiamine)	Nuts, brown rice, rice, legumes, fish, egg yolks, poultry, pork	Health of skin, mouth and eyes, carbohydrate metabolism, digestion	Tobacco, coffee, alcohol, sulphur drugs, anti-biotics, oestrogen
Vitamin B2 (Riboflavin)	Nuts, wholegrains, seaweed, organ meats, dairy products	Promotes healthy nervous system, brain function, synthesis of sex hormones	Sugar, alcohol, coffee, sleeping pills, oestrogen, food processing methods
Vitamin B3 (Niacine)	Nuts, dairy, wheatgerm, seaweed, poultry, lean meats, liver, dairy products	Promotes healthy nervous system, brain function, synthesis of sex hormones	Alcohol, coffee, heat, sulphur drugs, sleeping pills, oestrogen
Vitamin B5 (Pantothenic acid)	Wholegrains, cereals, mushrooms, egg yolks, organ meats	Health of adrenals, skin, immune and nervous system, growth, energy, healing	Alcohol, coffee, heat, sulphur drugs, sleeping pills, oestrogen
Vitamin B6 (Pyridoxine)	Wholegrains, cabbage, legumes, green vegetables, meat	Carbohydrate-fat-protein metabolism, healthy skin and nervous system	Sugar, alcohol, coffee, contraceptive pills, food processing, radiation
Vitamin B 12 (Cobalamin)	Nuts, miso, soy sauce, Marmite, pickles, fish, organ meats, dairy products	Red blood cell formation, healthy nervous system, metabolism	Coffee, alcohol, tobacco, laxatives, oestrogen, sleeping pills, sunlight
Biotin	Wholegrains, nuts, lentils, egg yolk, sardines, pork, lamb, liver	Carbohydrate-fat-protein and vitamin B metabolism, skin, hair and muscle health	Alcohol, coffee, raw egg white, sulphur drugs, oestrogen
Choline	Lecithin, wheatgerm, egg yolk, fish, liver, organ meats	Digestion of fats, liver, kidney, hair, thymus gland and nerve health	Sugar, alcohol, coffee, oestrogen, food processing, sulphur drugs
Inositol	Lecithin, citrus fruits, nuts, raisins, milk, wholegrains, vegetables (cabbage)	Fat and cholesterol metabolism, healthy hair	Sugar, coffee, alcohol, corn, anti-biotics, food processing, oestrogen
Folic Acid	Green leafy veg, beans, rice, sprouts, fish, liver	Reproduction and growth, red blood cell formation, liver and glands	Alcohol, coffee, tobacco, sunlight, food processing methods, oestrogen
PABA (para-aminobenzoic acid)	Rice, bran, wholegrains, liver, kidney	Helps form folic acid and assimilate vitamin B5, acts as a sun-screen	Alcohol, oestrogen, sulphur drugs, food processing methods
Vitamin C (ascorbic acid)	Citrus fruits, rose hips, strawberries, peppers, tomatoes, sprouted alfalfa seeds, broccoli	Healthy teeth, gums and bones, good immunity, better iron absorption, collagen production	Tobacco, hectic lifestyle, pollution, chemicals, anti-biotics, aspirin, steroids, radiation
Vitamin D	Sunlight, organ meats, fish (herring, sardines, salmon, tuna), eggs yolks	Healthy bone formation, healthy nervous system, normal blood clotting	Mineral oil, smog, working night shifts, clothes, dark skin
Vitamin E	Vegetables, seeds, nuts, soy beans, wholegrains, sprouts, green veg	Powerful anti-oxidant, protects red blood cells, healthy muscles, nerves, hair and skin health	Rancid fat and oil, chlorine, extreme temperatures, iron (ferrous sulphate), oral contraception
Vitamin K	Leafy green veg, broccoli, alfalfa, yogurt, egg yolk, kelp, fish liver oils	Blood coagulation, liver function	Mineral oil, x-rays, radiation, rancid fat, aspirin

mineral	sources	benefits / function	contra-agents	helpers
Boron	Fruit, vegetables, nuts, wine, cider, beer	Proper mineral absorption and bone health	Triglycerides	Calcium, magnesium, vitamin D
Calcium	Dark green leafy veg, canned fish with bones, peas, tofu, grains, seeds, nuts, seaweeds	Healthy bones and teeth, involved in blood clotting, heart rhythm, transmissions in nervous system	Lack of exercise, lifestyle magnesium, vitamin D, hydrochloric acid, phytic acid, fluoride, salt	vitamins A, C, D, F and iron
Chromium	Wholegrain cereals, corn oil, clams	Helps stabilize blood sugars, fatty acid, cholesterol and protein synthesis, enzyme activity and metabolism	Unknown	Unknown
Copper	Soy beans, raisins, nuts, legumes, fish, organ meats	Formation of red blood cells and bones, involved in enzyme activity, firms elastin with vitamin C	High levels of zinc, mercury, lead, vitamin C, sulphides	Amino acids and fresh vegetables
Iodine	Mushrooms, kelp, fish	Involved with metabolism and energy production, enhances thyroid function, healthy skin, hair, nails, teeth and digestive system	Unknown	Unknown
Iron	Green leafy veg (except spinach), dried fruits, legumes, nuts, seeds, fish, poultry, liver	Promotes growth and protein metabolism, skin, hair, nails and bone health, disease resistance, forms haemoglobin	Excessive coffee and tea, chocolate, zinc phosphorus ant-acids	Calcium, copper, vitamins C and E
Magnesium	Green veg, wholegrains, dried fruit, garlic, seeds, nuts, seafood	Carbohydrate-fat-protein utilisation, healthy bones, teeth, arteries, heart, nerves	Calcium, vitamin D Proteins and fats	Vitamins B6 and C
Manganese	Green leafy veg, peas, beets, nuts, egg yolk, wholegrain cereals	Enzyme activation, sex hormone production, vitamin utilisation	Excessive calcium, cobalt, phosphorus, zinc, iron	Lecithin, choline
Molybdenum	Legumes, grains, organ meats, dairy products	Proper amino acid metabolism and mental function	Unknown	Sulphur amino acids
Phosphorus	Nuts, grains, fish, poultry, dairy products	Aids in growth and repair, promotes healthy gums and teeth, carbohydrate and fat metabolism	Excessive iron, magnesium and sugar	Calcium, iron, manganese, vitamins A, D and F
Potassium	Dried fruits, pumpkin seeds, nuts, avocados, beetroot, potatoes, spinach, tomatoes, yams	Improves oxygen flow to brain, helps body remove waste products	Coffee, alcohol, sugar, diuretics, steroids, laxatives	Sodium, vitamin B6
Selenium	Nuts, broccoli, cucumbers, garlic, fish, meat, dairy products	Anti-oxidant, preserves tissue elasticity	Unknown	Vitamin E
Silicon	Unrefined grains, root veg, cereals	Health and repair of connective tissue	Unknown	Calcium
Vanadium	Shellfish, mushrooms, herbs (dill, parsley), black pepper seed	Inhibits absorption of cholesterol in blood vessels	Unknown	Copper, iron + zinc
Zinc	Wholegrains, wheatgerm, herring, pumpkin seeds	Promotes healing and digestion, supports growth, fertility and mental alertness	Excessive alcohol and calcium, iron, copper	Phosphorus, vitamin A

Liz Cook's famous nutrition (vitamin and mineral) wallcharts are really attractive and informative. (www.lizcookcharts.co.uk)

Vitamins and minerals are both better absorbed from food than from many supplements you can buy - although most of the better supplement firms do now produce 'food state' supplements. The body also uses vitamins and minerals in various combinations - and you can't just take a single vitamin to overcome a deficiency. They all work in a fine balance and too much of one can disrupt the others. A good and varied diet is the best form of vitamins and minerals. Taking supplements needs a certain amount of background knowledge to be effective and it's best to seek qualified advice, so's not to do harm or waste money.

Are supplements really necessary if I eat a BALANCED DIET?

Yes. Unless you are a full-time athlete, you can't eat enough food to provide sufficiently high levels of all the micronutrients you need. Government surveys carried out in America and Europe show that the vast majority of people don't even get the RDAs of all the vitamins and minerals from their diet – and are therefore suffering from multiple micronutrient depletion. If you eat a lot of processed foods, and/or smoke, or are elderly or diabetic, you are likely to be even more malnourished. Dr Paul Clayton

... again, this is an entirely personal decision, there is plenty of information available and you will find experts saying you can get everything in a good diet and experts saying you can't. It's just possible the experts who say you can't may be more independent. Governments aren't going to be keen to endorse the message that our food doesn't offer adequate nutrition. There is always going to be some scepticism linked to advice where people see a vested interest in supplement provision. I found it quite easy to find out who was saying what and why and assess the advice and what made sense to me. We all have to find the solution that makes sense to us.

If you want to know more about the content and nutrition of your diet - there is an ingenius product available called the Food Calculator. In their own words: 'The Food Calculator is a revolutionary new dietary analysis system allowing the comparison of dietary intake against Government guidelines and Optimum Nutrition recommendations. In simple terms, it helps individuals to determine how well-balanced their diet really is and provides guidance on how to correct any nutrient imbalances or deficiencies, which may impact upon health and wellbeing.' The Food Calculator can also interpret and explain the nutritional information with you to provide the help and understanding that is really needed. (www.thefoodcalculator.com)

Eating well

Lots of people think they have a healthy diet because they eat many common foods recommended by health professionals. It is still quite possible to do that and lack adequate levels of essential nutrients.

A good way to structure your diet is:

- **45% or less coming from carbohydrates (grains)**
- **45% or more from vegetables and fruits and**
- **10% from protein foods (fish, nuts, seeds, beans, pulses, eggs, free range meats, etc)**

The best diets are:

- **full of a huge variety of different foods**
- **colourful (not artificial colours)**
- **fresh**
- **foods as close to how nature produced as possible**

Widely held recommendations say:

- **minimize animal products**
- **avoid saturated fats**
- **as whole and unprocessed as possible**
- **minimize exposure to toxins (eg: chemicals)**
- **include a good quantity of raw foods as often as possible.**

IT IS VERY IMPORTANT TO EAT S-L-O-W-L-Y and CHEW VERY, VERY WELL

Some of the foods we need to eat are often not part of the average diet and we may need to be a bit more adventurous.

Good examples of quality, nutrient-rich foods are:
Nuts (almonds, brazils, cashews, pistachios, walnuts, hazelnuts)
Seeds (sesame seeds, sunflower seeds, pumpkin seeds, poppy seeds, linseeds)
Grains (wholewheat, brown rice, oats, rye, millet, quinoa, buckwheat)
All vegetables
All fruits
Pulses (red lentils, green lentils, puy lentils, brown lentils, black lentils, yellow split peas)
Beans (kidney beans, butter beans, broad beans, borlotti beans, black turtle beans, haricot beans, chickpeas, flageolet beans, aduki beans, beans and beansprouts of all types)
Fish (but not so much farmed fish, including salmon and prawns)
Free range meats and eggs
Olive oil for cooking (see Fats and Oils, page 107).
Other plant oils can be used in salad dressings but not heated.

Messages are sent from the mouth to the brain and the body about what we are eating and it takes about 20 minutes for the mouth and our digestion system to tell the brain that we are full up. So if we eat too fast, we will have eaten much too much by the time we get the message to stop.

Eating slowly sends different messages to the brain and the digestive system and gives time for the right amount of digestive juices to act on the right amount of food. Chewing well is the best aid to our digestive system that we can give. This breaks the food down, saving much more, much harder work further on in the stomach and intestines - the muscles at the back of our jaws, in our cheeks also send messages to the brain and digestive system. So the more we chew, the better that information system works.

You don't have to finish everything of every meal. Wasting things outside the body is a lot less expensive than the possible costs of wasting them inside the body. Anything above and beyond what we need is waste - we aren't saving ourselves any money by eating things we don't need. (We may be saving a lot of money by not eating it).

Eat small portions, slowly and become in tune with when it's time to stop.

If you are overweight/borderline overweight - don't eat when you aren't hungry! It's amazing how many people do. If you aren't hungry, don't need to eat - then don't - but eat regularly and sensibly. If you wait until you are too hungry it is easy to eat too much.

Stop eating when you have had enough!

If you are underweight/borderline underweight - give yourself reminders to eat - even if you aren't aware of being hungry – especially first thing in the morning.

Perhaps you know you'll lapse from the best of intentions – perhaps that is a reason you won't make any changes. Don't let that stop you. If you indulge in a few treats or lapse from time to time, you'll be like the rest of us. You can't invalidate weeks of nourishment by throwing in a few mouthfuls of rubbish. Jane Sen

Nutrition, Metabolism and the Whole Body

The topic of nutrition and metabolism has an easily seen role in human body function. Each cell in the body cannot remain alive without maintaining the operation of its metabolic pathways. Anabolic pathways are required to build the various structural and functional components of the cells. Catabolic pathways are required to convert energy to a usable form. Catabolic pathways are also needed to degrade large molecules into small sub-units that can be used in anabolic pathways. The basic nutrient molecules – carbohydrates, fats and proteins of the correct type – must be available to each cell to carry out these metabolic processes[1]. As well as the basic nutrient molecules, cells also require small amounts of specific vitamins and minerals to produce the structural and functional components necessary for cellular metabolism.

Several body systems operate to make sure that essential nutrients reach the cells, as needed, to maintain metabolism in a manner that preserves relative constancy of the internal environment. The nervous, skeletal and muscular systems help us obtain complex foods from our external environment. The digestive system reduces complex nutrients to simpler, more usable, nutrients – then provides the mechanisms that allow us to absorb them into the internal environment. The circulatory system, both the cardio-vascular and the lymphatic circulations, transports the absorbed nutrients to the individual cells either for immediate use or to the liver or other organs for temporary storage. The endocrine system regulates the balance between immediate use and storage. The respiratory system, working with the cardio-vascular system, provides the oxygen needed to transform glucose energy into the energy molecules used within the cell. These two systems also provide a mechanism for removing waste carbon dioxide generated by

[1] these processes include oxidative phosphorylation and the transformation of energy to ATP (adenosine triphosphate) via the Krebs (or citric acid) cycle

the catabolism of nutrient molecules. The urinary system provides a mechanism for removing waste urea generated by protein catabolism. Even the integumentary system (skin) is involved by producing vitamin D in the presence of sunlight.

Metabolism, with all the physiological mechanisms that support it, could be described as the essential process of life. It is the sum total of all the bio-chemical processes that distinguish a living organism from a non-living object.

Using Nutrition to treat illness also goes back to the Hippocratic School of Medicine that originated in Greece about 400BC. Hippocrates suggested that disease lay in air, water and food . . . and noted the body's ability to heal itself, given the right conditions.

Evolution, Diet and Design

Our bodies were not designed for many aspects of a 21st century lifestyle. The human body evolved over a period of approximately 2 million years. Our basic physiology has changed very little during that time and our diet and lifestyle changed very little and very slowly until relatively recently, in evolutionary terms. We lived very close to nature until the agricultural revolution 10,000 years ago. The most dramatic changes have taken place in just the 60 years since the second world war.

To understand these relative timescales, if you imagine 2 million years represented by 2 miles, then 10,000 years would be equivalent to 54 feet or 18 yards (about 4½ car lengths, or the 18 yard box in football) - and 60 years, about 3 inches (7.5cms). Think of our recent evolutionary history as a 2 mile journey, where 99% of dietary and lifestyle changes happened during the last 54 feet - but more significantly 50% of change happened during the final 3 inches (7.5cms).

The recent (in evolutionary terms) changes referred to include:

- massive increase in meat consumption - formerly around 5%
- factory farmed meat and dairy products containing anti-biotics and growth hormones
- consuming the natal milk of other species (dairy products) - only modern humans have developed this habit
- fruits and vegetables contaminated with pesticides and chemical fertilizers, whilst nutritionally more deficient due to depleted, intensively cultivated soils
- exposure to environmental toxins, including household cleaning chemicals and synthetic body care products
- self-inflicted potentially harmful substances from significant quantities of recreational toxins such as tea, coffee, alcohol, tobacco, drugs, etc

- steep increase of nutritionally poor refined carbohydrates such as sugar and white flour
- dramatic decrease in physical exercise together with dramatic increase in psychological stress
- extensive use of synthetic, toxic pharmaceuticals.

Many people get to the stage of going through life wishing they had as much energy as they would have thought of as normal, sometimes looking at people in their own age group who are more energetic and full of life. People who as far as they know treat themselves well and yet often struggle to get through the day.

Supporting the body to perform naturally, our bodies will often contain all we need to be well. It should be easy to be well and take years of dedicated effort to make ourselves unwell - but that is what can become the new norm, years of sub-conscious effort, inadvertently making ourselves unwell.

We now encounter the increased evolutionary, environmental and genetic challenges, or stresses that the significant changes of the last 50 to 100 years have brought, plus depleted nutrients and less favourable lifestyles.

The last 5 to 6 feet of the intestine tube, the colon, is where the most distress can occur. After just a quarter of a lifetime of inappropriate diet, the colon can become lined with mucous and toxins which impede efficient elimination, leading to periodic constipation and a feedback of toxins into the bloodstream, causing recurring headaches, tiredness and a weakened immune system. In turn a weakened immune system may lead to increased susceptibility to minor infections such as colds and flu, etc. Constipation, headaches, tiredness, colds and flu are amongst the most common symptoms we suffer.

The irony can also be that the increased use of synthetic pharmaceuticals is to address symptoms of modern lifestyle diseases, caused by the changes outlined above.

Fats and Oils

The fats and oils debate: whether to eat margarine or butter, which is the best oil to cook with and which are the healthier oils - and many other questions. As mentioned earlier, the answers depend on various factors, to do with molecules, molecular bonds, hydrogen and oxygen.

Plant oils are naturally runny at room temperature and one way to make them into a firmer product, eg: margarine or spreads, is to hydrogenate them. This became very common because it was a convenient way of making comparatively cheap oils into manageable, popular spreads and also gave the products a long shelf life. The longer shelf life was due to the product becoming more stable. During hydrogenation, unsaturated oils are pressurized with hydrogen gas at a high temperature, for a long period, usually with a catalyst which is usually a metal. We end up with a product artificially saturated with hydrogen atoms (and possibly trace metals). Natural properties of the oil are changed and destroyed in the process. Once these natural properties are lost, the oil is more dead than alive and so there's nothing much left to go off.

Completely hydrogenated oil products have been transformed from unsaturated fats into saturated fats and are then described as stable (long shelf life).

Partially hydrogenated products can be developed into many, many, many different compounds, not only the food products but all manner of polymers and plastics (containers, DVDs, CDs, road signs). It is often easy to see the same rainbow of colours in these products as we see in oil. Processing the food products, creates trans-fatty acids. The process allows oils to be turned into semi-liquid or solid fats with lots of different textures, convenient for spreads and baking, especially in the food industry.

The main concerns over hydrogenated and trans-fats are that they are altered substances, changed from a natural structure into an unnatural structure. They no longer act or interact with other substances in the same way. The body likes to know and recognize what it is dealing with. Altered substances can interfere with how the body can bio-chemically process those molecules and can cause and promote inflammation, excessive blood clotting and stickiness, increased cholesterol, interference with the liver detoxification system and form free radicals[1], which cause cellular damage. Cell respiration and other functions are impaired and the immune system inhibited. Every chemical reaction in metabolism requires specific interactions between specific, recognized molecules with specific enzymes, for predictable and precise results. The first few years of use or infrequent, occasional use of these altered fats, with altered molecules, may or may not have noticeable implications in the short term. Longer term, because of the interference with bio-chemical processes, it is more likely to have a cumulative affect and cell damage build up over time, even many years, which can lead to degenerative diseases and conditions. These conditions include the heart, cardio-vascular and cancer illnesses which have taken up such prevalent positions in health statistics.

Since these substances and products have been found to be harmful, manufacturers have amended many processes. Lots of products now say they are made without

[1] free radicals; page 112

hydrogenated or trans-fats.

Many oils can be used for low to moderate temperature cooking: olive oil, peanut oil, sunflower and safflower oil, sesame oil and avocado oil. So can the saturated fats like butter and coconut oil but the unsaturated ones would be deemed to be healthier.

For high temperature frying, only the saturated fats, eg: butter, coconut and palm oil are *stable*. At very high temperatures, when the oil or fat shimmers and smokes, that is oxidation and again the molecules are altered which produces substances that can interfere with our natural bio-chemical processes. Any goodness or nutrients of the oil are lost, eg: vitamin E or carotene; free radicals are produced, chemical changes take place and some trans-fatty acids are produced. The oils safest, most stable, at these very high temperatures are peanut and sesame – but they come with the general health provisos about frying and deep frying (oxidation, saturated fats, trans-fats, loss of nutrients, free radicals, browned food equals damaged molecules, etc).

All the oils, including the delicate, unrefined, pressed, plant, nut, seed and grape oils are great to use for cold preparations and salad dressings. The less an oil is heated, the more goodness it has.

Normal use of oils, at moderate temperatures, preparing good food is an important part of a healthy, balanced diet and provides valuable nutrients.

There are many reports and papers and findings and books on this, and Udo Erasmus's book: Fats that Heal, Fats that Kill is 443 pages entirely on fats and oils, with extensive whys and wherefores, figures, tables, diagrams and equations.

Anti-oxidants

Plants produce substances which protect them against viruses, bacteria and fungi. Many of these protective substances are beneficial to humans as well and can help us fight disease by supporting our immune systems. Some of the most beneficial substances are called anti-oxidants. These include Vitamins A, C and E and selenium, beta-carotene and cysteine (an amino acid) plus many others. They provide protection against oxidation of the vulnerable molecules and structures in the cell.

An anti-oxidant is a chemical substance that inhibits oxidation; a substance, such as vitamin E or C or beta-carotene, which protects the cell from the damaging effects of oxidation. In manufacture or processing, an anti-oxidant may be something added to a product to prevent or delay deterioration by the oxygen in the air.

They are called anti-oxidants because they protect against oxidants. Oxidants are electrically charged ions derived from oxygen and are capable of attacking membranes and structures of the cell and impair the ability of the cell to function. They can also cause modification of DNA which can produce mutation, or carcinogenesis[1]. The anti-oxidants protect against carcinogenesis. They can also help prevent arteriosclerosis[2] and atheroma[3]. In the nervous system, nerve cells can be attacked by oxygen bodies (free radicals) resulting in general deterioration. Anti-oxidants appear to be helpful protectors. They are not, strictly speaking, nutrients in themselves – they are valuable properties of nutrients (further examples given below).

Eating a high proportion of vegetables and fruits will give us the anti-oxidants we need for good immune function. Diets that have evolved over a long time span, as our ancestors would have had, tended to contain these powerful substances but modern diets have changed dramatically to include more processed, denatured and convenience food, often at the expense of our wonderful, wholesome, fresh vegetables. The proportions of our meals have changed too. Instead of small portions of protein and carbs accompanying a nice big plate of vegetables; we now often have a small portion of vegetables accompanying larger quantities of protein and carbs – or no fresh vegetables at all. This is leaving people more vulnerable to degenerative diseases that were less common 100 years ago and are now forming a large proportion of conditions we suffer from (cancer, heart and cardio-vascular disease, diabetes, neurological disorders, arthritis, rheumatism).

Some anti-oxidants and what they do

Lycopene is only found in tomatoes and watermelon. It seems to be active mostly when the food is cooked. It can help to protect against cancer, in particular prostate cancer and possibly other hormone related cancers and it has been implicated in protecting against pancreatic cancer.

Carotenoids – vegetables that contain significant amounts of B-carotene (the vegetable pre-cursor to vitamin A) also contain other carotenoids. There have been studies where increasing a group's intake of carotenoids by carrots, fresh green vegetables and fruit has had various reductions in incidence of cancer. The findings of these surveys and studies are changing all the time and for accurate and up to date findings, it is essential to do individual, current research. Beta-carotene is very strong and you can achieve an increase in intake of 1.7mg/day to 2.7mg/day by less than a quarter of an average carrot.

[1] carcinogenesis: the production of cancer; the process of initiating and promoting cancer (carcinogen – substance that causes cancer)

[2] arteriosclerosis: diseases characterized by thickening and loss of elasticity of arterial walls

[3] atheroma: deposit or degenerative accumulation of plaques on the inside wall of an artery

Indoles is found in the form of Indole-3-carbinol, found in cabbages, Brussels sprouts, cauliflower, broccoli and kale. Again, various studies have found these to be beneficial to health, including reduced incidence of breast cancer.
Quercitin is a flavanoid present in onions. Studies have shown anti-cancer properties of onions. Shallots and yellow or red coloured onions have higher concentrations of quercitin. Red grapes, broccoli, marrow and courgettes, which have yellow flesh, also have high levels. It is anti-tumour, anti-inflammatory, anti-bacterial and anti-viral. It affects many carcinogens by inactivating them and it protects DNA.
Co-Enzyme Q10 is an anti-oxidant but not a nutrient. It has a particular protective action for low-density lipoproteins in the blood. It is found in sardines, mackerel, peanuts, pistachio nuts, soya beans, walnuts, sesame seeds and some meats.
Glutathione is a tripeptide and a significant anti-oxidant. Glutemyl-cysteinyl-glycine is its active form and it is highest in asparagus but present in other foods too. It is particularly necessary for the liver to use in detoxification pathways.
Sulphorophane is found in broccoli and Brussels sprouts. It stimulates the body to produce its own protective enzymes and neutralizes free radicals.
Limonine boosts levels of naturally occurring enzymes that may break down carcinogens. It is found in oranges and lemons.
Polyphenols may neutralize free radicals to help block damage to DNA. They are found in Green Tea.
Lignans act as a phyto-oestrogen similar to soya isoflavones. They are found in flaxseed.
Isothiocyanates are found in radishes, mustard and horseradish and are thought to have anti-cancer properties.
Allicin and Allyl Propyl disulphide are in onions and seem to have a marked blood sugar reducing effect. The action is very much like the potent anti-diabetic drug tolbutamide.
Allicin is an anti-bacterial substance found in onions and garlic but as it is unstable it cannot be made into tablet form. Anti-biotics kill bacteria but they can also have side-effects and potentially damage the liver and allicin appears not to have these side-effects.
Pectin in apples reduces blood cholesterol.
Ellagic acid is present in walnuts, grapes, strawberries and raspberries and is thought to have an anti-cancer action – it may block the production of enzymes needed for cancer cells to reproduce.
Allyl propyl disulphide protects against duodenal and gastric ulcers by protecting the lining of the stomach and duodenum.
S-adenosyl-methionine in cabbage juice protects against gastro-intestinal ulcers.

Free Radicals

Free radicals are atoms or molecules in the body with an unpaired electron, making them highly unstable. They are like the nuclear waste of the body. Atoms like to be stable, with their electrons happily paired up, so if they have an unpaired electron they will search out and collide with other molecules in an attempt to steal an electron. If they do/when they do, that atom will then have an unpaired electron and become a free radical and this can start a chain reaction which can damage the cell and our DNA. Some free radicals arise normally during metabolism. Sometimes the cells of the body's immune system create them deliberately to neutralize viruses and bacteria. However, environmental factors such as pollution, radiation, cigarette smoke and herbicides can also create free radicals. Our free radical scavengers are anti-oxidants, they bind with the free radicals before they can do damage. When the unstable free radicals 'borrow' an electron from a normal cell in the body, the process is called oxidation. It's the same process as when metal rusts or a cut apple turns brown. Free radicals cause oxidation inside the body, which is why we want plenty of anti-oxidants to counterbalance them. Normally, the body can handle free radicals but if anti-oxidants are unavailable, or if the free radical production becomes excessive, damage can occur. Free radical damage accumulates with age. Over-consumption of processed foods, sugar and white flour products, or under-consumption of fresh whole foods, or excessive amounts of stress and chronic infections all increase the production of free radicals. This is a far-ranging chemistry subject all of its own and there is lots of excellent information available.

Free radicals are linked to very many diseases and conditions:

- Alcoholic liver and heart conditions
- Artherosclerosis/arteriosclerosis
- Arthritis
- Autoimmune diseases
- Cataracts
- Circulation disturbances
- Diabetes
- Emphysema
- Inflammatory reactions
- Liver Cirrhosis
- Malaria
- Multiple Sclerosis (MS)
- Parkinson's Disease
- Premature Ageing
- Retinal diseases
- Rheumatoid diseases
- Senile Dementia

Dairy

It would be difficult to cover nutrition without mentioning milk and dairy products - but it is also a difficult topic to include. Like many aspects of health and wellbeing, these subjects easily cross into areas that are very politically and commercially sensitive.

To cover the basics - the place to start is that cows' milk is very, very different in make-up to human milk. It has 3 times as much protein and far more calcium - both of which put a high burden on human kidneys, especially young human kidneys. As well as drinking milk - dairy products are everywhere in our diet - cream, ice cream, yogurt, cheese, cottage cheese, sauces, soups, dips, cakes, biscuits and more - and they are incorporated as dried products in many foods. They can easily make up around 40% of our modern diet.

If this is something we shouldn't be having - we are having an awful lot of it.

I studied this as someone brought up and always having lived in the countryside, who as a little girl of 6, 7 and 8 years old, would walk down the road with a huge, white pottery jug, to the dairy farm - and talk to the couple who ran the dairy and talk to the cows, I knew all the cows' names - and walk back with a jug brimming with fresh milk.

Milk of any species is designed for the nurture of young. It is a very rich food to promote fast growth and body development. It transports hundreds of different bio-chemical components. It varies according to species, time of feed and stage of nurture after birth - it is a powerful, bio-chemical cocktail packed with hormones. It is the ultimate designer drink. It is entirely, individually designed to the nth degree for exactly what it is for. Cows' milk is designed and intended for baby cows - calves. Calves grow much larger than humans, much more quickly and their hormone cocktail and what they need is very different to the concentrations of hormones in human milk, for humans. Hormones in human blood are in very small amounts, a few micrograms per millilitre (ml) of blood and the rate of secretion is very low. This is because they are so powerful and these tiny quantities have very large effects on the body. By drinking cows' milk we are having the wrong hormones, the wrong quantity of hormones and the wrong combination.

There are experts to say dairy products are an important part of a healthy diet - and experts who say the opposite. You have to take your own decision.

After an extensive amount of research and study we have come to be of the view that consumption of dairy products is not helpful to health. There is endless material on this subject, so if you are interested, there is no shortage of information to help you come to your own decisions.

One basic would be that we are the only species to continue to drink milk after weaning. No other animal does that. There is no scientific requirement to consume milk after weaning. It is uniquely strange to drink the milk of another species. We probably wouldn't be comfortable with the thought of drinking dogs', pigs', rats', horses' or giraffes' milk – but for agricultural and economic reasons we have become comfortable with drinking cows', sheep's and goats' milk.

A growing number of people are being diagnosed as intolerant to milk and dairy products. Some studies estimate that 70% of the world's population is unable to digest lactose – some of those people are aware of problems and others are not. At that sort of percentage, that would probably suggest that that is 'normal', ie: it isn't a deficiency, it isn't strange. The enzymes required to break down and digest milk are rennin and lactase and they are no longer present in most humans after the age of 3-4 years.

There is also an ingredient in cows' milk called casein – at 300 times the level in human milk. It coagulates in the stomach and forms large, spongey lumps or curds, well adapted for the 4-stomach digestive system of the cow. Our stomach and digestion are completely different. Once inside the human system these quantities of casein form a very thick, gluey goo which puts a tremendous burden on the body. It is excess, we don't need it, so it is a huge extra workload for the body to deal with to get rid of it – taking a large amount of energy to process it. The goo can harden and stick to the lining of the gut and trap other particles of waste – gradually slowing the all important transit time of the gut and elimination. It also reduces the absorption of nutrients through the gut wall. The most common result is lethargy and fatigue. By-products of milk digestion also leave a toxic mucous which is very acidic. The gooey mucous and slower transit time will also contribute to weight gain. Weight loss is made much more difficult if there is a lot of mucous in the gastro-intestinal tract. Casein is also used as the base for some of the strongest glues in woodworking.

Dairy foods are the most common cause of allergy in infants.

The milk from cows today has also changed significantly over the last 60 years. Cows are now bred to produce 4 times as much milk as not all that long ago. Wide ranges of chemicals are legally administered to dairy animals, generally to increase the rate of growth and milk production of the cow, plus anti-biotics, anti-parasitic drugs, prostaglandins, pituitary hormones, oxytocin, leutinizing hormones and follicle stimulating hormones – as well as any veterinary prescribed drugs. Intensive dairy farming has led to unnaturally forced, higher yield milk production per cow, year on year. Cows are made pregnant earlier, with shorter times between calving, the young are removed from the mother and the cows are milked for longer. This can cause increased cases of mastitis. There is a legal limit to which pus is allowed to be present in milk. In the EU it is 400,000 somatic pus cells/ml. (EU directive 92/46/EEC). That is 2 million pus cells per teaspoon. So, you can either have the pus cells, or the anti-biotics, or both. Anti-biotics are present in the food we eat and the milk we drink and can disrupt our own immune systems. It does mean we are taking secondhand anti-biotics. This can compromise the efficacy of any anti-biotics we may need to take ourselves. It also allows bacteria to become immune to some anti-biotics, making it more difficult to treat human diseases and will alter the balance of our own bacteria in the gut.

Of course there will be arguments that people have consumed milk and dairy products all their lives with no ill effect. Some people have smoked 40-60 cigarettes a day and lived to be 100, with the same sort of stories on consuming liberal amounts of alcohol. The problem here is risk – some people are more at risk than others, due to any amount of different factors – and as the habits develop, the odds against the risks are diminishing. As the odds change we may see it differently. Human behaviour is based on personal experience and emotions as well as mathematics.

The calcium in cows' milk is a much coarser substance than the calcium our cells like to absorb – and it is bound up with casein. It is designed for calves, not humans. All green leafy vegetables contain calcium – so do raw nuts – sesame seeds contain more calcium than any other food we know. A lot of fruit contain calcium. Eating fruit, vegetables and nuts, including concentrated fruit, eg: figs, dates, prunes, dried apricots – delivers lots of calcium and in a form we can absorb.

Where do cows get their calcium from? they need much more than us, they have much bigger bones to look after. They get their calcium from grass – perhaps some grains too, but mainly grass. Cows, rhinoceros, elephants, great big, strong animals – get their calcium from grass and plants – they don't eat milk or cheese. One of the main roles of calcium in the human body is to neutralize acid. All dairy products (except butter) are extremely acid-forming (butter is a fat, so it is neutral). It is quite easy for valuable calcium in the body, including from the bones, to be used up neutralizing the acid of the dairy products being eaten. So you can eat dairy products for calcium and end up with less calcium than you started with.

Nutritionists and doctors not restricted in what they can say by political constraints frequently link consumption of dairy products to heart disease, cancer, arthritis, migraine, headaches, allergies, ear infections, colds, hay fever, asthma, respiratory problems, abdominal pain, flatulence, diarrhoea, IBS.

NHS dieticians still generally defend including dairy in the diet. Most people paying for independent advice will be being advised significantly to reduce/remove dairy products from the diet – in the field of the prevention and treatment of cancer it has now become an accepted norm.

(There are many references and sources and papers for information on dairy foods and produce in our diet. I have listed two titles in the reading and reference: 'Your Life in Your Hands' by Professor Jane A Plant and 'Fit for Life' by Marilyn and Harvey Diamond.)

Cholesterol

(also see next section on Homocysteine)

Cholesterol is a fatty substance that the body uses for many things – to build and maintain cell membranes; build hormones, eg: testosterone and cortisol, the hormone essential for increased alerts, quick reactions and adapting to stress; in the coatings and functions of nerve and brain cells; for normal foetal and embryo development; for modulating oxytocin and serotonin receptors – and more. Cholesterol is found in the diet in variable quantities. If levels are too low, the liver manufactures more. If quantities are high then the liver makes less. Insufficient cholesterol has been linked to autism, behaviour and sleep problems, irritability and vulnerability to infections. High levels are typically linked to artherosclerosis, narrowing of the arteries, restricting blood flow, typically near the heart or brain and which can lead to heart attacks or strokes. These symptoms are also referred to as cardio-vascular[1] disease (CVD). Oxygen in the body is transported via the blood, so a restricted blood flow will also restrict oxygen supply. These conditions will often lead to a shortness of breath and/or chest pain, especially linked to physical or stressful exertion.

Deposits from fatty build-up on the wall of the blood vessel can also break off and form clots and block blood supply.

We seem to have become used to talking about good and bad cholesterol, or HDL and LDL[2]. Cholesterol has to get around the body and it isn't soluble in blood so it is transported on carriers. The carriers are called lipoproteins and they give their names to the HDL and LDL – high and low density lipoproteins.

Foods we eat that naturally contain cholesterol, dietary cholesterol, generally fall into the good (HDL) department, eg: nuts, seeds, avocados, oily fish, and plant oils – olive, sunflower, corn and walnut – excluding coconut and palm oil. HDL carries excess cholesterol from the tissues, to the liver, for elimination – so it actually helps reduce cholesterol. Monounsaturated and polyunsaturated fats are also HDL. Good levels of HDL help control cholesterol and insufficient/low levels of HDL can increase the risk of

[1] cardio – heart; vascular – blood vessels

[2] high-density lipoproteins and low-density lipoproteins

heart attack, stroke and CVD. Physical activity can also raise HDL levels.

Foods containing saturated fats fall into the bad (LDL) department, eg: meat pies, sausages and fatty meats, butter, ghee, lard, cream, hard cheese, cakes, biscuits and foods containing coconut and palm oil. Trans-fats, or hydrogenated fats, also fall into the bad (LDL) list and are often in ready made biscuits, cakes, pastry, margarine, spreads and processed or convenience foods.

High amounts of the bad LDL will deposit cholesterol on the artery walls forming plaques. More and more plaques will narrow and harden the arteries and may eventually block blood flow. Saturated fats and trans-fats are the most important factors that raise blood cholesterol, not dietary cholesterol. Keeping these foods to a minimum will help to keep blood vessels healthy, unrestricted and flexible, to avoid the risk of obstructed arteries, heart attack and stroke and so will good, regular exercise.

Dietary fibre helps to reduce cholesterol in the blood, eg: fruit and vegetables, oats, beans, peas, lentils, chickpeas.

Good HDL can also remove some of the cholesterol already attached to the artery walls, so HDL is considered the good cholesterol as high levels of HDL in the blood can decrease the risk of heart disease.

Homocysteine *– and its role in heart disease*

Cholesterol can lead to atherosclerosis[1] which can lead to heart attacks – one of the biggest killer diseases in the UK – but how does a substance that is essential to health, that the body manufactures in significant quantities, become a causal factor in disease? The relationship between cholesterol and atherosclerosis is known. Plaques that block arteries are formed from deposits of cholesterol – but some people form them and not others, although everyone has to have some circulating cholesterol.

More recently homocysteine has come under this spotlight. The deposits of cholesterol that occur act as masks over areas of damage in the arteries and these patches, once started, can continue to grow until an artery is obstructed and restricts blood flow and oxygen. The initial damage to the artery, before the build-up of cholesterol, may more accurately be the start of this process and the chemical frequently known to cause that damage is homocysteine. Once the arteries are obstructed, the restricted blood flow and oxygen supply and real possibility of heart attack and stroke are increased.

Homocysteine is an intermediate metabolyte (product of metabolism) formed when

[1] progressive hardening and narrowing of the arteries (sometimes also referred to as arteriosclerosis)

methionine, an essential amino acid from protein in the diet, is converted through several steps to cysteine, another essential amino acid. So homocysteine will be present in everyone whether healthy or not. Because it is only a stepping stone in a reaction from one metabolyte to another, it should only ever be present in very small quantities before it is changed to the end product in the reaction, cysteine (process = methionine, to homocysteine, to cysteine).

At each of the steps, enzymes are needed to make the reactions happen and the enzymes need certain nutrients to work. If the enzymes are absent or there is a deficiency of vital nutrients, the reaction will not happen completely. The nutrients necessary are vitamin B6, vitamin B12 and folic acid. In many people the reaction from methionine to homocysteine takes place – but the next step of the reaction, from homocysteine to cysteine, does not. This leaves a high level of homocysteine to build up.

The problems with homocysteine are numerous. It interferes with the way the arterial cells use oxygen so that there is a greatly accelerated accumulation of free radicals. The free radicals damage artery tissue proteins, such as elastin and the blood vessel wall. At this point the cholesterol can stick to the damaged areas of the artery wall making it narrower but the cholesterol isn't the initiating factor, the homocysteine is.

Homocysteine stimulates abnormal production of smooth muscle cells which are found in arteries so the artery walls become thicker and less flexible. It triggers various clotting factors which are a risk factor in heart attacks and it is also believed to be a significant factor in Alzheimer's Disease, osteoporosis and certain forms of cancer.

So homocysteine is a reactive and disease-forming molecule, produced in everyone but only appears to build up in people with vitamin deficiencies of vitamin B6, vitamin B12 and folic acid. These nutrients are present in reasonable levels in healthy diets but not in poor or restricted diets and not in many processed and convenience foods.

Vitamin B6 is present in wholegrains, bananas, avocados, nuts, seeds, some green leafy vegetables, fish, egg yolk and most meats.

Vitamin B12 is present in nuts, miso, soy sauce, Marmite, liver, organ meats, meat, fish, eggs, brewer's yeast and some dairy products. Absorption of vitamin B12 depends on a secretion of intrinsic factor from the wall of the stomach which then combines with B12 to aid absorption lower in the gut. If stomach secretions are low, which they often are in older people, or if someone is taking ant-acids over a long period of time they may become deficient in vitamin B12. A blood test from the GP should show if there is a problem.

Non-meat sources of B12 are very small, can be negligible and vegan prepared B12 supplements are derived from mineral enhanced yeast.

Folic Acid is present in green vegetables, wholegrains, liver, kidneys and eggs. It is destroyed by cooking, except when it is protected by the presence of vitamin C.

It makes good sense to keep cholesterol levels within the normal range but if there is a family history of heart disease, investigating diet and nutrients and ensuring sufficient vitamins B6, B12 and folic acid can make a valuable contribution to protection against the disease.

Again, there is extensive further reading on this. To name a few:
Homocysteine – the new cholesterol, Stephen Terrass MRNT;
Homocysteine – basic biochemistry, Dr Adrian Hunnisett BSC PhD MPhil FIBMS;
The methyl group cycle – its importance to health, Dr Paul Clayton PhD.

Sugar - the story

Sugar cane originated in the South Pacific and spread to China and India. In 325 BC Alexander the Great wrote about it during his conquest of India and Nero wrote about it in AD50. The Greeks and the Romans didn't spend long with sugar, the Persian Empire developed its cultivation and the centre of the sugar trade moved to Mecca.

The Western world discovered sugar during the Crusades (1076) - invading Arabs had brought it to Spain. It was taken from there to America and the New World by Christopher Columbus (1492), on the instructions of Queen Isabella.

At this time it was used in exceptionally small quantities and was seen as a spice and possibly with medicinal properties. It then started to be used in cooking - and was taken up particularly enthusiastically by the English, who became big consumers of sugar - it was still very expensive and so became a sort of fashion item to use, especially in sauces.

At the end of the 16th and beginning of the 17th century it was becoming more affordable and more widely used and medics started to link sugar to ill health and began to realize it was 'inappropriate medicine and upset bodily humours'. It was blamed for tuberculosis and the Great Plague in London, of 1666; and Dr Thomas Willis (1621-1675) the great British anatomist confirmed it definitely responsible for the illness, diabetes.

By the end of the 18th century the trade and appeal of sugar were widespread.

During the Napoleonic wars (1799-1815), sugar became very scarce in France, due to the blockades, and they looked for a substitute from beet crops. In 1812 Benjamin Dellesert developed the process that ensured the future of sugar, producing it much more economically from beet - the beet crops had a higher yield than sugar cane and the costs were considerably less.

Claude Bernard (1813-1878) - a French physiologist discovered that it was glucose that provided the energy for muscular activity - he unfortunately linked this to sugar and promoted it as a good food and energy source.

Sugar, which had been banished in the 18th century for its poor affects on health was suddenly reinstated and even recommended as a food for sportsmen (1897). France and England both reformed tax laws to encourage the consumption of sugar and 'increase the health of the people'.

Very soon afterwards, it emerged again, in Germany and in America that there were already very serious implications on health from consuming sugar, particularly intestinal disorders in children; the English thought it responsible for many forms of headache. A very few years after Claude Bernard's discovery, the French also realized the mistake and that the glucose metabolized in the body was very different from the glucose being eaten as sugar/saccharose, an industrial product – and again it was linked to ill health.

In the early 1900s it was pronounced responsible for obesity. In 1923 Dr Paul Carton criticized sugar and its cause of dependency and referred to it as a drug.

The sugar lobby fought hard to defend sugar and its popularity and the industry was more than rich enough to provide endless PR and advertising. Rationing during the 2nd World War also made sugar a more and more desirable commodity. In 1986 the US Food and Drug Administration decreed that except for some tooth decay, there were no contra-indications at all for the consumption of sugar.

From 1700–1800 sugar consumption was low and stable, said to be around 0.6kg annually per person, for those who had access to it.

By 1880 much broader availability had put annual consumption up to around 8kg per person, a 15 times increase.

By 1900 it had risen to 17kg per person, in 1930 to 30kg per person and by 1960 to 40kg per person.

Since 1985 consumption has stabilized in France at around 35kg per person; in the UK 49kg per person and in the US at 63kg per person.

. . . (and as some people don't use or like much sugar, that means some people are having an awful lot of sugar)

To understand this change we need to look at how quickly it took place.

- 1400s, sugar consumption negligible
- over the next 3 centuries to the 1700s, increase to 0.6kg per person
- the following 2 centuries to the 1900s increases of 50 times in France and 100 times in US.

Over 3 million years, the diet of man progressively evolved:

- from gathering food
- to hunting
- to primitive cultivation and raising crops, particularly cereals

each of these changes taking thousands of years.

The generally indiscriminate use of sugar evolved in less that 200 years, within the space of 5 or 6 generations. It is inconceivable that the human body could adapt that quickly to cope with perpetually high blood sugar levels; as well as other high glycaemic foods being introduced also destabilising the natural chemical balance of the body.

As this situation develops, diabetes and obesity is increasing plus cardio-vascular risk and high blood pressure – all of them share a common cause – hyperinsulinism.

Chocolate

The many mysteries of chocolate - chocolate seems to enjoy a unique reputation and attract phenomenol attention. So much has been said, written and claimed about the extraordinary produce of the cocoa bean.

Chocolate has been around for at least 3,000 years, apparently originating with the Aztecs and Mayans in America, and possibly before then. They ground the beans and made a bitter, hot cacao/cocoa drink which was believed to have stimulant and restorative powers, bestowing wisdom and vitality. This was generally reserved for VIPs; warriors, nobility and priests and the beans were high value currency. 100 cocoa beans could buy a slave. A Spanish explorer, Herman Cortez sent cocoa beans back to Spain in 1519 with recipes - and it is from there it is most likely to have begun its takeover of Europe and the rest of the world.

The physician, scientist and collector Sir Hans Sloane (1660-1753) most famous for his collections of plants, animals and many other objects of his time which went on to form the beginnings of The Natural History Museum, contributed to the story of chocolate. Towards the end of the 1680s he spent 15 months in Jamaica and there learnt about the cocoa drink of the local people. He added milk to it and probably sugar which he thought made it more palatable. He brought this chocolate recipe back to England where it was manufactured and initially sold as a medicine - and later, in the nineteenth century, Cadbury produced chocolate using Sloane's recipe.

Chocolate, in the solid bars as we know it today, was developed by Rodolphe Lindt, a Swiss confectioner, in 1879, who added the triglyceride cocoa butter which set the chocolate. Chocolate is made using beans from the cocoa tree, Theobroma - cacao. The beans are removed from the pod, fermented, dried, roasted and then ground to produce a soupy, cocoa liquor which is pressed to form cocoa butter and cocoa solids, which can be ground up for cocoa powder. Plain/dark chocolate is made from cocoa liquor, cocoa butter, sugar and flavourings. Milk chocolate is made from cocoa liquor, cocoa butter, sugar and flavourings with milk added - and white chocolate is made from cocoa butter, sugar, milk and flavourings, eg: vanilla.

Chocolate is linked to religious ceremonies, the Goddess of fertility Xochiquetzal, the Aztec Emperor Montezuma (c1519) who apparently drank 50 goblets a day and Giacomo Casanova (1725) who used to take it as an aphrodisiac. It has been studied in modern research on increased longevity, protection against heart disease, enhanced cognitive ability and mind altering experiences - and there have been other studies establishing that it is preferable to sex and more passionately-rewarding than kissing.

Chocolate is rich in carbohydrates, with high amounts of fat and sugar - and all its other wonderful powers are attributed to the comparatively tiny amounts of alkaloids and other chemicals. To take enough polyphenols, via chocolate, to lengthen life - we can probably safely estimate that we are talking about a vast quantity of chocolate and consuming very high levels of fat and sugar. The special properties are most associated with the dark chocolate, the product closest to the original powder from the bean. The more it is diluted and mixed with other things, to form different products, the less of these special properties the chocolate can have. In many chocolate products, the chocolate/cocoa content is negligible - especially the very sweet, highly modified products.

The two main methylxanthines in real chocolate are Caffeine and Theobromine, present in very small amounts - but which do act as subtle stimulants to the central nervous system. Caffeine, also in coffee and tea, has a stimulant action on the central nervous system and the heart and is associated with wakefulness and increased mental activity. It is a diuretic and can cause headaches and constriction of blood vessels. Theobromine is also a weak stimulant to the central nervous system. Depending on the type and quality of chocolate, 1.5%-3% is theobromine, the property which gives chocolate its bitter taste. It is diuretic and too much theobromine would cause nausea, insomnia, restlessness, hyperactivity, even delirium - but to get to that stage, most humans we would have to eat an awful lot of chocolate. *This isn't the same for young children who can often be sick from too much chocolate and it isn't the same for animals. Even small amounts of chocolate can make dogs very ill and be very dangerous. 2oz of chocolate can contain enough theobromine to kill a small dog.*

Chocolate also contains phenols. It is the anti-oxidants of the phenols that are associated with the claims of protection against heart disease. The phenols prevent the fat in the chocolate from becoming rancid. Again, there would be a dilemma here about taking a product containing a lot of fat, which has a comparatively very small amount of an ingredient that helps prevent the damage caused by the fat. There is a lot of information available on this and on all the various properties and claims about chocolate.

Phenylethylamine is found in chocolate, a chemical related to amphetamines which raises blood pressure and blood glucose. This is the ingredient associated with the pleasurable effects. It can make us feel more alert and give us a sense of wellbeing and contentment by acting to make the brain release beta-endorphins. It is a mood elevator and relieves depression. It is known as the 'love drug' and why chocolate is associated with its aphrodisiac powers.

Anandamide in chocolate produces the narcotic effect, the same ingredient as in marijuana. It is a cannabinoid, which are also naturally produced by the brain - our natural, feel good, 'high' neuro-transmitters. Chocolate contains significantly less than marijuana. The anandamide in the chocolate makes us feel good and stimulates our natural anandamide so we feel even better. Naturally these neuro-transmitters are associated with decreased perception of pain, changing perception of time and the increased sensory properties, responsible for the addictive craving.

The serotonin in chocolate has the relaxing effect, making us feel calm and is associated with increased gastro-intestinal transit, both vascular constriction and dilation, platelet aggregation and stimulation of the central nervous system. It is another ingredient that can cause nausea. As the level of serotonin decreases, this will also cause cravings for more.

The original fats in chocolate include stearic acid, which is believed to lower cholesterol, possibly by being converted into oleic acid, a monounsaturated fat. This results in the high fat content not necessarily raising blood cholesterol but this will depend on any other fats present in the chocolate. Unfortunately, the same process doesn't eliminate the calories. Excess fats will be stored in the body and cause weight gain and obesity.

The sugars in chocolate are typically in the form of glucose and fructose. Excess sugars will be stored in the body and are linked with weight gain and diabetes.

As well as the fats, carbohydrates, proteins, vitamins and minerals there is histamine, also possibly responsible for craving and mood change, magnesium and potassium and thyphyllline another central nervous system and cardio-vascular stimulant and diuretic.

As a food, chocolate isn't the most valuable or useful. It can provide quick energy - but that will be quickly followed by a low, not just back to where you were but lower. It will always have its many and mystical qualities and is very unlikely to be rivalled from its unique position in our passions and desires - but technically it is high in fats and sugars and not the most well balanced food in the world. It's a treat, it's special.

Average/typical food values are:

	dark per 100g	**milk per 100g**	**white per 100g**
carbohydrate	63.5g	56.9g	58.3g
fat	28.0g	30.7g	30.9g
protein	5.0g	7.7g	8.0g

The Importance of Water

Water is essential to life. If there is no water on a planet then there will be no life there.

It is part of all life form and humans are about 75%-80% water. In the body water forms the basis of blood and is the main constituent of lymph which bathes all the cells, and the fluid inside the cells. If the cells lose their water, ie: don't have enough water, unless drastic action is taken they will loose their shape and size and function. This happens as we become dehydrated so the body has emergency tactics to stop water loss. The layer that surrounds cells contracts in thickness, to toughen up. This forms a barrier that reduces further dehydration but will also obstruct the free movement of molecules in and out of the cell. The cell won't be able to absorb the nutrients it needs and eliminate the waste it needs to as well as it should.

The cell produces a waterproofing barrier around the cells and this coating is cholesterol.

Essentially, the cell moves into a survival mode of operation. A wide variety of symptoms can flare up when this happens, such as allergic reactions. Increasing your water intake will help the effective elimination of the accumulated rubbish you need to get rid of and also improve some chronic problems you may not have connected with water needs and dehydration. In order for the water to flow freely it must constantly be replaced and replenished. When it is not replenished it becomes sluggish and wastes build up affecting the surrounding cells.

As an emergency action against dehydration, cholesterol works well but it is not good to have around in significant quantities, when it may contribute to thickening of arteries. We can reduce the build up of cholesterol by drinking lots of water and rehydrating the body so that there is no longer a need to produce large quantities. Cholesterol is essential for health as it is needed to produce adrenal hormones, testosterone and the lining to all nerve cells including brain cells. If it is not present in the diet in sufficient quantities, the liver will manufacture it.

If we limit the transport of nutrients and waste products in and out of the cells this can produce stagnation and cause food molecules to putrefy inside us and reduce the secretions of fluids. As the cells hang onto the water, they obstruct the release of hormones and enzymes, so dehydration can then affect digestion by a lack of digestive enzymes. At the centre of many chronic health problems is a situation of dehydration. Once the flow of water is re-established cells can function properly again. Ideally everyone needs to drink about 4 pints or 2 litres of water every day to stay well hydrated. If we are taking rigorous exercise or work, especially in hot weather, then we'll need more.

Drinking water in frequent glugs is more useful to the body than drinking large quantities, say ½ pints and pints at once and having long intervals in between. The body wants to know that there is a water supply and no need to operate in drought mode. By not drinking enough water, we are telling the body that there is a shortage and so it will operate to conserve water - which will influence all the things described in these paragraphs. As plain and pure water as possible is best - but the important thing is to drink the water - so tap water is much better than not enough water.

Itchy, irritated eyes, especially in the evening, or itchy skin, are often tell-tale signs of dehydration.

One indication of dehydration is our pee. If we are well-hydrated it should be virtually clear - if it isn't then we are dehydrated and need to drink more water.

Fizzy or sparkling water is not helpful, it doesn't hydrate the body and the carbon dioxide creates acidity, this creates extra work for and can be harmful to the kidneys - and displace calcium. Fruit juice is treated like a food, not a fluid. The body has to process anything that is not water to extract the water and the process involved in that uses water - so we are using up extra water from the body, to separate and process fluids, to extract the water.

The body would also prefer the water to be ambient temperature, ie: not too chilled. Chilled water is a good way of cooling down if you are too hot - but for normal drinking and hydration, even in warm and hot weather, the body organs like unchilled water. It doesn't shock the organs so much and is more easily absorbed and doesn't use so much energy warming it up to body temperature. (So, on most water cooler machines, the white lever supply is better than the blue lever supply - or whatever other buttons and signage the machine indicates).

Because of the requirement for water throughout all the organs and tissues and systems of the body - a lack of water can be attributed to the cause of many different conditions and illnesses: headaches, allergies and asthma, diabetes, constipation, irritability, stomach ulcers, anxiety, gallstones, kidney stones, high blood pressure and obesity.

This is also a good place to mention that we have the same messaging system for being thirsty as being hungry - so quite often, when we think we are hungry and choose to eat some more food, our body is actually asking for water - and if we could take those regular drinks of water, we could eliminate a lot of hunger pangs when we aren't really hungry.

Water isn't only H_2O, natural water has valuable minerals. If we drank our 1.5 - 2 litres of water each day and that was good, natural, mineral water, that could provide about a sixth of our daily calcium requirements. Bottled mineral waters do vary. EU regulations say that only water from an uncontaminated spring with a consistent mineral level can be called 'natural mineral water'. This would have to mean water from a very deep spring, where it had been in contact with the natural minerals for a long time. Tap water will contain varying levels of minerals depending where it is from, region and geology, treatment, etc – but tap water may also have nitrates, trihalomethanes, lead, aluminium, chlorine and in some areas fluoride which would act as anti-nutrients. Some areas also have maximum admissible levels of pesticides. This is another area of personal preference and decision. There should be the minerals in tap water but there may also be the contaminants. If we use bottled water, it's worth remembering that we may need to substitute the minerals.

In June 2008 there were newspaper reports of health campaigners achieving remarkable results by encouraging residents of care homes for the elderly to drink more water. Dehydration was linked to dizziness, increased infections, confusion and falls. One lady who was 88 years old had found walking any distance very difficult and a struggle and later said that she felt 20 years younger after simply increasing the amount of water she drank to 8 or 10 glasses per day. She felt more alert and more cheerful. The care home reported dramatic results; significant improvements in health, fewer falls, fewer doctor call-outs, less use of laxatives, less urinary infections, better sleep and improved/lessened symptoms for dementia patients after making water more easily available and encouraging residents to drink more water.

Tea and coffee

These are such popular and staple items in so many people's everyday life. Whilst both these drinks are nearly all water, they do not help dehydration and may actually cause it. They both contain substances that are diuretics, meaning that we lose more fluid than we take in. For every cup of tea or coffee drunk, we need to drink an additional cup of water to maintain body fluid levels, some people say 2. In the case of many of the colas, it can be more than that. If we don't drink extra water, the body will steal and borrow from wherever it can and affect other functions. Tea and coffee are stimulants and affect brain function, so may make us feel better but also cause a subsequent low – so we have another cup. The caffeine in coffee, tea, cola and other products is addictive and we can live riding a wave of little highs and lows which can sap energy and affect mood – and like stress, these reactions require water and will be dehydrating. Tea and coffee are trusted friends and form an integral part of sharing time and company and relaxation – but it's worth being aware of how much of them we may drink and having sufficient water to counteract any dehydration. Being more conscious of having a tea or coffee can help make the switch away from the automatic reflex we may have developed to drink either of them without even thinking about it. We love our tea and our coffee – and our body loves water, so does our brain. This is also covered in the chapter on Mental Health, page 271. It's very noticeable, if you give up tea and coffee for 6 months or so and then have a cup of tea or coffee – you feel really thirsty between half an hour and an hour later. Some of the negatives associated with Tea and Coffee which we may or may not know or are easy not to think about, are listed here – but lots more information is available and easy to find. Day by day most of us get away with drinking tea and coffee – but we have to use our own judgement on whether we may be drinking too much of either or both. Reducing how much we have does make the ones we do have special. By giving up tea and coffee in the normal way, the occasional cup can be a real luxury.

Tea

1. Has an anti-thiamine action and destroys thiamine (vitamin B1).
2. Contains fluorine and also fluoro-aluminium complexes.
3. Inhibits the absorption of iron, especially from cereals (high levels of vitamin C minimize this action).
4. Has a diuretic action which can upset sodium/potassium (Na/K) balance in favour of sodium.
5. Tea tannins affect the heart.
6. Causes blood sugar levels to rise unnaturally and therefore upsets blood sugar balance.
7. There is some evidence of carcinogenic effects from tea tannins.

Coffee

1. Affects stomach secretions, including stomach acid.
2. Affects acid/base equilibrium in the body – makes us more acidic.
3. Upsets electrolyte balance, especially of sodium and potassium and upsets water balance; a definite diuretic.
4. Like tea, has anti-thiamine action.
5. Affects behaviour.
6. Adversely affects blood fatty acids and sugar.
7. Has been linked to duodenal ulcers.
8. Inhibits iron absorption.
9. Produces nitrosamines, which can act as cancer-causing agents.
10. Demineralizes the tissues.

Example Caffeine levels in some products

150ml/5 fl oz	Coffee, instant	40-105mg
medium	Espresso, cappuccino, latte	30-50mg
150ml/5 fl oz	Filter coffee	110-150mg
grande	Starbucks coffee	<500mg
150ml/5 fl oz	decaffeinated coffee	0.3mg
150ml/5 fl oz	tea	20-100mg
150ml/5 fl oz	green tea	20-30mg
150ml/5fl/oz	cocoa (drink)	10mg
1 slice	chocolate cake	20-30mg
28g/1Oz	chocolate (bittersweet)	5-35mg
350ml/12 fl oz	Coca-Cola Classic	45mg
350ml/12 fl oz	Diet Coke	45mg
8 fl oz	Red Bull	80mg
1	Pro Plus	50mg

YOU SHOULDN'T DRINK COFFEE AT WORK,
IT KEEPS YOU AWAKE IN THE AFTERNOONS.

Ronald Reagan

Detoxing and Routes of Elimination

Most health and fashion and beauty magazines have pages devoted to detoxing with different plans and diets and supplements all recommended for the complete detox experience.

These regimes and programmes are suggested as ways to improve our health and the way we feel.

Detox is a natural process and we are detoxing every day. Every metabolic process in the body produces by-products and many of these can be harmful if left 'lying around' in the tissues. Possible effects of toxins are to change the balance of neuro-transmitters, inhibit metabolic pathways, promote inflammation, induce free radical damage, change the balance of hormones and damage the energy-producing organ of the cell (the mitochondria). To protect itself the body has 4 main mechanisms. These are: elimination; to store fat-soluble toxins in fat cells; to activate free radical scavenging molecules, the anti-oxidants; and to change the toxins into less harmful substances in the liver.

The main detox organs are the liver and the kidneys. Elimination organs are the colon, the bladder, the lungs and the skin.

The liver is the body's waste recycling centre, where toxins produced in the body and others taken in from the environment are either recycled or detoxified ready for elimination. The liver has 3 major functions of detox. It filters the blood to remove large toxins, it synthesizes and excretes bile, which contains fat-soluble toxins and it breaks up unwanted chemicals. Typical toxins needing to be dealt with include caffeine, hormones, insecticides, alcohol, yellow food dyes, aspirin, oestrogen, diazepam and many others. In order to carry out these processes a large number of nutrients are required; vitamin C, vitamin E, vitamin B2, vitamin B3, vitamin B6, folic acid, vitamin B12, flavanoids and various amino acids[1]. If our diet is poor in nutrients the liver may not be very effective at detoxing with the result that more is stored in the tissues where it can cause damage and inflammation.

Once toxins have been processed they are either passed down the bile duct from the liver where they are eliminated with fibre from the colon in stools, or they pass into the bloodstream and are filtered by the kidneys and excreted in urine. The colon transports the waste away from the body. Like other waste removal systems it can become blocked or obstructed, especially if it isn't emptied frequently (constipation) and if the waste and

[1] including glutathione, glycine, taurine, and arginine

environment are too dry (dehydration). Our colon needs looking after and by eating the right foods with lots of fibre – wholegrains, fruits and vegetables, drinking plenty of water and supporting a population of healthy bacteria, the colon should function well.

If we don't do this, then the colon can become a breeding ground for pathogenic bacteria, a dumping ground for toxins. A toxic bowel is often the root cause of many health problems. If the bowel is sluggish, typically we won't feel well. This can be the cause of tiredness, headaches and migraines, other aches and pains, colds and flu.

Every minute of the day we also eliminate waste from our lungs. We tend to forget that when we breathe out, the carbon dioxide we are breathing out is a waste product. If we could not get rid of the carbon dioxide it would accumulate which would make our body fluids much too acidic. The carbon dioxide is a waste product from energy production in the cells. Occasionally we might breathe out other substances too, resulting in bad breath but a healthy body with low toxicity does not produce much smell. It is important to breathe deeply and fully to keep our lungs and respiratory system working properly (see later section on Breathing, page 180).

We can also eliminate some toxins through the skin when we sweat and often the smellier the sweat the more toxins we are excreting this way. Eating a lovely, healthy diet can be by far the easiest way of dealing with body odour. We should smell gorgeous. It has become accepted practice to use underarm deodorants and anti-perspirants, often every day, to prevent body odour. Deodorants can be relatively harmless, depending on their ingredients. Anti-perspirant products actually block the sweat glands so that we are actively preventing our bodies get rid of waste it is trying to eliminate. This can lead to a back up of toxic waste, especially in the lymph glands just under the skin of the armpits. The lymph glands are supposed to drain the tissues of the breast in both men and women and we need to avoid that toxin accumulation in breast tissue.

If any of the organs of elimination or detoxing pathways are blocked or not working well, toxins will start to accumulate and cause the conditions necessary for disease to start. Ensuring a good quality diet with all the nutrients necessary is the best protection against this. The body is detoxing all the time and the more healthily we eat, the more we are helping the body do what it is designed to do – and in turn, the better we'll feel.

Whilst a structured, deliberate detox can be highly effective and helpful for people who are chronically ill, it is always best carried out under the supervision of somebody professionally qualified to advise.

Structured detox regimes need to be planned by professional, qualified advisers and the regime properly discussed and understood. They are usually just based on very simple foods, or juice only intake for a few days whilst using something fibrous to continue the operation of the colon and mop up toxins, supported by vitamins, minerals and plenty of fluids. For someone not used to detox regimes, an initial detox would start off with a week of strict detox followed by 2 or more months of simple foods, avoiding extra toxins. Benefit would normally be achieved after 2-4 months. A week's or a month's worth of detox won't usually make a big difference unless someone just happens to have had an exceptionally good diet. For people who do have an exceptionally good diet, or detox regularly, a week or a month can make a significant difference. If we haven't had the best diet for years and years and years – we can't just miraculously put that right with a quick detox. We can work with the system to help it function as it should. They are an effective 'optional extra' for people who find that sort of thing helpful. The main thing is to help your body operate its normal detox system, day by day.

Energy

So now, we are eating well, our body has all the nutrients it needs for structure and function, we have a great supply of energy and we aren't inhibiting any of that by toxins or overload. If all the organs and systems in the body are happy and working well – so is our energy.

The amount of energy we need is expressed as units of heat (calories).

An average man at rest uses about 1,700 calories per day just for vital functions. This is called the basal rate. For every extra activity whether it is reading, walking, manual labour, mountaineering, skiing or typing at a computer, extra energy is required. A sedentary worker may only need up to 2,500 calories per day in total but someone on a polar expedition may need in excess of 6,500 calories. (This is equivalent to huge volumes of food which would be difficult to get through in a day).

If we eat more calories in a day than we need then the body can store the extra calories in the form of glycogen (stored sugar molecules) or as fat. This can be useful in the short to medium term if needed to build up reserves before some strenuous activity such as running a marathon or going on an expedition. If you don't need to build up reserves for special activity, the extra fat can cause health problems and we function better when we match our calories in to calories out.

Either directly or indirectly all hormones have an effect on energy. They may cause the release of more energy such as by adrenalin as it prepares the body to run away from danger, or the thyroid as it increases metabolism.

Day by day what we are most likely to notice about energy is whether we have enough energy and feel good, mentally and physically – or not – and feeling tired. This is generally explained by nutrition, keeping the body working well and having sufficient exercise to work the body and sufficient relaxation and rest for the body to detox, repair and replenish. Anything not working as well as it should and any underlying illness will divert the energy from where we would like it to be. Following nutrition, health and exercise advice should restore energy levels. If we do have problems with lack of energy and tiredness, then this is probably trying to tell us something and we need to diagnose what may be causing it. It is often an early warning signal to make some changes.

Energy levels and blood sugar

Sugar, in the form of glucose, from good carbohydrates, is the preferred fuel for all our cells but especially the brain. Other cells can use fats and proteins if they have to. All cells need a constant supply of glucose at an optimum level to turn into energy storage molecules. If sugar levels are too low, cells will not work so efficiently and we may feel tired. The effects on the brain are greater than on the rest of the body and can produce lack of concentration, irritability, headaches, lack of co-ordination, anxiety, panic attacks, mood swings and depression. If glucose levels are too high then both body and brain can be in a state of agitation, which may also lead to a state of anxiety.

So the body needs to keep levels steady at around the optimum – not too much and not too little. It does this by secreting hormones that either release glucose from stores of glycogen in the liver and in tissues, or by secreting insulin which causes glucose to flow into cells to be used or stored.

What works best for keeping sugar levels constant, is food containing sugars that are closely bound together and take time for digestion and absorption – 'time release' sugars. These foods are called complex carbohydrates and they are found in wholemeal products like wholemeal flour, wholemeal bread, brown rice, peas, unrefined cereals (millet, large porridge oats, quinoa), wholemeal pasta, kidney beans, rye bread, carrots, lentils, chickpeas, soya, aubergines, courgettes, garlic, onion, dried apricots, dried figs, etc. The sugar present in fruit is in a simpler, more quickly digested form but it is not present in the concentrated amounts that appear in sweets and cakes, so it only produces a medium rise in blood sugars.

Sugary foods and foods high in glucose are not good at keeping blood sugars level because the glucose is absorbed very rapidly and the level rises too high and too fast. We then have to release insulin to control the blood sugar, which the body sees as a danger – that happens as an emergency reaction and we then experience a blood sugar low. If we responded to that with another hit of sugary food, that pattern would continue and we would be feeling high and shakey, followed by low and sleepy. This is the mechanism which can eventually wear out and give way to diabetes. We can quickly fix occasional and emergency blood sugar lows with a moderate amount of a quick release, sugary, glucose food – but it is not a medium to long term solution.

The fast and slow release sugar foods are now often referred to by 'The Glycaemic Index' (see page 137). High GI foods are fast-releasing sugar foods, which wear off and leave us wanting more food – and Low GI foods are slow-releasing sugar foods, which keep blood sugars level and keep the appetite level, so that we aren't seeking food all the time and our bodies aren't trying to tell us we are hungry all the time (see table for high and low GI foods, page 137).

If carbohydrates are not available, then the body can burn fat and protein to produce energy but it is less efficient and has some unwanted side-effects, such as increased levels of acidity.

The hormones and enzymes that process and control sugars in the body need a good supply of chromium, magnesium, manganese and zinc. These nutrients are found in good quantities in vegetables and whole foods but not in refined or sugary foods. When these nutrients are deficient, blood sugar control is poor.

Any food that stimulates release of sugar, even if it contains none itself, raises blood sugar levels. Drinks containing caffeine, such as Coca-Cola, Redbull, coffee and tea, all increase the amount of glucose in the blood. Alcohol is classed as a sugar in bio-chemistry and increases sugar levels – hence heavy drinkers may become obese. Chocolate also contains a stimulant similar to caffeine.

When we eat these stimulating foods and high sugar foods repeatedly, the pancreas is over stimulated and starts to produce too much insulin which causes a significant drop in blood sugar levels with the sort of symptoms mentioned earlier. The steep rise and then steep fall in sugar levels can lead to mood swings, depression and panic attacks.

Over a prolonged time, over-production of insulin leads to the pancreas being overworked and unable to react properly to blood sugar levels leading to a form of diabetes and/or other chronic health problems. It is very important to keep blood sugars stable and insulin production constant in order to stay in good health.

The detection of high blood sugar levels and the release of insulin is seen as an emergency by the body. High blood sugar is very dangerous, including the quick peak immediately after a chocolate, sweet snack or drink, so the reaction is a full emergency response, every time. We weren't designed to encounter high sugar levels in the normal way, so when we do, that is the mechanism we have to manage it. This is why the mechanism can become damaged. We are asking a lot of our body and taking it outside its normal method of operation. The levels of acceptable blood sugar we can tolerate are within a very narrow scale.

The glycaemic index is based on the glycaemic level of glucose being arbitrarily set at 100 and other foods plotted from there. The glycaemic index of a particular food is established by measuring the increase and then the decrease in blood sugar levels at regular intervals after eating the food (this has been painstakingly researched by scientists.

GI is a well-researched and successful way of weight-loss dieting – and so is GL.

GL is Glycaemic Load.

In GI measurements, you want foods that are high GI.

In GL measurements, you want foods that are low in GL.

For more information see 'Eat yourself slim ...and stay slim' by Michel Montignac and 'The Low GL Diet' by Patrick Holford.

High Glycaemic Index Carbohydrates

maltose (beer)	110
glucose	100
roast potatoes	95
chips	95
rice flour	95
modified starches	95
mashed potato	90
crisps	85
honey	85
hamburger buns	85
carrots (cooked)	85
corn flakes	85
pop corn	85
easy-cook rice	85
rice cakes	85
puffed rice	85
broad beans (cooked)	80
pumpkin	75
water melon	75
refined sugar/sucrose	70
white bread	70
sugar-coated cereals	70
chocolate bars	70
boiled potatoes (peeled)	70
colas, sodas	70
biscuits	70
modern maize	70
normal white rice	70
noodles, ravioli	70
raisins	65
brown bread	65
boiled potatoes (unpeeled)	65
beetroot	65
jam with sugar/grape juice	65
refined semolina	60
long-grain rice	60
bananas	60
melon	60
white spaghetti (well cooked)	55
cheese biscuits	55

Low Glycaemic Index Carbohydrates

wholemeal bread	50
bran bread	50
brown rice	50
long-grain Basmati rice	50
tinned peas	50
sweet potato	50
wholewheat dry pasta	50
white spaghetti (al dente)	45
fresh peas	40
unrefined cereals (no sugar)	40
unrefined porridge oats (large)	40
kidney beans	40
natural fruit juice (no sugar)	40
pumpernickel (black bread)	40
whole rye bread	40
bread (100% unrefined flour)	40
ice cream made with alginates	40
100% unrefined flour dry pasta (al dente)	35
dried apricots/figs	35
Indian maize	35
wild rice	35
quinoa	30
carrots (raw)	30
lentils (brown/yellow)	30
chickpeas	30
fresh fruit	30
French beans	30
soya vermicelli	22
jams (no sugar or grape juice)	22
lentils (green)	22
split peas	22
black chocolate (>70% cocoa)	20
fructose	15
soya	15
peanuts	15
apricots (fresh)	<15
green vegetables	<15
tomatoes	<15
aubergines	<15
courgettes	<15
garlic	<15
onion	

Food Labels

Labels were introduced following consultation and advice from the FSA - Food Standards Agency - to give information to consumers on the ingredients contained in a food or food product and the quantities of the ingredients. They were also to give information to help people know what was in food, how it should be kept, how it should be prepared and guideline daily amounts. The information is worked out based on average adult requirements.

Labels list ingredients in descending order of the amounts in which they are present in the food or product, so the item which there is most of comes first. The information should tell us how much of each ingredient is present and give a comparison against the GDA - guideline daily amount - for each of the ingredients, in the following categories: calories, fat, carbohydrate, protein, sugar, salt.

Information is given per 100g of food - and many manufacturers also give the information per serving, or per pack.

There is a degree of discretion in food labelling and some suppliers give more information than others. As well as the nutritional information required or recommended by the FSA, there will be information on the label from the manufacturer trying to persuade us to buy the food - so there is a combination of fact and advertising and promotion.

As well as the energy/calorie, protein, carbohydrate, fat, sodium and fibre categories, a lot of food now also carries GI information - glycaemic index. This is generally because the GI diet has become popular. Low GI foods are digested slowly and release energy slowly helping us to control food intake. Often this does indicate or endorse healthy food but some ice creams and chocolate are indicated as low GI. It does not mean they are low in calories or recommended as good for us. It means that the fat present in the product slows down the digestion of the sugar. Many of the foods will still be high in calories, which is shown in the calorie information.

(There is further explanation on GI in the chapter on Nutrition: Energy pages 134-137.)

Calories

The energy measurement for food is calories (kcal).

A 20% variance is allowed either way on the calorie count stated on labels, so 100 calories could be 80-120 calories.

The GDA (guideline daily amount) for women is up to 2,000 and for men up to 2,500.

Protein

Most adults will consume more than enough protein in their food everyday for the body's needs, to grow and repair. It isn't governed by guideline daily amounts on food labelling – presumably because it is unlikely that a typical diet would be too low in protein and up to now we haven't put much emphasis on the disadvantages of too much protein. The government recommends that we obtain 15% of our total daily calorie intake from protein. Another guide is approximately 35g per day. A typical diet today tends to be high in protein, around 30% of daily calories which can be a huge struggle for the kidneys.

(Nutritionally it is a very good idea to have proteins from as wide a variety of sources as possible: beans, lentils, soya and other vegetable proteins, peas, broad beans – and not too high a proportion from animal sources alone, ie: meat, fish, eggs and dairy).

Fat

Fats are high in calories.

20g of fat per 100g is a lot. 3g of fat per 100g or less, is relatively low.

As a general average, women shouldn't exceed 70g of fat per day; men shouldn't exceed 90g per day.

Saturated Fat

Sometimes saturated fat will also be indicated. Saturated fat is what has been found to raise levels of 'bad' cholesterol which can be responsible for heart disease.

3g of saturated fat per 100g of food is a lot. 1g per 100g is relatively low.

Women shouldn't exceed 20g per day; men shouldn't exceed 30g per day and that is as part of the total fat GDA, not as well as other fats.

Sugar

Sometimes the label will give total carbohydrate amount, sometimes it will give a figure for carbohydrate also indicating the amount that is added sugar. The best guide is to look where sugar, or sugars, appear on the list of ingredients. The nearer they appear to the beginning of the list, the higher the quantity. Sucrose, glucose, glucose syrup, golden syrup, maple syrup, treacle, invert sugar, honey, dextrose and maltose – are all sugars.

10g of sugar per 100g of food is a lot. 2g is relatively low.

Women shouldn't exceed 28g per day (7 tspns); men shouldn't exceed 34g per day (8 tspns).

Sodium

Salt is often listed as sodium on food labels. Salt = sodium x 2.5.

So if the sodium on the food label reads 1g, the salt figure is 2.5g.

Sodium is added to our foods in the form of sodium chloride, which is what we call salt.

Salt can raise blood pressure and significantly increase the risk of heart disease or stroke (see page 146).

GDA for women: 6g; for men: 6g.

Fibre

Fibre is good for the digestive tract, to keep digestion and bowel function and elimination operating smoothly. It is shown on some food labelling and not others. To have enough fibre in the diet we need to choose lots of fruit, vegetables, pulses, nuts (raw, not roasted or salted), wholemeal bread, wholegrains and baked beans. It is very unlikely we could have sufficient fibre per day from prepared foods, processed and convenience foods and food carrying labels, which is why we are recommended to have as much fresh food as possible, especially fruit and vegetables.

Trans-fats – are made from vegetable oils which are thickened and hardened by hydrogenation. Trans-fats increase levels of bad cholesterol and decrease levels of good cholesterol, which increases risk of heart disease and stroke. They don't appear on our food labels yet but are already compulsory information on US food labels. Trans-fats and hydrogenated fats and oils should definitely be avoided and the only way to do this is to look at the list of ingredients.

Low Carbohydrate – probably means that in these foods some of the sugar has been replaced with substitutes like maltitol and sorbitol because they don't raise blood sugar as rapidly as standard sugar. The substitutes very often contain the same number of calories as sugar but the manufacturers may have chosen not to include them. So low carbohydrate does not mean low sugar.

Reduced sugar – means contains 25% less sugar; the sugar content has been reduced by 25% – it does not mean 'low'. If you want to know how much sugar is in the product, check the sugar content by referring to the nutrition label.

Pesticides, Hormones, trace elements, anti-biotics and other veterinary medicine residues – do not have to be given on food labels. Organic foods will have less or none of these. Organic food production doesn't use these unless organic equivalents are not available and then they have to be stated on the label.

Organic – organic food needs to be certified by an organic authority, eg: the Soil Association and to be organic 95% of the ingredients must be organic. Pesticides and various chemicals are not used in production, as above.

Use By date – self-explanatory – use the food before this date; usually appears on foods that have a short life before they go off, eg: milk, soft cheese, dips, yogurt, cold meats, some breads and pastries.

Best Before date – self-explanatory – to consume the product at its best, use it before this date, after which the food could deteriorate in flavour, appearance or texture – it won't or may not be at its best. This is more a quality indicator than one of safety. Usually found on tinned, frozen or dried foods. The foods may remain safe to eat for some time. For many years tinned food didn't have best before dates on – but the best before dates on these foods are long term and after that presumably what they are saying is, it's up to us.

Always eat eggs before the best before date. Although they last a reasonably long time, eggs can contain salmonella bacteria and if present the bacteria would start to multiply after this date to levels that may be dangerous to human health.

Display Until and Sell By date – are information to the seller of the food to indicate when the food needs to be removed from sale.

EXAMPLE OF FOOD PRODUCT LABEL

per pack				
Calories 476	Fat 20.1g	Saturates 5.1g	Salt 2.1g	Sugars 9.0g
Nutrition				

Typical values	per pack	per 100g
Energy	1998kj	826kj
	476 kcal	197 kcal
Protein	24.2g	10.0g
Carbohydrate	49.6g	20.5g
of which sugars	9.0g	3.7g
Fat	21.1g	8.3g
of which saturates	5.1g	2.1g
Fibre	7.0g	2.9g
Sodium	0.85g	0.35g

EXAMPLE OF TRAFFIC LIGHT INFORMATION

	GREEN	YELLOW	RED	RED
	LOW per 100g	MEDIUM per 100g	HIGH per 100g	HIGH per portion
Fat	3g or less	3.0 – 20g	more than 20g	more than 21g
Saturates	1.5g or less	1.5 – 5g	more than 5g	more than 6g
Salt	0.3g or less	0.3g – 1.5g	more than 1.5g	more than 2.4g
Sugars	5g or less	5 – 15g	more than 15g	more than 18g

GUIDELINE DAILY AMOUNTS FOR AVERAGE ADULTS

	Women	Men
Calories	2000	2500
Fat	70g	95g
Saturates	20g	30g
Salt	6g	6g
Sugars	90g	120g

The Traffic Light System

The traffic light system was designed as an easy to recognize system indicating for each product where the food/product comes in the low to high ratio of GDA for different ingredients; for example, whether it is relatively high in salt, or low in sugar. The same food/product can be low in one category and high in another - so it is still up to the consumer to gauge whether that product, in addition to other foods and products bought and consumed that day, keeps overall food consumption within the recommended range. The idea would be that if we had chosen something relatively high in salt at lunch time, in a packet of sandwiches for example - we need to choose things low in salt for anything else eaten on the same day. They try to encourage healthy eating.

NB: The other way to do this is to make and prepare your own food from the individual ingredients. Then you can choose fresh ingredients without additives, preservatives and pre-selected, processed ingredients and dressings, etc.

What food labels do tell you

- Labels do list the ingredients, in order of quantity but they do not tell you how much there is of all the ingredients in the food/product.
- The weight of the food.
- All the ingredients, including additives.

What food labels don't tell you

- Food labels rarely give you the vitamin and mineral content, except where they have been added to the product by the manufacturer, eg: breakfast cereals, soya milk. (Added synthetic vitamins and minerals are not usually as effective as the real thing).

- Labels won't tell you whether the food/product has anti-oxidants in.

- Traffic light labels don't tell you which fats are present, so the product may be high in fats that have health benefits, or fats which don't.

- Labels won't tell you what storage and processing methods have been used, eg: fumigants, lubricants or solvents, or what packaging the food has been in contact with. Our food can contain or have come into contact with a huge number of very strange ingredients, such as: chlorine, paraffin – and many, many others.

All the major supermarkets have very good websites with information about labelling.
plus: www.eatwell.gov.uk www.nutrition.org.uk

Blank Brand Houmous

INGREDIENTS:
Cooked chickpeas (42%), Vegetable oil, Water, Sesame Seed Pulp (13%), Concentrated Lemon Juice (3%), Salt, Garlic.
Cooked Chickpeas contain: Water, Chickpeas.

Home Made Houmous

INGREDIENTS:
Cooked Chickpeas, Olive Oil, Garlic, Lemon Juice, Tahini (Pulped Sesame Seed), Ground Black Pepper, Salt (optional)

Blank Brand Prawn Sandwich

INGREDIENTS
Oatmeal bread 48% (Wholemeal flour, water, oatmeal, wheat bran, wheat gluten, yeast, salt, spirit vinegar, soya flour, emulsifiers (E472e, E471, E481), Vegetable oil, Flour treatment agent (E300)
Prawns 33% (Prawns, Water, Salt)
Mayonnaise (15%) (Rapeseed Oil, Water, Pasteurized Whole Egg, Pasteurized Egg Yolk, White Wine Vinegar, Spirit Vinegar, Dijon Mustard (Water, Brown Mustard Seeds, White Wine Vinegar, Salt, Citric Acid), Dextrose, Sugar, Salt, Stabilizer (E415), Citric Acid, Modified Maize Starch)
Blended Spread (Vegetable Oils, Water, Butter, Buttermilk Powder, Salt, Emulsifier (E322) (from Soya), Colour E160a).

NUTRITION
Typical values per pack
Energy Value 1585kJ/378kcal, Protein 16.8g, Carbohydrate 33.5g, of which sugars 1.0g, Fat 19.8g, of which saturates 2.2g, Fibre 2.5g, Sodium 1.1g, Salt 2.8g.
Typical values per 100g
Energy Value 955kJ/228kcal, Protein 10.1g, Carbohydrate 20.2g, of which sugars 0.6g, Fat 11.9g, of which saturates 1.3g, Fibre 1.5g, Sodium 0.7g, Salt 1.7g.

Blank Brand Seafood Sticks

INGREDIENTS:
Water, Surimi (35%) [Textured White Fish Protein (94%), Sugar, Stabilizers, (Polyphasphate, Diphosphate)], Wheat Starch, Humectant (Sorbitol), Salt, Crab Flavouring (from Shellfish), Sugar, Soya Bean Oil, Soya Protein, Rice Wine, Egg White Powder, Colours (Cochineal, Paprika Extract).

Sodium and Salt

Historically our bodies are designed to hold onto sodium as a precious, possibly rare commodity, to make sure that we have enough of it. There would not have been large amounts in our diet. In original whole foods, sodium is only present in tiny quantities. We would have been more likely to have a salt deficiency than an excess.

Sodium is now present in many foods and in much higher quantities so can easily become dominant. As well as the natural sodium content food may have, it is now added in the form of sodium chloride – salt – to an enormous number and variety of the foods we eat.

95% of ingested sodium is absorbed. It is common nowadays for it to be present and absorbed in excessive quantities. When the amount of sodium absorbed is high, because of the way our electrolytes work, in balance with each other, it can increase the excretion and loss of potassium and our cells can easily become deficient in potassium.

On the other hand, our bodies were traditionally used to liberal amounts of potassium, present in whole foods. On a bio-chemical, cellular level, the body used to be able to afford to lose significant amounts of potassium because there was a plentiful supply of it and no shortage in the diet. There was no special mechanism to hang onto potassium and as yet we still haven't evolved one, although now a typical modern diet is lacking in potassium and increased salt leaves us prone to eliminating and losing what valuable supplies there are.

Potassium is needed because it enables nutrients to pass into our cells and waste to be passed out. It promotes healthy nerves and muscles and maintains fluid balance in the body. It relaxes muscles and helps the secretion of insulin to control blood sugar. It is involved in metabolism, maintains heart function and stimulates gut motion to help proper elimination. To function well we want to have adequate potassium. Deficiency signs include: rapid irregular heartbeat, muscle weakness, pins and needles, irritability, nausea, vomiting, diarrhoea, swollen abdomen, cellulite, confusion, mental apathy – but these can also be attributable to other causes as well – so as with any other symptoms, always check with a qualified professional, don't self-diagnose. And yes, I'm sure you've guessed this – good sources of potassium are: fruit, vegetables and wholegrains.

If sodium is present and absorbed in excessive quantities, which is very common nowadays:

- it will encourage plaque type deposits in the blood stream, which restrict blood flow and increase pressure

- it will affect the elasticity of the blood vessels and muscular walls, which will also restrict flow and increase pressure

- and it will throw out of balance the electrolyte and mineral balances that we should have, that our body likes.

Sodium is a normal constituent of urine and the amount excreted is regulated by a hormone (aldosterone, from the adrenal cortex).

Cells in the kidney detect high sodium[1] and are stimulated to produce renin. Renin converts one of the proteins produced by the liver (angiotensinogen, to angiotensin 1).

Another enzyme[2] converts that protein (from angiotensin 1 into angiotensin 2) which is a very potent vaso-constrictor and by squeezing the blood vessels like that, increases blood pressure.

The renin and raised blood potassium levels also stimulate the adrenal gland.

Water is reabsorbed with sodium and together they increase blood volume, leading to reduced renin secretion. When the reabsorption of the sodium goes up the excretion of potassium also goes up - and this is where we indirectly, unintentionally reduce the intracellular potassium.

Eating a lot of salt and so increasing blood sodium, draws calcium from the bones to counterbalance the sodium. If we have high blood pressure we may excrete more calcium in urine, increasing calcium loss. So high sodium intake is also linked to osteoporosis.

Magnesium is sometimes known as the ‘anti-stress’ mineral. It helps relax and smooth muscles, including the muscle surrounding the heart and it helps to relax the blood vessels, which will in turn lower the blood pressure.

The arteries are surrounded by a layer of muscle and an excess of sodium, or a lack of magnesium (or calcium, or potassium) can increase the muscular pressure.

Adults should have no more than 6g of salt a day but on average people are having about 9g of salt a day.

People with high blood pressure are 3 times more likely to develop heart disease or a stroke, than if they had normal blood pressure.

The salt we add to food ourselves is estimated to be about 25% of the salt we eat. The other 75% is already in food we buy. It really is important to try and know what our overall salt consumption may be - it is very easy to be having high salt levels without even thinking about it and salt = sodium x 2.5.

[1] in the afferent arteriole of the nephron, of the kidney

[2] angiotensin converting enzyme (ACE)

Babies and Children

Babies need less than 1g of salt per day and then from 7 months to 12 months, no more than 1g per day. Breast milk has optimum levels of sodium and so do the infant formulae on the market.

It's important not to add extra salt to food for babies and children. It will very easily damage their kidneys which won't be able to cope with the high salt content. It's also important not to give babies and infants pre-prepared, processed, convenience foods marketed for adults. They are very likely to have too much salt. Foods especially designed and made for babies and infants should be within advised salt intake levels but always check the labels to make sure that they aren't too high in salt and choose the ones with the least salt.

Maximum salt amounts per day for children

1 – 3 years	2g per day	(0.8g sodium)
4 – 6 years	3g per day	(1.2g sodium)
7 – 10 years	5g per day	(2.0g sodium)
11 and over	6g per day	(2.5g sodium)

There are a number of sources of material and information on salt and sodium. Some I used were:

Optimum Nutrition Bible – Patrick Holford
Anatomy and Physiology in Health and Illness – Anne Waugh, Allison Grant
British Heart Foundation, The Blood Pressure Association, British Hypertension Society
CASH – Concensus for Action of Salt and Health (BP unit St George's Hospital, Tooting)
www.eatwell.gov.uk

DRINK YOUR FOOD AND CHEW YOUR DRINK.

Ghandi

NOTHING WILL BENEFIT HUMAN HEALTH
AND INCREASE THE CHANCES FOR SURVIVAL OF LIFE
ON EARTH AS MUCH AS THE EVOLUTION TO
A VEGETARIAN DIET.

Albert Einstein

LET FOOD BE YOUR MEDICINE AND
MEDICINE BE YOUR FOOD.

Hippocrates (4th century BC)

AS I GET OLD, I'M TRYING TO EAT MORE
HEALTHY FOOD, SO I'VE BOUGHT GORDON RAMSEY'S
NEW COOK BOOK – "TAKE 2 EGGS AND ****** OFF".

Jack Dee

MAJOR ENDOCRINE GLANDS

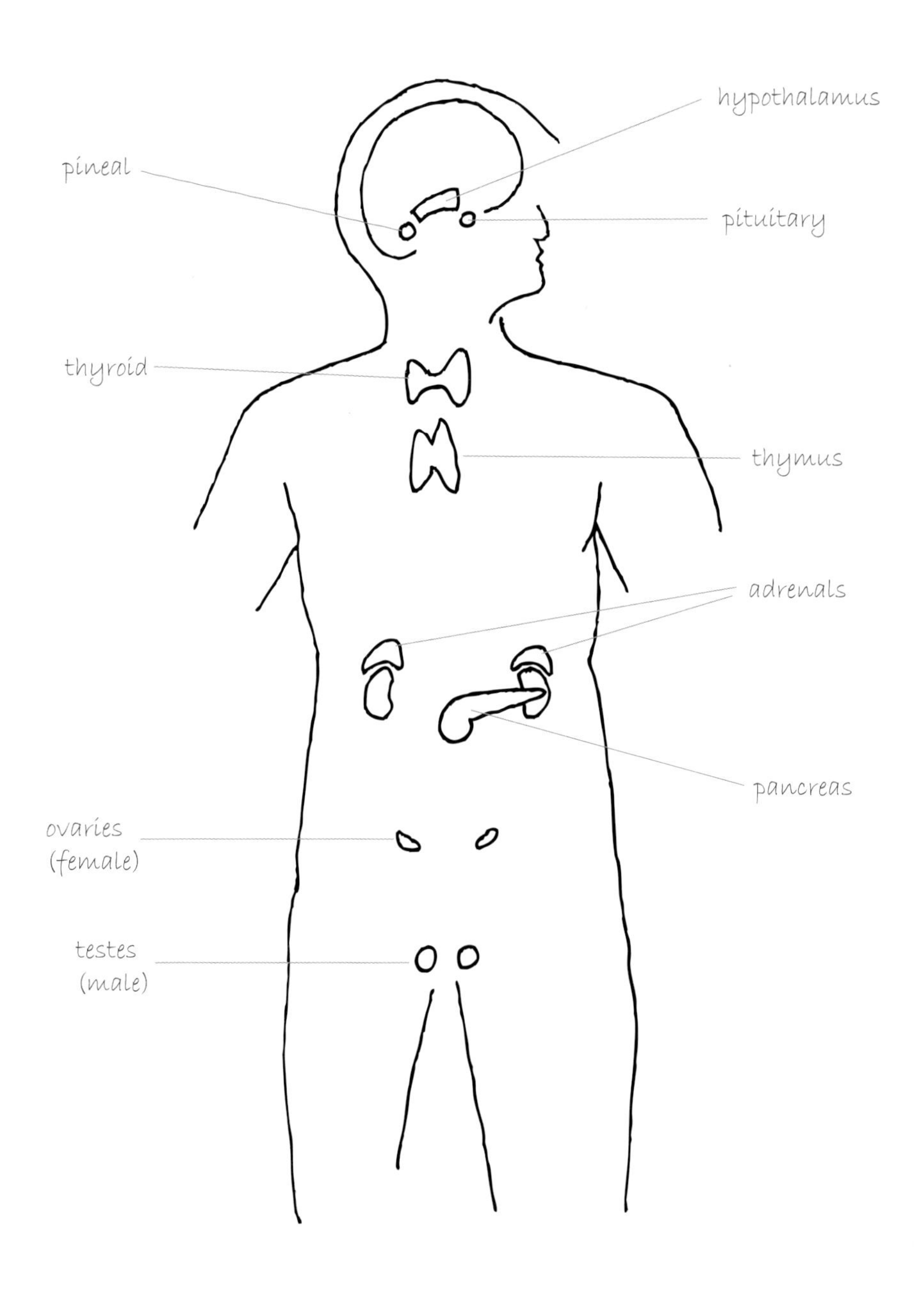

Hormones

Hormones are the chemical substances that regulate and affect the activity of our cells, tissues and organs - our body - physically and mentally. Biologically they are substances secreted from endocrine glands (ductless glands), directly into the bloodstream, transported and distributed by the bloodstream to their target organs.

The word is from the Greek, meaning to arouse to activity, to excite. Hormones stimulate other hormones or tissues at the target cells, or work in combination with neuro-transmitters of the nervous system; they cause and enable things to happen.

Neuro-transmitters sent out by the nervous system cross very short distances, from one neuron/nerve cell, to another. Hormones diffuse into the blood and can be carried the length and breadth of the body. The two work together, the nervous system and endocrine system. Nearly every process in the body is kept in balance by a fantastic, intricate interaction of the different nervous and endocrine regulatory, chemical reactions and processes.

As well as physically carrying out the role they are designed for - hormones are of course also famous for our feelings. When adrenalin is enabling us to respond to something, step up to a challenge, face a difficult situation - for that time it may also make us feel good - because, for that time - we are operating at an elevated level. We aren't only actually physically stronger, we also have the feelings that we are physically stronger. We feel strong, good, important. We are not only actually thinking more quickly and being more decisive, we feel as though we are thinking more quickly and being more decisive. It's very easy to like those feelings, feel more confident and good about ourselves. We can experience an adrenalin 'high'. This is why people can get addicted to the adrenalin kind of stress, whether being under pressure from timescales or workload or strenuous exercise and work-outs - always pitching against higher, harder performance targets. Other people may be very uncomfortable with the experience and not like it at all. These reactions and responses are where it is easy to see that the things going on in our body are directly connected to the brain and to conscious and sub-conscious information systems. We may consciously think a response and cause a response, or our body may respond without conscious input.

Our hormones are involved in all the aspects of our life. The immune system's defence and repair processes, maintaining homeostasis, blood sugar control, digestion, reproduction - all our metabolic functions. A large amount of our renewal and repair processes take place at night. Our hormones are influenced by the time of the day and darkness and light and in turn influence other bio-chemical reactions. This is information that our body uses to know what time it is, what needs to happen and the hormones regulate and control the roles they are involved in, what needs doing. If our hormones are out of balance, many physical and mental aspects of our lives can and will be affected; we may not sleep well and we may not carry out renewal and repair well.

The chemistry between our brain and our body keeps us alive and enables us to do what we do, all the time. Building new tissue, repairing tissue, flexing muscles, moving, thinking, producing energy are all bio-chemical reactions. Something is reaching and entering our cells, reacting with something, causing something else to happen, causing something to be produced. The nervous and hormonal processes are all chemistry and imbalance in our chemical make-up will affect these systems. Many of the drug treatments taken for physical and mental conditions are based on restoring chemical balances, or overcoming chemical imbalances. The balances are often very delicate.

Hormones do what they do by reaching the target tissues and cells and then activating the specific role, at that place, at that time. This may be synthesis of new hormones, activation or de-activation of enzymes which are in turn regulating metabolic reactions, opening or closing specific channels in the plasma membranes, starting something, stopping something, making sure something happens.

There are many different kinds of hormones, eg:

trophic hormones –	stimulate other endocrine glands and their hormone secretion
sex hormones –	target reproductive organs and tissue
anabolic hormones –	stimulate anabolism, making something, building something, in their target cells and tissue
steroid hormones –	are manufactured from cholesterol, including: cortisol, aldosterone, oestrogen, progesterone, testosterone
non-steroid hormones –	are manufactured primarily from amino acids, there are far more of them, including: insulin, parathyroid hormone, prolactin, oxytocin, adrenalin.

Hormones can only do what they do at specific target sites. If a cell doesn't have the right receptor site, it won't respond to the hormone. The molecules of the hormone will only fit the molecules of the specified, target, destination cells – like fitting a coded lock and being allowed through. Although hormones are travelling throughout the body, they will only affect the tissue they were produced and destined for. How they operate when they reach the site is also further chemical reactions and processes. As an example – the hormone reaches the target cell, fits the lock/entry system, passes into the cell to the nucleus, binds with hormone receptors, activates a gene sequence with RNA in the cell, the newly formed RNA moves into the cytosol of the cell and synthesizes protein molecules. The new protein molecules are made because of the steroid hormone – they wouldn't have happened without the hormone. There is a table of the different hormones and what they do on pages 316 and 317.

Lots of our hormones work in combination with one or many other hormones. As shown in the list of hormones in the table, there are x-releasing hormones and x-stimulating hormones, and x-inhibiting hormones. The mechanisms that influence secretion of hormones may be x-releasing hormones, or direct nervous input triggers. There is a very close, inextricable relationship between the endocrine and nervous and other systems.

It is nervous impulses reaching the brain (the medulla) that trigger the secretion of adrenalin to respond to situations. The excited buzz of meeting someone or the fear and anxiety of meeting someone – and taken through to extreme, the fight or flight response. In a breast-feeding mother, when milk production uses available calcium, from the blood and consequently lowers blood calcium levels, the parathyroid glands sense the change and increase the hormone (PTH) to stimulate osteoclasts, to release more of the calcium stored in the bone. The blood calcium level is restored. Insulin lowers blood glucose levels, so after a meal, especially a meal high in carbohydrates and sugars, our insulin levels are increased to reduce the blood sugar level. When the blood sugar levels lower again, the level of insulin decreases. The hormones work on the feedback principles explained in homeostasis (page 84).

Things we encounter – people, situations, food, environments – affect us. That affect is produced by hormones. We've sent signals to our body and our body has reacted. Those reactions then cause further reactions. Our mood, our emotions, our physical ability and our mental ability are all caused by the trigger and ongoing sequence of hormone messengers. We can get into loops of very pleasant, enjoyable hormones – and we can get into loops of difficult, sad, unhelpful hormones. We can play a significant, conscious part in how we are and what is happening. Our thoughts influence our hormones and our hormones influence our thoughts.

Endorphins were discovered almost by accident, in the 1970s. Research was being carried out into drug addiction and why, specifically, the brain would have receptors for opiates, molecules from a poppy plant. The findings were that the brain had its own set of neuro-chemicals, with their own neuro-receptors and because of similarities in the chemicals, these receptors were also receptive to the poppy opiates. The naturally produced, human, neuro-chemicals are far more potent than morphine, opium and heroin and aren't harmful. We may not inject them or ingest them or inhale them but they are there and very effective. If we have overridden them by life events or other chemical imbalances which may have taken place, we can learn, or re-learn, how to use them, how to make them available.

Endorphins and enkephalins in our body are produced in times of stress. They blunt the pain or anxiety we may otherwise experience from over-exertion or injury, in an emergency. They have analgesic properties which turn off the pain and strong calming properties which is why we can sometimes astonish ourselves how well we cope with or respond in an emergency. Whether in a crisis situation or not, these hormones can induce a heightened sense of wellbeing, or euphoria. The name endorphin is derived from the words endogenous and morphine - meaning a morphine-like substance originating from within the body. The way many prescription or recreational drugs work may be from their own active ingredients, or by increasing the effects of our own natural endorphins, or both.

Oxytocin is involved in social recognition and relationships. It is released in men and women during orgasm. It is also associated with homeostasis in body temperature, activity levels and sleep and waking patterns.

Melatonin forms part of the circadian (24 hour) cycle, causing drowsiness as a pre-cursor to sleep. Melatonin naturally occurs associated with darkness at the end of the day and reduces as daylight increases. If our eyes and brain are stimulated by light, during the hours of darkness, or when we are trying to sleep, melatonin production will respond and be reduced, making sleep more difficult. Melatonin is also a powerful anti-oxidant and prevents damage to DNA which will in turn prevent mechanisms that cause harmful conditions, including cancer.

Dopamine is associated with behaviour, movement/motor activity, motivation, attention, sleep, mood, cognition and learning. It is commonly known as the hormone involved in the pleasure system of the brain. We are typically motivated to do things either because we want to, we are attracted towards something - or to avoid something, that we don't want. Dopamine motivates us towards activities we want, that we like, that are rewarded by pleasure, satisfaction and achievement; experiences such as eating or sex. Some of the addictive properties of drugs work by having the affect of increasing the concentration of dopamine influencing brain cells.

Serotonin is associated with aggressive behaviour, anger, depression, bi-polar disorder, migraine, anxiety, obsessive-compulsive disorder. Physiologically it plays a role and influences many functions - constriction of the blood vessels, stimulation of the smooth intestinal muscles and regulation of body processes related to the daily/circadian cycle.

Adrenalin is a very powerful stimulator of the nervous system in times of fear or arousal. Elevated amounts of adrenalin are released into the bloodstream to prepare the body for energetic action. It increases blood pressure, stimulates the heart, increasing heart rate and cardiac output, dilates respiratory airways to increase breathing capacity and increases the release of glucose from the liver. It is released and works in partnership with noradrenalin.

Noradrenalin's primary function is to help maintain a constant blood pressure, stimulating certain blood vessels to constrict when the blood pressure falls below normal. Our normal, everyday reactions and responses work on a certain amount of adrenalin, as well as when we are in heightened, more intense situations.

Action of Adrenalin and Noradrenalin

Effect on the body	Advantage during stress
pupils of eyes dilate	increases visual sensitivity, especially to movement
sensory threshold lowered	increases perception of external stimuli
mental awareness increased	'decisions'/reactions made faster
bronchioles dilated	more air inhaled into lungs
heart rate increased	increases delivery of metabolytes to and waste from cells, tunes performance
vaso-constriction of most arteries	increases blood pressure
vaso-constriction of vessels to brain and muscles (only adrenalin)	increases supply of metabolytes and removal of waste products
glycogen converted to glucose in liver	more glucose available for energy production
digestion and peristalsis inhibited	allows blood to be diverted to more urgent or life–saving processes
hair raised – goose pimples	inherited, evolutionary feature – in feathered or furry animals changes appearance either for courtship display – or to appear larger, to deter attackers.

The effect of many recreational drugs is to artificially enhance the production and secretion of our hormones. These alterations can and do have a disruptive affect on the natural chemical balance which is why they can bring about long term imbalances and disorders.

Many of the North American Indian rituals and those of other ancient cultures are excellent examples of how to combine our physical, mental and spiritual powers – how to honour knowledge and understanding and how to be a part of our lives and performance, via our hormones. Wisdom, intuition, feelings, emotions and communication play essential roles in how we operate successfully. These are often incorporated in symbolism and tradition, from groups pow-wows to harness learning, purpose, belonging and celebration and beating chests to motivate and awaken/fire up for action. It is strongly debated whether beating the chest can stimulate the thymus and its role in our immune system and production of T-cells. Humans do it, gorillas and apes do it – a display of dominant behaviour or a useful way to feel good, awaken ourselves and boost the immune system – or both – who knows? Many successful people have personal rituals that they go through either on a routine basis or before special events. Much of our folklore and music and dancing is based on preparing ourselves for something or celebrating something – changing or influencing our feelings. We have rituals for good times and sad times, managing feelings and emotions. We can stimulate and sedate our moods and emotions. Hormones are immensely powerful things.

Our happy hormones are stronger than opiates, completely tailor-made for us, don't do any harm and are constantly available, free. Accessing them should be natural – if we don't override that mechanism. We can literally think our hormones in and out of existence, we manufacture them. Exercise is known to boost the release of extra endorphins. When exercise may be helpful, it is interesting that other hormones may depress us and prevent us wanting to do things that are good for us. It is a fascinating subject and there is almost endless information on our hormones. It is why anticipation can feel as good as the real thing; why smelling a particular food – baking bread, lemon, coffee, chocolate – or imagining a special event can be as wonderful as the thing itself. Just the thought of things can instigate a whole change in chemistry. One title, particularly popular and often referred to, is *The Endorphin Effect* by William Bloom.

Over-production of a hormone is called hypersecretion and too little is called hyposecretion and either can be due to many and various causes.

Hormones are manufactured from what we eat and so the balance of the food in our diet will affect our production and balance of hormones, how we feel and what we can do. How we think affects our hormones and exercise affects our hormones – and our hormones affect how we think and our performance.

Enjoying company, enjoying music, a walk, spectacular views, a play, a really good, long laugh – are all very good for us and a good work-out for our happy hormones.

Hypothalamus

growth hormone releasing hormone (GRH)
growth hormone inhibiting hormone (GIH)
corticotrophin releasing hormone (CRH)
thyrotropin releasing hormone (TRH)
gonadotropin releasing hormone (GNRH)
prolactin releasing hormone (PRH)
prolactin inhibiting hormone (PIH)

Pituitary

growth hormone (GH)
prolactin (PRL)
thyroid stimulating hormone (TSH)
adrenocorticotropic hormone (ACTH)
follicle stimulating hormone
luteinizing hormone (LH)
antidiuretic hormone (ADH)
oxytocin (OT)

Pineal

melatonin

Thyroid and Parathyroid

triiodothyronine (T3)
tetraiodothyronine (T4)
calcitonin (CT)
parathyroid hormone (PTH)

Adrenals

aldosterone
cortisol (hydrocortisone)
adrenal androgens
adrenal eostrogens
adrenalin (epinephrine)
noradrenalin (norepinephrine)

Pancreatic islets

glucagons
insulin
somatostatin
pancreatic polypeptide

Ovaries

eostrogens
progesterone
'pregnancy promoting steroid'

Testes

testosterone

There is a table of our hormones and what they do on pages 316 and 317.

Stress

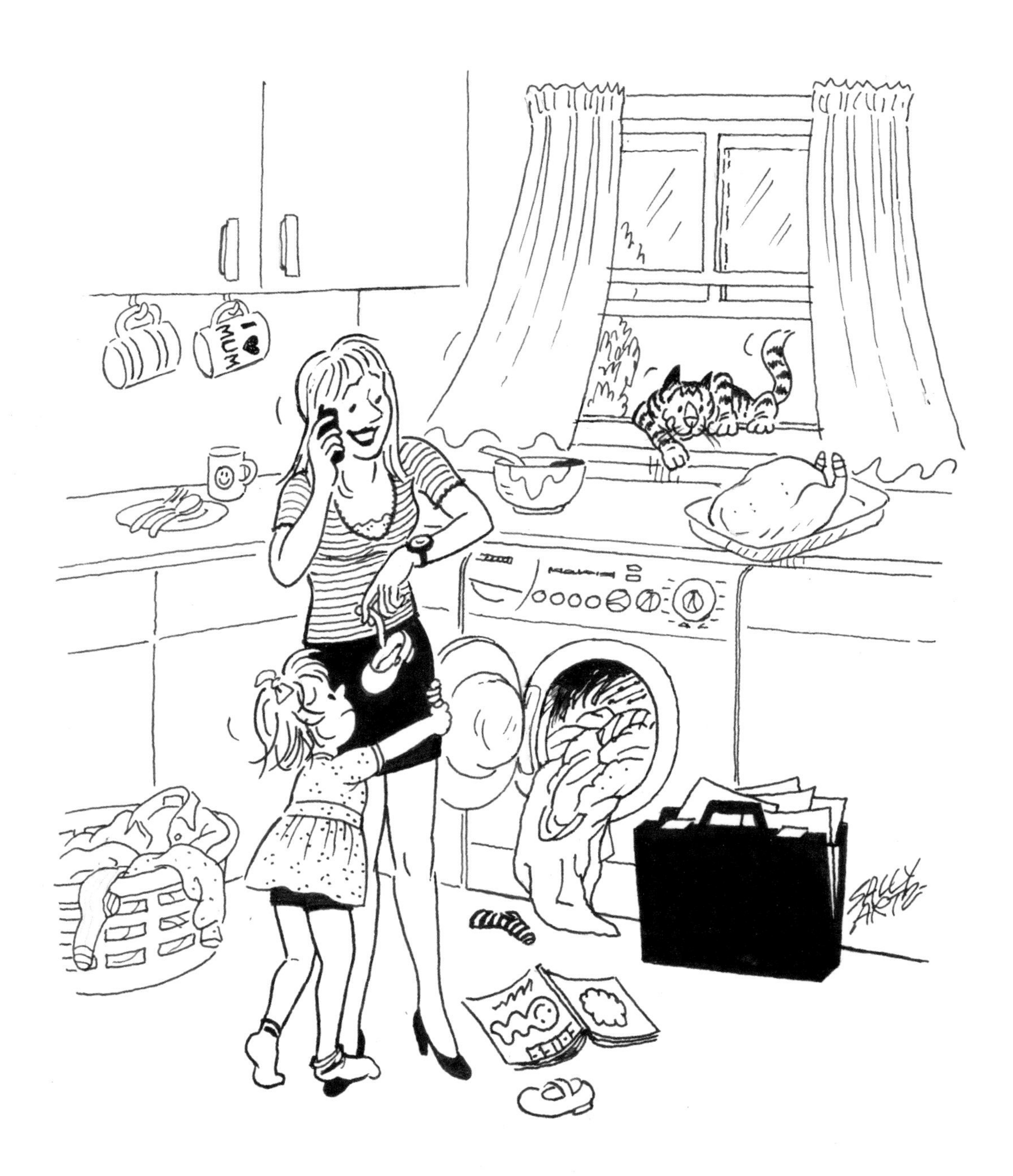
I ♥ MUM

Definitions of stress

A state or condition of the body produced by 'diverse nocuous agents', or mental, emotional or psychological events, perceived or real, which are threatening or undesirable, manifested by a syndrome of changes.

Any influence that disturbs the natural equilibrium of the living body.
A fundamental rule of physiology is that the cells of the body need a constant environment and that the primary function of any organ is to maintain this internal environment despite changes in surroundings. Stresses in this sense include physical injury, exposure (eg: hot, cold), deprivation (eg: thirst, hunger), all kinds of disease, emotional disturbance – any of which can disturb the normal regulation of the internal environment.

(Penguin Dictionary of Medicine)

A non-specific response of the body to any demand made on it. (Hans Selye)

Differs from one individual to another.
Can result from any situation that exceeds the individual's capacity to cope.
Comes mainly from interpretation of events. (Jerome Frank)

Short term activation is fine and is a crucial part of the fight-flight response.
Long term, the increases in blood pressure and platelet stickiness and the suppression of the immune system increase the risks of heart disease, stroke, infections, cancer, dementia and osteoporosis.
Chronic stress genuinely makes people very ill. It makes you ill because it over-activates a part of the brain called the hypothalamus, resulting in the sustained release of high levels of adrenalin and cortisol in the circulation. (Dr Paul Clayton)

Stress is a response to internal or external processes which reach levels that strain physical and psychological capacities to, or beyond, their limit.

Stress: any stimulus that disturbs the stability of the internal environment.
(External – temperature change, lack of oxygen, lack of nutrients, loud noise.
Internal – low blood sugar, increased acidity (ECF), pain, unpleasant thoughts).

Why does it happen?

The physiological changes brought about by stress are designed to improve our performance: the adrenal glands release adrenalin and cortisone, together these two hormones gear the whole body for action. Our blood supply to the brain is increased, initially improving judgement and decision-making; the heart speeds up, increasing blood supply to the muscles, breathing rate and function improve; glucose and fats are released into the bloodstream to provide additional energy. As part of the physiological changes, digestion shuts down, blood pressure rises and blood is drained from the stomach and intestines, as well as the skin – the body is diverting focus to the front-line heart and muscles and away from anything that isn't immediately essential. One-off stress alerts are usually easily coped with by the body. If stress alerts recur frequently, side-effects can build-up; extra nutrients are used up which can leave us a bit depleted, digestion is slow and disrupted and resistance to infections can decline. Minor problems can develop such as headaches, stiffness, insomnia or moodiness.

Being able to have a stress response is not only normal, it is essential. A certain degree of stress is how we learn, grow and create meaning. What is becoming more common now though, for some people, is obtaining a stress state and instead of it being a short term, appropriate response, we are sustaining that stressed state, staying stressed and accumulating further stress. We aren't designed to do that. We are designed to have stress, respond, then return to 'normal'. Sustaining stress is when something has to give. To keep that kind of the stress response going, we will be stealing energy, water, and resources from different parts of the body and that will stress those parts of the body affected. At this stage there is not only the original, initial stress – there is the additional inflicted stress caused by not returning to a normal state.

Like the 'high' mentioned in the chapters on Hormones and Exercise – the state can even become a desired state, it can be addictive. Some people may think they like being stressed but the body doesn't – especially when staying there requires synthetic support, eg: coffee, alcohol, drugs, continual stimulus.

These geared-up changes are the result of the role of the sympathetic branch of the nervous system. The parasympathetic branch induces a state of relaxation and tranquillity. Some people who spend much of their time in an over-anxious or tense state have difficulty in bringing the parasympathetic branch into action.

Others may have the significant response from the parasympathetic branch – they don't step up to the challenge – they have the opposite reaction, the mental blank, the over tiredness, the heavy limbs – the lack of response. And of course, there is any combination of the two as well; over-energized, then not, hyper-mental activity, then the blank, over-eating then skipping meals, erratic, unpredictable responses.

Originally, our initial fight or flight ability was in direct response to situations – to survive a quick, physical response to danger – a life or death struggle or a dash to safety. We have retained the hormonal and chemical defence mechanisms but often today our lifestyle does not allow physical reactions to the stress agents we face. Attacking the boss or throwing computers through windows, aren't considered appropriate. We are generally restricted from that action, which may be why lots of people find that kind of portrayal very appealing when it appears in physical acts on the TV and films. The flight, non-aggressive reaction is also now not usually appropriate. Walking out of tricky meetings, going home in the middle of the day, refusing to respond to things, won't usually be judged a successful solution. This means the body has strong chemical and hormonal responses that are primed and roused but thwarted, frustrated, they can't go into action. A mass of strident, pumped up chemistry on the loose, full of anticipation and excitement, let down and ignored. For many people finding an alternative outlet is very successful – exercise, sports, hobbies, social groups and activities, lots of things.

In prolonged or extreme cases, if not managed, the initial minor problem symptoms of stress can develop to serious problems, including heart disease, diabetes, gastric ulcers, inflammatory conditions, arthritis and cancer.

Finding alternatives – coping – is management. This is yet another of the things we have to *manage*, at work and in our lives generally. We manage time, priorities, budgets, communication, people, projects, presentation and we manage stress.

Stress is also a shared responsibility. We have a responsibility in managing our stress levels but so do people who can affect our stress, especially in working environments – which makes sense because as well as affecting our health, stress affects working performance. Employers particularly can risk serious litigation proceedings. This not only costs money and management time, it also carries the risks of liability for damage and loss of public relations and reputation.

How stress affects us and how we deal with it is very strongly influenced by our own individual *perception*.

What someone finds stressful and threatening – somebody else will not.

It is important to try and gauge things as objectively and accurately as possible. Over-reactions and mis-judged reactions can lead to stress we don't need to have. Keeping calm, a couple of deep breaths, thinking and assessing the best response, can save a lot of stress and be much better for us.

'Do I really need to stress? What may be more helpful, here, now?'

This is worth doing because stress can be cumulative. Once stressed about something, additional situations which may have been quite simple and straightforward, will become drawn into the stress and whip-up a spiralling effect. We can quite quickly have our own mini tornado – and then a maxi tornado.

It can be very useful to keep things separate. Keep dealing with as many of the simple and straightforward things as we can, outside the stress. This gives a sense of achievement and control, which helps manage the stress.

Having said that, we have to be careful of a very common behaviour pattern during stress, which is to focus on simple things to the extent we never get anything else done. It is so much easier to do the easy things that we can spend all day doing that, or staring into space. I believe the professionals call this 'displacement activity' – doing anything other than what we need to do. We know we have to do the tax return – but we'll just put the dustbin out, wash the car, clean out the kitchen cupboards, anything – and keep that going for days if necessary. We know we have a big report to write but we'll just do some filing, remind other people what they are supposed to be doing, go through the last 3 years worth of e-mails deleting unnecessary messages. Mechanical, repetitive, almost mindless tasks are so appealing when the brain really doesn't want anything else to do. Watching the tele can be very appealing too, whether it is something we want to watch or not, it becomes trance-like, almost mesmeric – and much better than whatever it is we actually need to do.

We may not be able to change or remove the stress – but we may be able to, probably can, change our reaction to it. A lot of our responses and reactions to things are conditioned or pre-formed and become automatic. We react to something in a particular way, without really thinking about it. Some people find children playing annoying – but children play, it's what they do – so having a different response would be a really good idea. We can teach ourselves different responses. We are likely to meet aggravating people – so agree with yourself that that is likely to happen. They are aggravating and you have decided not to have a reaction – do a deal with yourself. You know they are aggravating and you know you have decided not to react – and you've got everything under control. Have an intelligent response. Save your energy for something much more worthwhile.

There are various stress management techniques and I have tried to cover just a few through the rest of this chapter.

Most important: Stop, Breathe, Think.

So, there is a stressor – the thing that starts the stress, then there is the response and then the return to 'normal'.

A *stressor* is any agent or stimulus that produces stress. The reaction or interpretation is what defines whether the event is stressful or not. The perception of the individual is critical.

The Stress Process

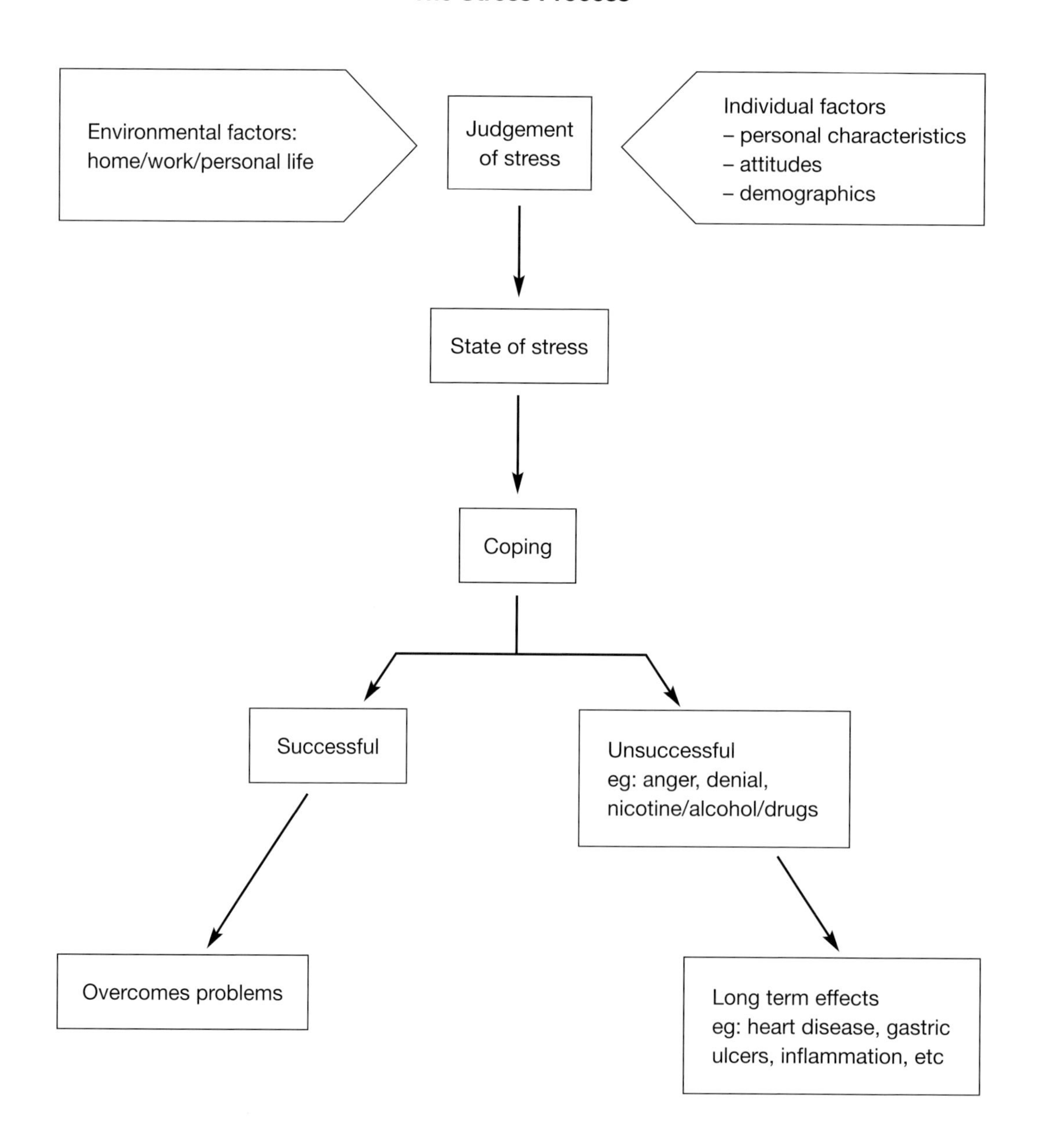

Most stressors are minor and/or routine: mild pain, an annoying noise, the alarm clock, the supermarket queue, not finding the keys or your glasses or taking the wrong turning.

Moderate stressors are often: pain, uncomfortable temperatures, noise, being put in hostile situations, undue pressure, experiencing inappropriate behaviour, loss, grief, hunger, thirst.

Extreme stressors can be: poisoning, trauma, extreme temperatures, infection, intense pain or noise, stressors outside the body's ability to resolve – homeostasis[1] will fail.

Coolness, warmth and soft sounds are non-stressors.
Extreme heat or cold and loud sounds are stressors.
Extremes, ie: too much or too little of almost everything will be a stressor.
Solitary confinement will be a stressor, so will overcrowding.

Typical stressors include: infection, injury, burns, temperature, hunger, blood sugar dips, thirst, lack of sleep, exhaustion, anaesthesia, loud sounds, fear, frustration.

Apparently we are only born with two instinctive fears: loud noise and falling – all the others are learnt, as are phobias.

Emotions are stressors – and emotions are hormones – and the stress reactions/ responses are hormones.

We need to keep our hormones in balance to be well – and production and management/balance of hormones require us to be well, they require nutrients – to be capable of producing the hormones and the environment for the hormones to work in.

Whilst the stress reaction is operating – it will be diverting energy and hormones from where they would normally be and what they would normally be doing – which is why what they are trying to do is return you to the unstressed state – to get back to what they should be doing.

Stress responses are OK – it is what is supposed to happen. Too frequent stress

[1] Homeostasis:
The constant state of balance in the internal environment.
Maintenance of temperature, blood pressure, oxygen, carbon dioxide, water and electrolyte concentrations and pH concentrations, despite external events and changes.
Maintained by positive and negative feedback mechanisms.
Homeostasis is maintained by control systems which detect changes in the internal environment and respond to / rebalance/ correct the change.

responses or, worse, prolonged states of stress, are what cause problems – because we don't return to balance.

Stress responses should enable the body to adapt successfully to the stressors.

It is only when we, or events, have overridden them that they can no longer be successful. Even when overwhelmed, they will keep on trying. That is one of the amazing things about the human body. All the time, whatever we do to it, it will keep trying to survive. That is a good thing and works very well a lot of the time – but we need to meet ourselves halfway and not take it for granted. Our bodies have a lot to do and appreciate our help.

Stressors produce a state of stress. In turn, this instigates a series of responses – it activates the organs that respond.

Typical stress responses are:
increase in rate and strength of heartbeat
rise in blood pressure
altered breathing patterns
hyperglycaemia (high blood sugar)
pallor
coolness of skin
sweaty palms
dry mouth
water retention
physical tension
shallow breathing.

Symptoms of stress can be:
upset stomachs
excess tiredness
comfort eating
over-sensitivity, over-emotion – crying, over-reacting to events
withdrawing, emotionally cutting-off, closing down
severe headaches
clenched jaw, teeth-grinding
mood swings
irritability
skin eruptions (various), complexion changes
difficulty making decisions

confusion
inclining to cigarettes, alcohol, drugs
denial
depression
uncharacteristic behaviour.

Daytime or work related stress will affect personal or home life, typically:
tiredness
irritability, moodiness
moaning about work/stress, or not speaking about work/stress
being over-dependent, shutting others out.

Stress and disease

In physiological stress, whether it is good or bad for us seems to depend on our own body's responses to it rather than on the severity of the stressors inducing it – which is why it can be and often is, a very individual thing. Stress responses should usually enable the body to adapt successfully to the stressors. Sometimes the body's adaptive mechanisms fail to meet the challenge and disease can result.

Decrease in number of white blood cells of the immune system (eosophinols and lymphocytes) indicate that the individual is responding to stress stimuli.

Example situations:
anticipation, exams, a rowing contest, a new situation
heart patients being informed they are being moved to a less-monitored ward
exciting movies, the fun fair.

Soldiers on prolonged marching are found to have fewer circulating eosophinols than normal.

Psychological stress
state of mind as opposed to state of body; caused by a perceived threat; a threat to survival or self-image; produces a syndrome of subjective and objective responses:

subjective	–	anxiety, anger, hate, depression, fear, guilt
objective	–	restlessness, fidgeting, criticizing, quarrelling, lying, crying, uncharacteristic behaviour.

Both states of response are related to each other.

A scientific discipline, psychophysiology has evolved and accepted research and detailed analysis confirm links between the immune, nervous and endocrine systems.

General Preventions and Cures to Stress include:

attention to health and fitness: diet, nutrition, exercise, sleep, relaxation
family: enjoy your family, let them enjoy you, balance and manage your responsibilities
work: regular reviews, development, promotion and working hours
self improvement: reading, discussion groups, study courses
hobbies: active and relaxing – balance the work or other aspects of life
relaxation: walks, weekends away, yoga, Pilates, breathing exercises, massage, aromatherapy, reflexology, music, peace and quiet, stillness
bodywork: exercise, fitness programmes, dance, stretching
talking: it's good to talk, the right amount to the right people – not too much, not too little
flexibility: of body and mind and schedule, give and take – at work and at home
assessing the situation: can you remove yourself from the stress or reduce your exposure to the stress?

along with, in some instances, specific drugs and counselling from professional, qualified advisers.

Counselling and help is a very individual thing and highly dependent on who we work with. The wrong help or counsellor can make things worse and the right help and counselling can be very effective. The difficulty is that when we are stressed we are often less able to take the right decisions and make the right arrangements for ourselves, judgement can be affected and we can be very vulnerable. Counselling and help is covered a little more in the chapter on Mental Health page 273 (see page 289).

Summary
Stress affects the entire body – physiologically and psychologically.

Responses involve numerous mechanisms and nearly every system of the body. The nervous system detects the signals that trigger the response – which then passes the signals on directly or via the endocrine system. Neuro-transmitters, hormones and regulatory chemicals influence the function of the skeletal muscles, the digestive system, the urinary system, the reproductive system, the respiratory system, the cardio-vascular system, the integumentary system – perhaps every system, organ and tissue in the body.

Because the chemistry at work affects the blood cells, stress can have a profound effect on the function of the immune system. There is an emerging field within human biology studying the mind-immunity link – the field of neuroimmunology and psychoneuroimmunology (PNI) – studies and research overlap significantly with endocrinology, psychology and haematology.

The level of adrenocorticoids in the blood plasma of disturbed patients having acute psychotic episodes has been found to be 70% higher than in normal individuals or in calm patients.

Stress also takes a huge amount of water, it's very dehydrating.

Every function – every single chemical reaction and function in your body uses water and many of these are going to be significantly increased and exaggerated during stress. Drinking extra plain, still water will be of fundamental help, physiologically and psychologically.

Dealing with Stress and Ways to De-stress

For quick fixes – to reduce stress instantly, as things happen, distraction and diversion tactics can be very effective. You can put up with whatever is going on because you know in xx time you will be somewhere different, or doing something different. You can give yourself a feeling of superiority by telling yourself how ridiculous and silly someone, or something is – and that can enable you to put up with how things are. The situation isn't controlling you, you're dealing with the situation. If you can think of things humorously, that is a great antidote. Humour and laughing can dissipate stress very quickly – but if a situation is tense, we have to be careful with humour. If it's not appropriate, it's just going to make things worse. You can still promise yourself a laugh later. If you can, remove yourself, go outside, have a quick walk, breathe. Try and break the spell of the stress, do something, move, get a drink, go to the loo.

For the more chronic type – when stress has become more to do with how you are, the first step on the route to recovering from being in a stressed state, is to recognize it.

The stressed state may have taken quite a while to develop and so may take some time to resolve. It doesn't have to – we may be able to make changes and resolve things quickly – but we may need to be patient and track good, gradual progress. Either is fine.

The most effective key to recovery is to establish some time to do so – some time away from the pressures, some peace and quiet, some time for yourself – to give yourself a chance to make whatever changes are necessary. Ideally this will be large enough amounts of time to come away from the pressure, to think, or perhaps to get used to not thinking, to establish what you need to do and not do. Walking is a great therapy and good for thinking and daydreaming, switching off – but so is listening to music, total peace and quiet, sitting still, going to special 'feel good' places – anything which helps that essential 'switch off'. This is a step beyond diversion or distraction tactics. Diversion and distraction tactics are temporary, quick fixes but very unlikely to be solutions. Lots of things can serve to avoid or delay solutions and when stress is real, real solutions are the important priority.

For many people taking an outside look at things will help. If or when you are aware of becoming stressed, try and view what is going on from outside the picture. Look at the situation as though you were an observer. This can help take the pressure off, mentally remove you from the chaos for a moment and help think more clearly. This is effective in high-stressed moments, at the time and in overall management and assessing different aspects of life when you are able to take some time to yourself.

If you can't secure large amounts of time, at first, then any switching off time will help – but depending on the level of stress – you will probably need to build those times into larger intervals to be effective and bring about lasting, long term change. If you start to establish even short amounts of time to have some space – then you will generally find that extending those to larger intervals becomes easier, more possible. You aren't trying to do anything extreme – just restore normality – but to begin with that may feel quite extreme. This may even be annoying to start with and if it is, that's the point, that's a good indicator of why it is so essential.

There are other things you can do generally around nutrition and relaxation. This isn't something else to worry and stress about – it's things to work towards to help yourself, make things easier.

1 Breathe.

2 Drink lots of water.

3 Eat little and often; perhaps 3 very small meals and 2-3 snacks, containing a little protein per day. Chew thoroughly. Eat good food (avoid junk which is extra work, uses precious energy, produces toxins and gunks up the system, ie: adding to the stress).*

4 Don't overload the digestive system with heavy or rich meals.
Exclude any foods you know you are intolerant to.
Exclude refined carbohydrates, caffeine, sugar, alcohol, red meat, cow and pork products, wheat products and yeast products as much as you possibly can – all are pro-inflammatory – but don't get stressed about it, that's important – do what you can.

5 Exercise – change position, change heart rate, change body chemistry.
One of the most effective anti-stress strategies.

6 Manage your breathing (see section on Breathing, page 180).
Breathing slowly in for the count of 4 and slowly out to the count of 9 a few times helps to trigger relaxation mechanisms, calms you down and can give a more grounded effect.

7 Ensure you have a reasonable intake of the anti-stress nutrients; vitamin C, vitamin B5, zinc, vitamin B3, chromium, calcium and magnesium by good diet and taking a good multi-vitamin and mineral supplement. (The products from specialized suppliers in 'food state' preparations are significantly superior to high street brands. Many supplements on the market are poor quality and not in a form easily absorbed by the body. It's worth shopping around). Don't DIY medicate, follow qualified advice.

8 If you have been under stress for some time, to re-charge your adrenals Vitamin C, Vitamin B complex and Rhodiola and Siberian Ginseng are recommended to support the recovery of the adrenal glands. (Take advice, don't self-medicate).

9 Try and introduce time for yourself into the day. If you don't think you can – then you have your answer and that is what you need to try and work on. Relaxation is

key to de-stressing. Saunas, steam baths, massage, walking are great ways of relaxing. Find relaxation techniques that help you switch-off for a while, which is a good deal for you; it helps being more effective when you switch back on.

10 If you can, indulge yourself with some treatments, some pampering, something therapeutic – massage, aromatherapy, reflexology, yoga, a concert (depending on type!), an art gallery – whatever suits you, whatever relieves tension. Anything that helps switch off will also help be more effective when you switch back on.

11 If you are experiencing burn-out, exhaustive type of stress, a high energy eating plan would include: good quality, organic protein from fish, eggs, nuts, seeds, pulses and good grains (oats, rye, brown, red and wild rice, buckwheat, millet, quinoa), vegetables – vegetable and fruit juices or smoothies – fruit, especially berries. You can make soups, stews and casseroles from lots of combinations of these ingredients.*

12 Avoid TV unless you are sure that a programme is going to be a relaxing, feel-good experience. Especially in the evening avoid news, thrillers, violence and programmes with stressful content and angst.

13 Don't fill every hour of every day – book gaps into the schedule.

14 Laughing is wonderful – an excellent remedy.

*On the above items to do with food and nutrition, remember, these are in relation to routine eating patterns – they are not additional. We are trying to give the body easily digestible foods, in easily managed quantities.

If you are overweight, it is important not to increase food intake. Change to smaller meals and more easily digested food with better nutrient value.

If you are underweight, it is important to remember to eat. Eat good quality food, little and often, easily digested food with high nutrient value.

Some work-related circumstances, solutions, strategies

Overwork
Delegate work, negotiate with boss and/or team on workload. Identify source of work, source of increased work. Assess any duplication or unnecessary work. Identify any areas of work that could be removed, done elsewhere – without negative impact. Share excess workload. (An unsuccessful strategy would be to accept the work so that your overall performance deteriorates. The short term measure will be much more difficult to sort out in the medium or long term).

Don't know what to do
Ask! Consult company policy. Consult procedures. Talk to people. Share information. (An unsuccessful solution would be to guess, inappropriately; or to leave something not done and hope for the best).

Poor working relationship with someone
Act early. Think about the situation objectively. Are either you or the colleague acting unreasonably? Prepare some thoughts and a friendly, informal way of approaching the subject – talk to the person concerned.

If there is good reason not to speak directly to the person themselves, consult the person who is in the right position to do so. Is it a work problem or a personal problem? – separate the two. Establish the appropriate relationship to work together – you don't have to be best friends. (An unsuccessful solution would be to fall out with colleague, have a huge row, attack the colleague or criticize or bad-mouth the colleague through a third party).

Work vs family
Negotiate with boss. Assess family time and requirements. Again, think objectively and have some practical, constructive ideas. Why has it happened? When did it happen? What can be done? Flexible solutions. Regular review. (An unsuccessful strategy is to blame the company for the family discontent without seeking a solution).

Questions to do with role
Clarify with boss or team, what is being done and who is doing what. (An unsuccessful solution would be to adopt a unilateral, unagreed tactic or neglect areas of the work).

In all cases of stress, the above are just a few very simple examples: act early, be objective, identify why the situation has arisen; is it new? is it real or perceived? be prepared to compromise, negotiate to general and mutual benefit – eg: 'if you do this, then I can do this and we can do this'. Remember 'we' – it's not 'them' and 'us'. Think. Have constructive, positive suggestions. Don't moan.

Become used to talking to other people about specific and general situations. Asking advice and sharing ideas doesn't have to have a hierarchy, it's just good to look at things together, assess different points of view – and then take a considered, informed decision. Once you know what you are going to do – be sure you know why. Identify a situation that may be causing problems for someone else – suggest going to talk about ideas you have had about it and ask them what their thoughts are on something that affects you. Trading ideas often comes up with more solutions than trying to solve everything yourself.

This has happened. This is what I think. This is what I think we can do about it. This is why.

Some stress states can result in depression. Studies of depression have shown that it is linked to, and probably caused by, low concentration or impaired transmission of neuro-transmitters – noradrenalin and serotonin. Exercise increases the concentration of those transmitters and can lift the mood away from depression.

Illness conditions recognized to have a stress background include:

Hypertension (high blood pressure)
Coronary thrombosis, heart attack
Migraine
Hay fever and allergies
Asthma
Pruritis (intense itching)
Peptic ulcers
Constipation
Colitis
Rheumatoid arthritis
Menstrual difficulties
Nervous dyspepsis (flatulence and indigestion)
Hyperthyroidism (overactive thyroid)
Diabetes mellitus
Skin disorders
Tuberculosis
Depression.

These symptoms and illnesses can be caused by a number of things but stress can very easily exacerbate them – and stress management can very often significantly help to improve them.

Wayne Dyer from his book 'Your Erroneous Zones'

You are immobilized when . . .

You can't talk lovingly to your spouse or children though you want to.
You can't work on a project that interests you.
You don't make love and would like to.
You sit in the house all day and brood.
You don't play golf, tennis or other enjoyable activities because of a leftover, gnawing feeling.
You avoid talking to someone when you realize that simple gesture would help both of you.
You can't sleep because something is bothering you.
Your anger keeps you from thinking clearly.
You say something abusive to someone you love.
Your face is twitching, or you are so nervous you don't function how you would like to.

Again, there is almost endless material written and available on stress.

Professor Cary Cooper has written many books on stress and related subjects and he and Dr Paul Clayton are both well known and popular authors on this subject and write excellent articles, papers and publications.

Stress – background history

According to the Canadian physician Hans Selye and many others, prolonged stress provokes first an immediate reaction, then a more or less balanced state in which the stress is resisted and finally a breakdown of resistance. Many organs are involved but most of all stress affects the adrenal glands. If the resistance to change/the response to the stress, is depleted by any other kind of stress, there is less chance of resisting other stresses. So a serious injury increases susceptibility to infection and worry aggravates physical illness. Helye also called stress, General Adaptation Syndrome.

Stress can come from an external stimulus, or an alternative concept is that the stress comes from the person's response to a disturbance. Stress isn't new. In 1910 Sir William Osler explored the idea of stress and strain causing 'disease' when he saw a relationship between chest pains and a hectic pace of life.

In the 1930s Walter B Canon studied the effects of stress upon animals and humans, especially 'fight or flight' - choosing whether to stay and fight or try to escape when confronting extreme danger. Subjects experiencing cold, lack of oxygen or extreme challenge had physiological responses such as emergency adrenalin secretion - which Cannon described as being under stress.

In the 1970s Richard S Lazarus suggested that an individual's stress reaction depended on how the person interprets or appraises (consciously or unconsciously) the significance of a harmful, threatening or challenging event. The intensity of the stress experience is determined by how well a person feels they can cope with the identified threat. A person unsure of their coping abilities is likely to feel helpless and overwhelmed.

There are different categories and definitions of stress; the worst is helplessness.

In both animal and human research, the importance of one specific form of stress emerged repeatedly. That form is helplessness, including perceived helplessness. While immunosuppression occurs as a result of various forms of stress, it occurs more markedly in situations of helplessness, in which there is no possibility of controlling the stressor.

'These are stressful times. According to our very own Health and Safety Executive, 5 million people in the UK alone feel very or extremely stressed by their work. This is 1 in 6 of the entire work-force. Not surprisingly, stress is thought to be responsible for about a fifth of all sick-leave.

'Chronic stress genuinely makes people very ill. It makes you ill because it over-activates a part of the brain called the hypothalamus, resulting in the sustained release of high levels of adrenalin and cortisol in the circulation.

'Short term activation is fine and is a crucial part of the fight-flight response. Over the long term, however, the increases in blood pressure and platelet stickiness and the suppression of the immune system increase the risks of heart disease, stroke, infections, cancer, dementia and osteoporosis.

'Over the last century the relationship of blood glucocorticoid concentration to disease has been significantly studied. The reasoning emerged that if stress was adaptive and helps the body combat effects of many kinds of stressors, eg: infection, injury, burns, then possibly various diseases might be treated by adding to the body's natural output of glucocorticoids. Consequently cortisone has become very commonly used and referred to.'

Dr Paul Clayton

Hans Selye, 1935, McGill University in Montreal – made an accidental discovery that launched him on a lifelong career and led him to conceive the idea of stress.

He developed his stress concept and described mechanisms of stress.

He was trying to discover whether there might be another sex hormone, other than those already known. He had injected rats with various extracts made from ovaries and placenta, expecting to find that different changes occurred in animals injected with different preparations. He found the same 3 changes in all the animals:

the cortex of their adrenal glands were enlarged
lymphatic organs – thymus glands, spleens and lymph nodes – were atrophied (shrunken)
bleeding ulcers of the stomach and duodenum had developed in every animal.

He tried injecting many other substances, extracts from pituitary glands, kidneys and spleens and even a poison, formaldehyde. Every time he found the same 3 changes; enlarged adrenals, shrunken lymphatic organs and bleeding gastro-intestinal organs. Because of this Selye felt the symptoms were a specific syndrome (a set of signs and symptoms that occur together and that are characteristic of one particular disease). These 3 symptoms – the 'stress triad' – had been observed together but not of any one particular kind of injury but of all kinds of harmful stimuli. More experiments confirmed the same findings – and confirmed for him that they were a syndrome of injury.

First paper: 'a syndrome produced by diverse nocuous agents' July 1936 published in 'Nature'

1956 'The Stress of Life' – his monumental technical treatise.

Walter B Cannon had used the term 'emotional stress' in 1914 when discussing his theory of homeostasis. They were both convinced stress had both psychological (emotional) as well as physiological origins. It was Selye who brought the knowledge of stress and its importance in health and disease to the forefront of modern medicine.

Stressors produce a state of stress. In turn, this instigates a series of responses – it activates the organs that respond. How stress, a state of the body does this, is still not clear. Selye's best guess was that these unknown alarm signals acted through the floor of the brain, presumably the hypothalamus – to stimulate the sympathetic nervous system and the pituitary gland.

Effects of Stress on the Body

(A Melhuish – Executive Health)

	normal – relaxed	under pressure	acute pressure	chronic pressure/ stress
Brain	blood supply normal	blood supply increases	thinks more clearly	headaches and migraines, tremor and nervous tics
Mood	happy	serious	increased concentration	anxious and loss of sense of humour
Saliva	normal	reduced	reduced	dry mouth, lump in throat
Muscles	blood supply normal	blood supply increases	improved performance	muscular tension and pain
Heart	normal heart rate and blood pressure	output rate and blood pressure increases	improved performance	hypertension and chest pain
Lungs	normal respiration	respiration rate increases	improved performance	coughs and asthma
Stomach	normal blood supply and acid secretion	blood supply decreases, acid supply increases	reduced blood supply, reduces digestion	heartburn and indigestion giving ulcers
Bowels	normal blood supply and bowel activity	blood supply decreases, motility increases	reduced blood supply, reduces digestion	abdominal pain and diarrhoea
Bladder	normal function	frequent urination	increased nervous stimulation gives frequency	frequency and prostatic symptoms
Sexual organs	(m) normal sex (f) normal periods, etc	(m) impotence (blood supply decreases) (f) irregular periods	decreased blood supply	(m) impotence (f) menstrual disorders
Skin	healthy	dry skin, blood supply decreases	decreased blood supply	dryness and rashes
Bio-chemistry	normal oxygen consumed, glucose and fats liberated	oxygen consumption increases, glucose and fat consumption increases	more energy immediately available	rapid tiredness

Brian Clough, on dealing with players who disagree with him:

"WE TALK ABOUT IT FOR 20 MINUTES AND THEN WE DECIDE I WAS RIGHT"

Brian Clough

COMPUTERS LET YOU MAKE MORE MISTAKES, FASTER, THAN ANY OTHER INVENTION – WITH THE POSSIBLE EXCEPTION OF TEQUILA.

Mitch Ratcliffe

Breathing

Breathing distributes air throughout the body, delivering oxygen and taking carbon dioxide away. It also influences the sound of our voice.

In the normal way we take our breathing pretty much for granted and rarely pay any attention to it. Good breathing makes us feel good, energized, grounded, helps with confidence and thought processes. We need good posture to breathe well. Standing or sitting tall, letting our lungs fill with air, taking a few especially deep breaths from time to time are all good things to do and a basic tool of many people; actors, trainers, singers, public speakers and people in high profile roles. Breathing acts as a regulator in the body, physically and mentally. Being aware of our breathing can be a big influence in how we are. Breathing properly helps get the blood pumping, fully charged with oxygen and stimulates the cells of the body. Overall health is affected by the efficiency of our breathing.

In a lifestyle of less physical activity it is very easy to induce conditions of shallow breathing which makes lots of functions harder work for the body. Because there isn't an essential demand for large amounts of oxygen, if we aren't doing tough, physical work – we can 'get by' with a much reduced breathing pattern and form restricted breathing habits. Poor posture will also compromise breathing, making it more difficult to fill the chest cavity and pull in the fresh air we need and push out the old carbon dioxide. This can give an overall feeling of tiredness and lack of energy.

If we open a window, we can ventilate a room but if we open our mouth it is not enough to ventilate our lungs. We have actually, deliberately to draw the air into our lungs. We do this by using the muscles of the diaphragm, breathing and expanding our rib cage. Inhaled air is mixed with the stale air already in our lungs; so although the air we inhale contains about 20% oxygen, by the time it reaches our lungs it only contains about 14% oxygen.

All the stale, used air which needs to come out won't come out just by opening the mouth, it must be pushed out. This happens when the diaphragm relaxes and the muscles of the abdomen push up on the lungs. The rib cage can also be pulled down and in and we exhale. Although air from the lungs only contains about 14% oxygen, it gets mixed with fresher air in the trachea so that exhaled air may contain 16% oxygen.

It is quite easy to practise good breathing exercises – and good breathing techniques can improve lung capacity and stamina, strengthen core muscles and super-charge the body. People who use breathing techniques will also say this naturally strengthens internal organs and the immune system as well as improving mental clarity and concentration – all of which makes good, logical sense.

On the other side, incorrect breathing can be the cause of health problems and can lead to panic attacks, anxiety, headaches, migraines, palpitations, increased blood pressure, fatigue and chest wall pains. Many people with stressful lifestyles suffer from these symptoms and often wouldn't realize that it is due to incorrect breathing. There may be several wrong diagnoses and many other possibilities investigated before it is discovered that improving breathing alleviates these conditions very quickly.

It helps to be aware of our breathing – sitting and standing well and being aware of posture. We need to give ourselves time to breathe, take pauses and breathe properly – not leave our breathing to be squeezed in around everything else. There are some notes on breathing techniques and exercises in this chapter.

Breathing and stress

In a stressed situation, to help regain balance and control, taking a couple of deep breaths is often going to be the most effective, immediate response – and in a sustained period of stress, remembering to breathe is also really important. It sounds simple but very often we don't think and we shorten our breathing which will add to physical and mental stress.

Breathing exercises are some of our best defences in times of stress.

Unless a situation is a medical emergency needing professional treatment, slowing the breathing down will be effective quite quickly – and then trying to maintain a regular, calm, deep breathing pattern. In acute cases, some of us will have seen people who are hyperventilating being asked to breathe with a paper bag over their nose and mouth, to restrict the excessively fast, snatched breathing.

Singing, acting and elocution breathing techniques

When we are born our breathing is naturally correct, babies can breathe, yell and scream with optimum effect because they use their lungs and tummy without conscious thought. As we grow older, we can become lazy, only using the upper part of the lungs, taking a shallow breath instead of a normal one.

Surrounding our lungs is a muscle system called the diaphragm. When we breathe in the muscle lowers displacing the stomach and intestines. When we breathe out the diaphragm helps to manage the abdominal muscles around the lungs, controlling how quickly the breath is exhaled.

If we breathe out quickly, the diaphragm does very little but when we breathe out slowly the diaphragm resists the action of the abdominal muscles. A singer learns to use this muscle system to control the breath as it is being exhaled. In singing and public speaking this enables us to deliver long phrases and sustain a long note, without running out of breath.

If you hold a finger close to your lips and breathe out very slowly, the breath should be warm and moist and you should notice the action of the diaphragm as you exhale. This is the correct amount of breath used when singing normally. A singer does not need to force or push air through the vocal cords to produce a good strong sound, doing so creates too much pressure against the cords, preventing them from operating correctly and which can cause damage.

The tummy/abdominals area should move naturally inward toward the end of the breath, not be sucked in, as that prevents the diaphragm from working effectively. Instead the abdominal area should remain expanded to the level it was when you inhaled and allowed gradually to decrease naturally at the end of the breath.

This is where the control comes into play - the singer expands the lungs by inhaling and controls the amount of air expelled when singing a note by allowing the muscle support system to remain expanded for longer and deflate more gradually. This doesn't mean the stomach is pushed out but that the air goes in and the singer slows down the natural rate at which it goes down. In many people the breathing is shallow and only the top half of the lungs are used. Breathing correctly uses the whole of the lungs, as much as possible, so that more air is available, the singer, or speaker then uses the natural action of the muscles surrounding the lungs (diaphragm and abdominals) to control the amount of air that is exhaled when singing or speaking.

Good breath support requires good posture, abdominal breathing and breathing during natural pauses. This does not require great physical strength - but having toned abdominal muscles helps and also supports the other organs and systems of the body.

Important

It is also important not to hold your breath when doing something difficult or strenuous. Many of us do - for some reason. The principles are to breathe in to prepare to do something and breathe out as you move, reach, lift, bend, stretch, whatever it is. Moving on the exhale enables your muscles and body to move easily and prevents tensing up and strains - it also prevents stressing blood pressure and heart. So when you want to lift heavy bags, from the shopping trolley, or from the floor, into the back of the car: breathe in, stabilize your feet, balance and posture, loosen your arms and shoulders and breathe out as you move and lift the bags; the same for picking up a child, reaching a vase or a book off a high shelf, shifting a piece of furniture, etc.

Breathing Exercises

1 Stand or sit up straight. Breathe in for 5 counts and out for 5 counts, expanding the lungs at the bottom of the rib cage, rather than pushing the chest up. Feel the chest filling and emptying. Repeat a few times.

2 Stand up straight with your arms by your sides. Breathe in for 5 counts whilst lifting your arms straight in front of you and on up straight until over your head. Then breathe out for 5 counts whilst lowering them, straight out in front of you, then on down to by your sides. This action just helps think about filling with air/drawing air in and pushing air out.

3 Do the same exercise, lifting your arms straight out to each side, and then on up to over your head; and down straight to either side and on down to by your sides. Again, you are just emphasizing the movement of the muscles and being more aware of your breathing.

A bit more advanced, traditional acting and singing technique:

The following exercise may make you feel tired at first. If you continue to practice, you will begin to notice that it takes less effort to breathe, less energy is used when breathing, plus it helps you learn to co-ordinate the diaphragm and abdominal muscles when breathing.

Lie flat on your back.

Place your hands on your abdomen, just underneath your ribs.

Taking a slow, deep breath in, focus on filling up your ribs from the bottom. The aim is not to fill yourself to bursting but just to inhale enough air so that you can feel the difference between taking a full breath from the abdomen, to a shallow breath taken when just breathing from the chest.

You should feel the expansion, not only at the front of the body but also to the sides and back as well.

Breathe out slowly to a count of 5 – and repeat 10 or more times.

Practise a couple of times a day, morning and night for 5–10 minutes gradually increasing this to 3 or 4 times a day. Remember to breathe in to the bottom and back of your lungs.

Once you get it right, try and do this as often as possible, sitting, standing and whilst at work, or driving, until you are breathing naturally from your abdomen.

When comfortable with that, the next exercise is to increase breath control.

Take a breath in – and as you exhale, sing numbers out loud, counting from 1 to 7 – at any comfortable pitch. Start with counting up to small numbers like 7 or 10 and increase this gradually until you can manage 25 or more without straining, tensing or running out of breath.

These are very useful for anyone wanting to go on X-Factor or who is involved in public speaking.

(In all these exercises, try not to be influenced by the unnatural, misplaced exaggeration we used to put on sticking our chests out, previously associated with gymnasts and sergeant majors, which encourages shallow breathing from the top of the chest – pull air in at the bottom and back of ribs).

Pilates Breathing Technique

Pilates is based on working with the body to support and improve, muscular tone and strength, flexibility, breathing, joint mobility, co-ordination, alignment, body control, posture and core stability (see page 200).

To concentrate on the muscles you want to use in the breathing exercises, wrap a small-ish towel around your ribs, with the ends crossed over at the front. Sit or stand, holding each end of the towel. Breathing in let your hands move with the towel as it expands around your ribs and gently draw back as you exhale. Let the chest rise but don't consciously lift the chest up, the action should be lateral, opening out, especially from the back rather than up – and toward the bottom of the ribs.

In relaxation mode, lying on the floor, with your hands by your sides or lying gently over the bottom of your ribs – as you breathe in allow the breath into the lungs, expanding the ribs, opening the back of the ribs and opening out to the sides. As you exhale, allow the ribs to close, knitting together at the front, keeping shoulders relaxed and shoulder blades sinking into the floor. Let the out breath be as long and full as possible and let the next breath in follow naturally, to re-fill the lungs. Do this several times - at least 10 - and much longer if you can. As well as breathing technique, it's excellent relaxation, body therapy and wonderful for the mind and mental faculties too.

In exercise mode, the breathing principles are the same, with the core stability muscles engaged/switched on - the breathing patterns then depend on the exercises.

Breathing exercises are both calming and invigorating.

Think about what the lungs are, what they do, where they are, how they are positioned in the rib cage and how the diaphragm works.

To prepare for anything unpleasant, or which makes us nervous - a blood test, medical examination, dental appointment, injection - deep breathing techniques calm the nerves, relax the muscles, minimizing pain, helping us to think of something else and overcome the anxiety. A few deep breaths and it's much easier to visualize the sandy beach and crystal sea to take our minds off what we're anxious about.

Exercise

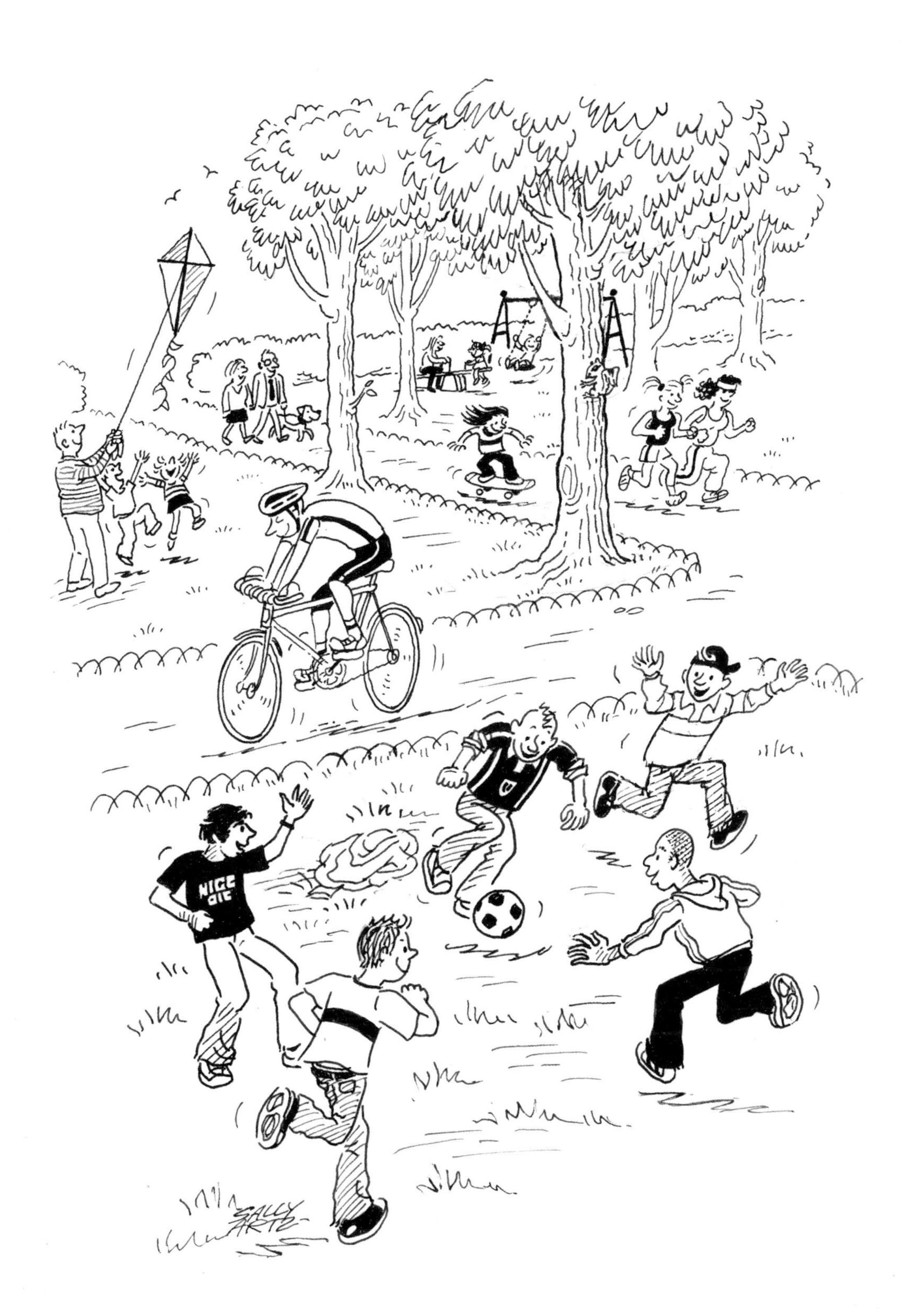
SALLY
ARTZ

Exercise

Exercise and physical fitness affects the entire body.

Exercise moves lymph around the body taking nutrients to cells and rubbish away. Muscles are designed to work by contracting and relaxing and that action works like a pump, taking blood, nutrients and oxygen to the tissues and muscles and taking de-oxygenated blood and waste products away, including lactic acid. Using muscles properly keeps them healthy. Exercise stimulates the thyroid gland which increases metabolic processes and metabolic efficiency. Sweating as a result of exercise enables the body to rid itself of toxins through the skin.

It stimulates the immune system (unless you overdo it in which case it can suppress the immune system). It helps prevent obesity, cardio-vascular disease, diabetes and much more, including protecting against cancer.

The most important aspect of exercise is to move the body more. For anyone who has a sedentary job, or sedentary lifestyle, it's especially important to try and find ways of incorporating more movement into the day. We may not have time to get to the gym 3 times a week but we can do lots of things to get moving. We need to think activity, not just exercise.

When you start to take up more activity, it's best to gradually build up to more strenuous exercise to give the body time to adjust.

Don't try to do too much too soon.

You can't regain fitness in a few days that you have lost in years of sedentary living.

Check your health. Either be sensible yourself about what you know – or see your doctor or someone properly qualified to assess how you are and what you should do.

Generally speaking, vigorous exercise involves minimal health risks, whereas habitual inactivity poses far greater health risks.

Fitness is a condition that helps us look, feel and do our best.

Physical fitness involves the performance of the heart and lungs and the muscles of the body – and our minds. It is influenced by age, sex, hereditary condition, lifestyle, exercise and eating practices. Not a lot most of us can do about the first three – but quite a lot we can do about the others.

Fitness can be thought of by 4 basic exercise categories:

Cardio-vascular Endurance – the ability to deliver oxygen and nutrients to the tissues and cells of the body and to remove wastes, over sustained periods of time. Good examples are long runs or swims.

Muscular Strength – the ability of a muscle to exert force for a brief period of time, eg: weights.

Muscular Endurance – the ability of a muscle or group of muscles to sustain repeat contractions, eg: press-ups, sit-ups and several gym equipment exercises.

Flexibility – the ability to move joints and use muscles through their full range of motion.

How often and how long you exercise and what kind of exercise it is best to do depends on what you are trying to achieve; your goals, your present fitness level, your age, your health, your skills, your interest. You can either decide for yourself what suits you or discuss different fitness programmes with the doctor, fitness coach, trainer – whoever you want to work with. This has to be done using an appropriate level of common sense, and/or professional and qualified help.

Ideally we should try and include some exercise for each of the four basic categories.

Each work-out should begin with a warm-up and end with a cool-down – or as seems more fashionable to say these days 'warm-down' – and as a general rule, space the work-outs through the week.

A typical example of a personal schedule could be:

warm-up	5-10 minutes (walking, slow jogging, knee lifts, arm circles, exercise bike – low to medium)
cardio-vascular endurance	three 20 minute sessions per week bouts of continuous aerobic exercise: brisk walking, jogging, swimming, cycling, skipping, rowing, many sports
muscular strength	two 20 minute sessions per week all major muscle groups; eg: weights, some gym equipment exercises

muscular endurance	three 30 minute sessions per week all major muscle groups: push-ups, sit-ups, weights, some gym equipment exercises
flexibility	10-12 minutes of daily stretching can be included after a warm-up or during a cool-down.
cool-down	5-10 minutes slow walking, low level exercise bike.

This equals 30 minutes a day, on the warm up, stretching and warm-down; plus another 2 hours 50 minutes through the week – and just that small amount of time can make a significant difference. Those are the basics and hopefully when you have started to incorporate those, you will find that you want to do more and enjoy doing more.

We can't hoard physical fitness. It doesn't work to have one mega exercise session once a week, or once a fortnight and nothing in between. Most people will need 3 balanced work-outs a week to maintain a reasonable level of fitness.

The 3:1 guide: after 3 months of training, if you stopped for 1 month – you'd be back to where you started.

Some activities will achieve more than one of the basic exercises at once.

Running, for example, involves cardio-vascular endurance as well as muscular endurance, mainly in the legs. Swimming involves cardio-vascular endurance as well us muscular endurance for the arms, shoulders and chest whilst also working out and strengthening the torso and back.

When

When you exercise is determined by your timetable and personal preference. Popular times for training are:

- early morning – before the tasks of the day interfere too much – and some say this makes them more alert and energetic for the day
- early evening, at the end of the working day – as a useful gear change after work and can be useful to throw off some of the mental stresses and tension, invigorate yourself for your own personal time.

It is not good to exercise strenuously within 2 hours of eating, if you can avoid it. Digestion makes heavy demands on the circulatory system. So does hot weather.

Excuses

We are never too unfit, too young or too old to start to work on physical fitness. Exercise, combined with sensible diet will affect our overall sense of wellbeing and can help prevent chronic illnesses, disability and premature death. Take advice from a qualified adviser if you have any doubts at all.

Benefits

Benefits of increased activity include:

Improved Health

- increased efficiency of heart and lungs
- reduced cholesterol levels
- increased muscle strength
- reduced blood pressure
- reduced risk of major illnesses, such as diabetes and heart disease
- if overweight, weight loss
- if underweight, weight control/management, from improved appetite, circulation, stimulation, strength and fitness

Improved sense of wellbeing

- more energy
- less stress
- improved quality of sleep
- improved ability to cope with stress
- increased mental acuity

Improved appearance

- weight loss, if overweight; weight control/management, if underweight
- toned muscles
- improved posture

Increased stamina

- increased productivity
- increased physical capabilities
- less frequent injuries
- improved immunity to minor illnesses.

In Marilyn Diamond's book 'Fit for Life' she describes that when she first started exercising, her resting heartbeat was 72 beats per minute. One month later it was 54. In one month she had strengthened and improved the function of her heart by 18 beats per minute. That's over 15,000 beats a day. This translates to millions fewer beats a year – somewhere around 5,475,000.

Aerobic describes activity that exercises the heart and stimulates the respiratory and circulatory systems. This way, fresh oxygenated blood reaches all areas of your body – carries the good stuff in and the rubbish out.

Putting increased activity and fitness into practice

Most health experts would recommend 30 minutes of moderately intense, physical activity on all or most days of the week, for non-professional sports people to maintain an average level of fitness. Examples of this would be brisk walking, cycling, swimming, and active gardening. If one 30 minute bout is difficult for any reason, then two 15 minute sessions or three 10 minutes sessions will do nearly as well. However, for weight loss, periods of exercise really need to be 40 minutes plus. All exercise will help fitness but for weight loss, longer periods are better because our bodies can perform 30-40 minutes of exercise without having to dip into and convert energy reserves, which is what we are looking for in trying to burn off excess. 40 minutes and longer sessions will start to make a difference if combined with an appropriate eating plan. Sessions of less than 40 minutes will help fitness but won't be as effective for weight loss.

Psychologically a good stage to reach is to think of your health and fitness as a permanent change in your lifestyle, not a separate, extra thing you have to do. The exercise and any other changes and regimes are part of the day.

As well as specific times and activities you introduce for your exercise in life generally, try and include incidental activity – you've probably heard of these before:

- using the stairs instead of lifts and escalators
- parking further away from the office or workplace and walking a bit further
- getting off public transport a few stops early and walking further
- getting up from sitting from time to time, stretching and having a walk around
- taking a brisk walk when you fancy a snack (instead of the snack)
- increase your pace when doing housework or gardening, walking, etc
- getting stuck into mowing the lawn or raking up the leaves
- go out for a walk – just for the sake of it.

The ultimate aim is also to enjoy improving your fitness:

- try and choose activities you enjoy where possible
- set realistic goals
- don't get discouraged if you don't see immediate results. Depending on the degree of unfitness, we have usually put a lot of time and effort into getting unfit – the good news is, it doesn't take nearly as long to get fit, if you want to
- don't give up if you miss a day – just get back to it the next day or as soon as you can – and don't cheat yourself with excuses – you know which ones are real and which ones aren't – you aren't kidding anyone
- listen to your body. This is very important. If you have difficulty breathing, if you have pain, if you experience faintness or prolonged weakness during or after exercise – talk to your doctor or someone medically qualified to advise you.

Consider trying more than one type of exercise to give you and your body a thorough work-out and prevent getting bored and fed up.

The rules

- Always warm up – and warm up slowly and gradually.
- Drink plenty of water.
- Stop at the first sign of muscle cramping or dizziness.
- Take special care of your feet and regularly check your feet, especially if you have a diabetic or vascular condition.
- Always cool down/warm down.
- Listen to your body: if you have pain, if you experience faintness or prolonged weakness during or after exercise – if you think there is something wrong – talk to your doctor or someone medically qualified to advise you. (Yes, this is repeated, it's important).

Stretching

Stretching before and after physical activity helps prevent injury and improves performance by increasing your range of motion and improving co-ordination. Stretching helps free your body of muscular tension, improves circulation and enhances muscle tone. Stretching also helps avoid some aspects of ageing, such as decreased flexibility, poor balance and stiff joints.

Calories

Calories burned vary in proportion to individual body weight but some typical averages would be:

Calories burned per hour

bicycling	6mph	240	
bicycling	12mph	410	
jogging	5.5mph	740	
jogging	7 mph	920	
skipping		750	
running on the spot		650	
running	10mph	1,280	
swimming	25 yds/min	275	(22.86 metres)
swimming	50 yds/min	500	(45.72 metres)
tennis singles		400	
walking	2mph	240	
walking	4mph	440	

Core Strength and Core Stability

Another essential aspect of activity, exercise and fitness is core strength and core stability. Many, many different forms of exercise overlook this very important/crucial element. I'm sure we could all but eliminate back problems and many musculo-skeletal conditions and injuries if we could just pay core strength and stability the respect it deserves. Many gym regimes, especially those advised by skilled, qualified trainers will now include exercise for core strength and stability and I have included a section on Pilates, later in this chapter which bases all its exercise and movement on core strength and stability.

This engages, tones and reminds us to use the deep core muscles it is all too easy to get by without using. We are wonderfully designed with very strong core muscles and wrapped in protective layers of muscles to support our internal organs, our spine, our hips, pelvis and abdomen and to take the strain when elevating limbs or exerting pressure. In a less physical lifestyle, if we aren't engaging and using these muscles all the time, they can relax and weaken and we don't consciously remember to engage them when they are needed. This puts a greatly increased strain on the other muscles, tissues, ligaments and tendons. Many lower back problems, from sedentary jobs, driving, lifting and carrying or poor posture, can be caused if we aren't correctly using these muscles.

It is best to learn the exercises with an experienced, qualified trainer or at least a professionally produced, reputable book, CD or DVD. Basically, it is like zipping up the muscles deep inside, between the pelvic bone and your ribs and your hip bones. It is often described as a triangle between the tips of the hip bones and the pelvic bone, pulling the tummy button towards the spine. This isn't the same as 'holding your tummy in' although it is along those lines, and you engage the muscles breathing out, not holding your breath. When we do this it creates a really strong core and the exercises are designed to switch these muscles on to support and protect us all the time, sitting, walking, whatever we are doing. They are excellent exercises with remarkable results. (There's more about Pilates on page 200.)

Body fat myths and misconceptions

Myth number 1 is that fat can be turned into muscle and muscle can be turned into fat. Muscle and fat are different things and cannot create one another. You can lose fat and build muscle and vice versa – and you can do it at the same time – but one is being lost and the other built up – they can't convert one to the other.

Myth number 2 is that weighing more on weighing scales means you must be overweight. This isn't strictly true. Muscle weighs approximately 75% more than fat so you can increase your body weight without increasing your body fat. You can increase your body weight and decrease your percentage body fat.

Myth number 3 is that weighing yourself is the best way to determine if you are overweight. Weight is a useful fact to know and to monitor – but to know whether you are losing body fat, keeping an item of clothing from your original size and checking the fit is probably a more accurate measure of body fat loss.

There are various ways of measuring body fat ratios at gyms and medical centres and different people have different preferred methods. If you are losing body fat and becoming fitter and have more energy – you will know – and you will feel better.

Outdoor Exercise

It is also a good idea to incorporate some outdoor exercise. Fresh air is our life force and changing and re-charging the air in our lungs is really invigorating. Sunshine is also the source of all life and energy on the planet. We may be warned off over-exposure to the sun – but it is as important to see enough sunshine. Having a window open in the room when you are sleeping is also supposed to aid the assimilation and elimination cycles, helping the body to be more effective.

Pregnancy

Exercise during pregnancy can have the following benefits:

- fewer leg cramps, backaches and other pregnancy-related pains
- increased sense of wellbeing and control during pregnancy
- reduced weight gain
- larger placenta (the nutrient base for the baby)
- shorter labour and easier delivery
- speedier recovery.

Recommendations include the following:

- regular exercise
- mild to moderate intensity routines
- measure working heart rate to ensure staying within the desired range
- extremes of joint flex and extension, such as deep knee bends, should be avoided
- avoid exercising on your back (supine) after first 3 months
- be aware of decreased oxygen available for aerobic exercise and modify exercise intensity
- stop exercising when fatigued – and do not exercise to exhaustion
- avoid exercises where loss of balance could be detrimental to mother or baby, especially at 6-9 months
- avoid any type of exercise involving the potential for even mild abdominal trauma
- ensure an adequate diet
- gradually increase exercise intensity after delivery.

Exercise and Evolution

Our origins and hereditary disposition have set us up for an active life which includes periods of endurance exercise. This potential level of activity would have been necessary for our ancestors to cover many miles in search of plant foods and to run great distances to hunt animals for meat. It is not so long in evolutionary terms since we lived the hunter-gatherer existence for which we evolved and adapted and it will take some time yet before the body adapts to a more modern lifestyle. The changes in lifestyle have been radical and taken place in a very short space of time, so in the meantime we need to consciously manage those changes.

The disposition for periods of endurance exercise does not stop with the onset of middle age. It is taken as fact that our abilities and performances deteriorate quickly with the onset of middle age at about 40. Not only is this not proven but plenty of people have shown that you don't have to be young to be an athlete and in fact exercise delays ageing. Dr Mike Stroud[1] illustrates this in his book 'Survival of the Fittest'. He entered a race of 300 miles over some of the most difficult terrain in the world as part of a team. One of his other team members was a 72 year old grandmother who only started running marathons at age 55 and has since run 75 marathons and 150 ultra-marathons. Some years later he persuaded his 70 year old father who had never run in a distance event before, to join him in running 7 marathons in 7 days on 7 continents, which they did. Many people have the ability to run a marathon if they had to, they just don't realize it.

In his book he also discusses how sport, performance and challenge are activities that men and women have evolved to take the place of hunting and gathering. There are advantages and disadvantages of our evolutionary inheritance. On the positive side there is resilience and physical strength that far exceed people's expectations. On the negative side there is a propensity to develop serious health problems.

[1] Mike Stroud completed a degree in anthropology and genetics and qualified as a doctor in 1979. He became a Member of the Royal College of Physicians in 1984 and a Fellow in 1995. He has travelled widely. He was the doctor on the 1984-86 "In the Footsteps of Scott" Antarctic expedition. In 1993 he was awarded the OBE in recognition of their first unsupported crossing of the Antarctic continent from coast to coast with Ranulph Fiennes. In the 1990s he was Senior Research Medical Officer for 6 years advising the MoD on nutrition, exercise performance and survival. He returned to hospital medical practice with particular interest in nutrition and metabolism. He and Ranulph Fiennes completed 7 marathons, in 7 days on 7 continents. He has contributed to many international publications.
Dr Mike Stroud – Survival of the Fittest: Understanding Peak Physical Performance

' . . . the heart attacks, strokes, diabetes, and other illnesses that arise from our modern lifestyles and diets that are far from those for which evolution designed us.'

' . . . by taxing some of our hidden evolutionary strengths we can avoid many of our inherited weaknesses, and so remain active and healthy well into old age.'

In July, August and September 2009 Eddie Izzard ran 43 marathons in 51 days. This was truly remarkable - someone with no previous athletic training, who had never run a marathon before, with minimal (approximately 5 weeks) preparation and training. He ran at least 27 miles a day, for 6 days a week, for 7 weeks and covered over 1,166 miles. 'He should be commended for showing that anyone can unlock that running potential. Our bodies are designed to run because that's genetically how we developed' - Sports Scientist, Professor John Brewer, University of Bedfordshire. He will have benefited from reshaped muscles, more efficient organs and boosted blood vessels. These extreme tests of endurance also demonstrate how powerful the combination of mental and physical capabilities can be. They are extraordinary physical accomplishments but also demand ultimate mental strength - fierce, relentless determination - physical and mental stamina.

The benefits of exercise are becoming increasingly apparent through research. There are connections between lots of chronic disease and inactivity.

More and more studies are accumulating more and more substantial evidence to support the role of physical activity in promoting good health. Regular physical activity decreases the risk of coronary heart disease, stroke and diabetes and the associated risk factors such as hypertension and obesity. Physical activity also seems to help in preventing falls of older people.

- Diseases of the heart and circulatory system, cardio-vascular disease (CVD) are the main causes of death in the UK accounting for almost 198,000 deaths each year. 48% are Coronary heart disease (CHD) around 94,000 deaths in the UK in 2006 and 28% from stroke, 55,400 deaths - according to the British Heart Foundation figures (2008). (www.heartstats.org)
- there are around 1.8 million people in England with diagnosed diabetes
- each year 110,000 people in England and Wales have their first stroke, and 30,000 people go on to have further strokes
- over 400,000 older people in England attend A&E Departments following an accident and up to 14,000 people a year die in the UK as a result of an osteoporotic hip fracture
- 41% of men and 33% of women have high blood pressure

- levels of obesity have tripled in the last 20 years. If the trend continues over a quarter of adults in England will be obese by 2010 and the National Audit Office's report outlined significant costs to the NHS and the economy.

In 1998, obesity accounted for:

- 18 million days of sickness absence per year
- 40,000 lost years of working life
- 30,000 deaths - of which 9,000 related to obesity before state retirement age
- £0.5 billion cost to the NHS
  £2.0 billion indirect costs to the economy
  totalling £2.5 billion costs annually

- obese men are 33% more likely to die of cancer
- obese women are at 50% greater risk of getting breast cancer.

General health and work absence stats:

- 164 million days a year lost to the UK economy through ill health
- costing the UK economy £13bn a year
- the most significant causes of absence, for manual and non-manual workers, are back pain and musculo-skeletal injuries
- smoking causes half of all premature deaths
- 1 in 4 of us die prematurely of cancer and 2 in 4 of heart disease but these diseases are 75% lifestyle related and may well be preventable
- half a million people each year experience stress at a level that will make them ill.

Sources:
CIPD - National Survey of Absence
CBI - Confederation of British Industry
ONS - Office of National Statistics
WHO - World Health Organisation
Cancer Research UK
HSE - Managing sickness absence

http://www.dh.gov.uk/en/Publicationsandstatistics/Publications/PublicationsPolicyAndGuidance/DH_4080994

A diet rich in saturated fats and processed foods, smoking, stress, alcohol and lack of exercise are all contributory factors to these statistics.

Experts advise that physically inactive people have about double the risk of CHD.

Physical activity is comparable to reducing that risk with other lifestyle factors, such as not smoking.

Pilates

I have tried throughout this book to be objective and not to promote favourites - but in covering exercise and fitness, especially as we go on to talk about joints, muscles and posture later, I have to include a few paragraphs dedicated to Pilates. There are so many different kinds of sports and hobbies and martial arts and different practices, far too many to cover - but I do believe that Pilates comes into a class of its own. It works the whole body and anyone can do it. It's practical and it works on body awareness - thinking about what you are doing, how you are doing it, preparation, alignment, balance and breathing - these are essential basics to all exercises. It is so important to think about how the body works and what we are doing.

The simple methods are excellent at preventing back and posture problems and improving, very often curing, any existing problems, for all ages and all bodies. Following Pilates' methods prevents injuries and stress-related conditions. Pilates retrains the body and mind to work together. We then aren't only incorporating the methods into the exercise but in how we move and work, all the time.

Joseph Pilates was born in Dusseldorf in 1880 and was a frail, sickly child. Obsessed with physical fitness to improve body image, he became a keen sportsman, taking up diving, skiing, gymnastics, boxing and wrestling. He was in England at the outbreak of the first world war and worked teaching self-defence to police detectives. He had to be interned because of his German nationality and during that time he developed physical fitness programmes for himself and others detained to maintain their health whilst they were confined. When he returned to Germany, after the war, he worked with ballet companies and the Hamburg Police Force. Between the two world wars, he was asked to train the new German army but refused and relocated to America. He married and set up his first fitness studio in New York working with top ballet dancers, actors, sports people and the rich and famous, including Gregory Peck and Katharine Hepburn. His work grew very fast in popularity and he trained people to teach, eventually making Pilates more accessible to everyone.

Pilates depends on the approach to the exercises, the preparation - training us to consciously control the body movements. Nothing is left to chance, it is all thought through – a sense of body awareness, co-ordination, balance and alignment. Before starting a movement, positioning the body, engaging the right muscles and breathing pattern are an important part of all the exercises. It teaches how core posture muscles stabilize the trunk, how to strengthen weak muscles, stretch and lengthen short, tight muscles, increase flexibility and joint mobility. There is no use of force. The exercises are smooth, flowing movements, avoiding strains and working with the design and construction of the body to give an extensive work-out without causing damage. They aren't 'easy' exercises. Experienced sports people and professionals have described them as some of the most difficult and demanding exercises there are. You use your head, your brain, your skeleton, your deep core muscles, your balance, your alignment and co-ordination altogether. This works the whole body and emphasizes core strength and stability – which personally, I would now have to say, I think is the secret to overcoming the vast majority of back complaints. Even when you think you have tried everything for persistent back problems, including physiotherapy, chiropractic and osteopathy treatments, I would say Pilates will still work in most, if not every case – as it will for any problem areas – shoulders, back, thigh, knee, wherever.

The general principles are concentration, co-ordination, alignment, breathing, balance and centring and relaxation. More contemporary followers have included the Australian Rugby Team, Pat Cash, Jodie Foster, Patrick Swayze, Glenn Close, Joan Collins, Madonna, Honor Blackman, Britt Eckland and Wayne Sleep.

As with all purchases, practices, pursuits and activities, seek recommendations and referrals. There is bound to be some variance in skills of Pilates teachers. The method and concept are excellent and it shouldn't be difficult to find someone to work with.

The psychological effects of exercise and hormones

Exercise also affects us mentally. Most scientific research on this looks into hormonal responses to physical activity. Levels of endorphins, enkephalins, catecholamines and serotonin have been studied.

Hormone comes from the Greek word meaning 'arouse to activity'. Hormones are produced by endocrine glands throughout the body which secrete the hormones to be carried into the bloodstream and to all the various cells and organs. They then stimulate physiological changes, wherever they are. There are 4 types of endorphins and it is beta endorphins which seem to show the greatest increase in plasma concentration during times of exercise.

Endorphins are thought to be released from the pituitary during times of pain or stress.

Prolonged or hard activity causes anaerobic respiration which causes lactic acid accumulation and a decrease in oxygen flow to the muscles. This state of acidosis is thought to stimulate the pituitary to release endorphins.

The endorphins enter the neural pathways, bind to opioid receptors and have the effect of blocking the pain signal molecules from the nerve terminal. The effect is that no, or reduced, pain signals reach the brain and the endorphins are said to have had an analgaesic effect.

Whilst having this analgaesic effect on the body, endorphin release results in a state of euphoria. As well as reducing pain this also aids the reduction of stress. Endorphins are known as the body's natural painkillers. Because they have a similar action to opiate drugs they are also known as the endogenous opioids.

The endorphins also stimulate the immune system by activating natural killer cells and can postpone ageing.

During a prolonged exercise or activity, of say 30 minutes, blood levels of beta endorphins have been found to increase up to 5 times. This varies from person to person and on how much exercise you regularly do.

In the same way as our body builds up a tolerance against opiate drugs, it also gets used to regular levels of exercise – so to experience the same endorphin affect, we would have to increase the amount of exercise. This is why exercise can become addictive – and the analgaesic effect is sometimes called 'the runners' high'.

Enkephalins are very similar to endorphins and are also released during periods of exercising. They are released from the thalamus of the brain and enter the bloodstream. They also bind to receptors and are thought to block the release of the neuro-transmitter, substance P involved in the transmission and sensation of pain.

Catecholamines are adrenalin and noradrenalin, their synthesis begins in the catecholinergic or sympathetic nervous system. It starts with an amino acid called tyrosine being taken up into the nerves, which produces dihydroxyphenylalanine, which produces dopamine, which produces noradrenalin which passes to the adrenal medulla, part of the adrenal gland which sits just at the top of the kidney, which produces adrenalin.

During times of stress and exercise, we activate our sympathetic nervous system. Increased stimulation of the endocrine glands produces increased noradrenalin and adrenalin, (ratio 20:80). When they are released into the bloodstream, they affect various different parts of the body and act as hormones:

- they increase heart rate
  (due to the affects of noradrenalin on the sino-atrial node of the heart)

- they restrict the flow of blood to other parts of the body not directly involved in the exercise

- they allow the muscles to receive more oxygenated blood, increasing our ability to use those muscles and allow the liver to convert more stored glycogen to use for energy.

Studies of depression have shown that it is linked to and possibly caused by, low concentration or impaired transmission of neuro-transmitters - noradrenalin and serotonin. Increasing the concentration of those transmitters when we exercise, lifts mood away from depression.

And if we were feeling OK anyway, we just feel even better.

Lots of study goes on into this and as well as the physiological work-out which makes the body feel better and we feel better, there are 3 additional theories as to why we would feel good:

- exercise can enhance mood because of the feeling of accomplishment, sense of achievement - especially if we are mastering something new or improving at something we like or want to do.

- exercise can act as a constructive distraction from other things, things we may have to do or have on our mind - so it gives us a break, renews and refreshes our state, invigorates us. This is an excellent example of the 'balance' we so often talk about. Stopping what we are doing and doing something different.

- the exercise may have a social aspect to it, interacting with peers, being in a team. The socialising may be as effective in making us feel better as the exercise - but both together are doubly effective.

William Bloom[1] has written a very popular book called *The Endorphin Effect* which goes into this in much more detail, skilfully describing the powerful effects of endorphins, heightened experiences and sense of connection - an awesome power of the biology of the human body. Amongst the effects he includes:

[1] William Bloom – Doctorate in Psychology from LSE, lecturer in Psychological Problems in International Poitics LSE, 10 years work with adults and adolescents with special needs, deliverer of many trainings, including NHS.

- a sense of personal integrity, not dependent on material success or the opinion of others
- inner strength
- long-term vision
- stable foundation for personal and career development
- clearer moral and ethical sense
- improved health
- better company to family and friends
- leadership qualities – specifically quiet leadership qualities
- feel more alert and intelligent
- increased sense of being in the driving seat of your life
- genuine enjoyment of life, whilst being solidly present to the challenges and suffering.

THERE IS NO SUCH THING AS BAD WEATHER.
GET YOURSELF A SEXY RAINCOAT
AND LIVE A LITTLE.

Billy Connolly

I DON'T EXERCISE. IF GOD HAD WANTED
ME TO BEND OVER – HE WOULD HAVE PUT
DIAMONDS ON THE FLOOR.

Joan Rivers

HOW ENDORPHINS AFFECT OUR MOOD

Endorphins are released into the bloodstream by the pituitary

↓

Endorphins enter nociceptive afferents
(neurons which carry pain impulses to the brain)

↓

Endorphins then bind to opioid receptors in the neurons –
these receptors are the same as the receptors which drugs such as morphine bind to

↓

Endorphins have an antagonistic effect on the receptors
and therefore block the release of neuro-transmitter molecules from the nerve terminal

↓

Pain signals are stopped from reaching the brain.
The endorphins are said to have had an analgaesic effect
and this produces a state of euphoria

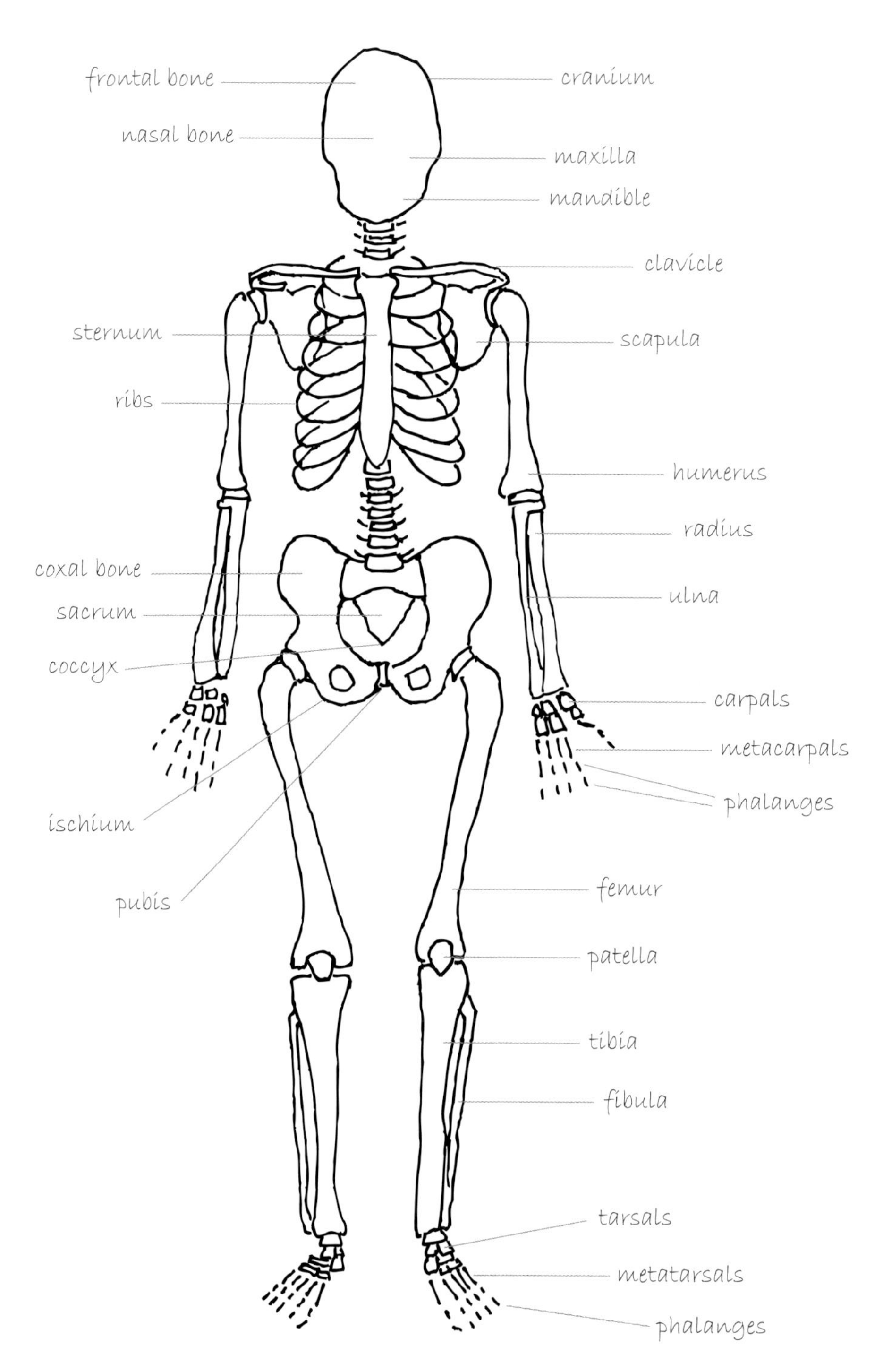
SKELETON
frontal bone
cranium
nasal bone
maxilla
mandible
clavicle
sternum
scapula
ribs
humerus
radius
coxal bone
ulna
sacrum
coccyx
carpals
metacarpals
phalanges
ischium
pubis
femur
patella
tibia
fibula
tarsals
metatarsals
phalanges

Bones

The Bones of the Skeleton: 206 in total

Skull		28 bones	
Cranium	8 bones		
Face	14 bones		
Ear	6 bones		
Hyoid bone	1 bone	1 bone	
Spinal column	26 bones	26 bones	(inc sacrum and coccyx)
Sternum	1 bone	1 bone	
Ribs		24 bones	
True ribs	14 ribs		
False ribs	10 ribs		
Upper extremities		64 bones	
Clavicle	2		
Scapula	2		
Humerus	2		
Radius	2		
Ulna	2		
Carpals	16		
Metacarpals	10		
Phalanges	28		
Lower extremities		62 bones	
Hip girdle/pelvic girdle	2		(inc pubis and ischium)
Femur	2		
Patella	2		
Tibia	2		
Fibula	2		
Tarsals	14		
Metatarsals	10		
Phalanges	28		

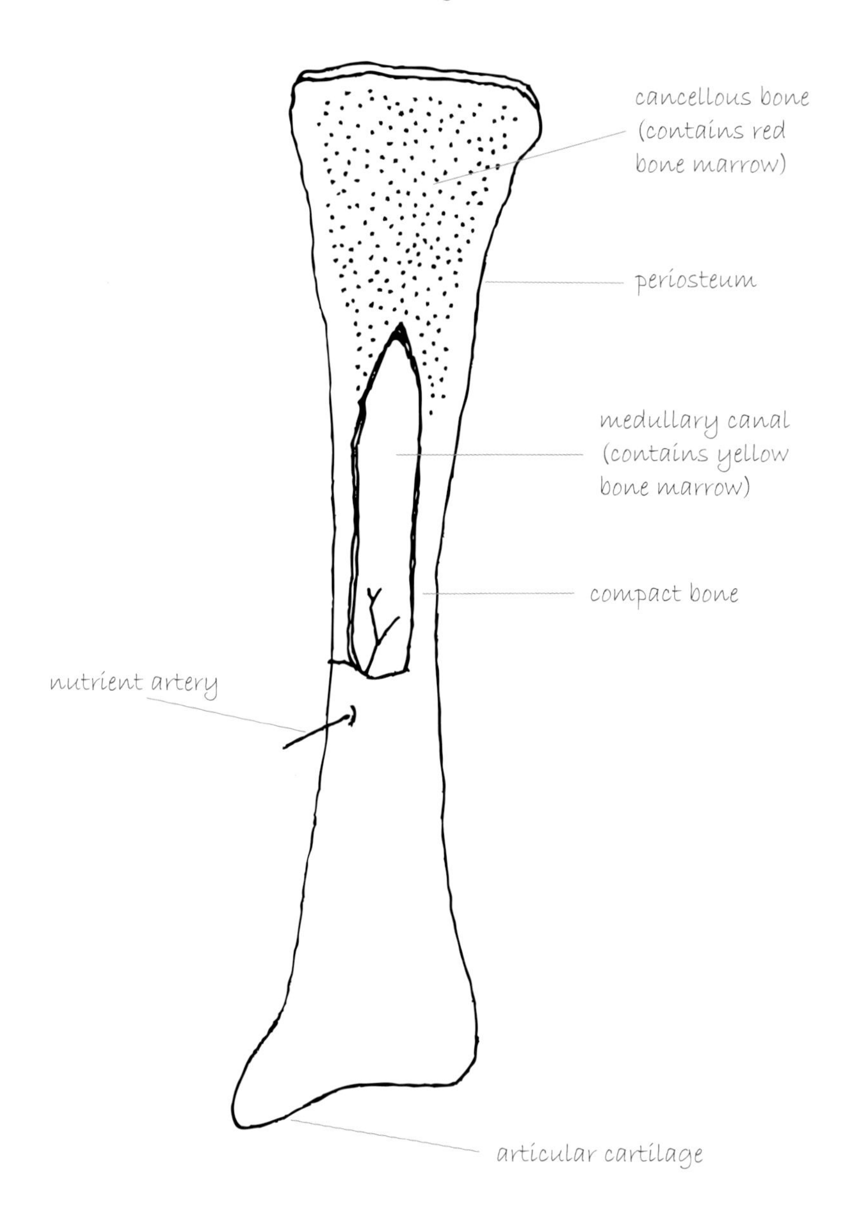
BONE STRUCTURE
(mature long bone)
cancellous bone
(contains red
bone marrow)
periosteum
medullary canal
(contains yellow
bone marrow)
compact bone
nutrient artery
articular cartilage

Bones, Bone Health and Spine

Structurally we have 4 types of bones: long bones, short bones, flat bones and irregular bones.

The size and shape of our bones differ according to what they do. Bones have 5 general functions:

- support - they are the framework for the body; torso, arms, legs, fingers, toes
- protection - eg: skull, ribs
- movement - hips, knees, shoulders, elbows, etc
- mineral storage - reservoir for calcium and phosphorous
- haemopoiesis - blood cell production.

Bones consist of bone cells, fibres and extracellular structure, usually referred to as the bone matrix. The bone matrix is the hard, calcified part of the bone which makes up most of the bone (see diagram page 208).

Bone can have a strength comparable to cast iron whilst about a third of the weight.

The best way to look after our bones is through activity and exercise which trigger the renewal and regeneration of the skeletal system - and to make sure that all the nutrients needed to form the new bone tissue are present and available from our diet.

The hard, calcified nature of bone comes from the deposits of special crystals of calcium and phosphate and this part of the bone matrix also contains magnesium, sodium, sulphate and fluoride. The rest of the bone matrix is made of connective tissue, collagen fibres and proteins which is where the growth, repair and regeneration take place. These nutrients, minerals and tissues all need to be provided by, or formed from, the constituents provided in the diet. Large areas of hard bone may also have inner softer or spongey bone. Spongey bone is found at the expanded heads of long bones, eg: hip - and fills most irregular bones.

Bone marrow is a special type of soft connective tissue in the central cavities of some of our long bones and some areas of spongey bone, where red blood cells are made.

The skeletal system stores approximately 98% of the body's calcium reserves. Calcium is present in the bone tissue and in blood and moves from blood to bone and from bone to blood depending where it is needed. During bone formation, calcium is required by the bone cells and so will pass from the blood to the bone. When there is high acidity in the body and blood calcium is low - calcium will move back from the bones to the blood. The teeth hold a lot of the rest of the calcium in our body and then the blood, muscles and nerves.

Production of bone tissue takes place when we are growing as our bones become larger and continues after they have stopped growing for repair and renewal. Throughout our life our bones are being continually worn away and destroyed and renewed at the same time. During the first 20 years of our life bone formation occurs faster than bone loss. Anytime around the age of 35-40 the process reverses and gradually bone loss exceeds bone formation.

Our diet needs to provide sufficient nutrients to minimize and protect us from bone loss over time.

Fracture and repair

If we break a bone, when the bone fractures, the tiny blood vessels in the bone matrix where the bone breaks will tear and the bleeding that occurs clots, forming a specialized callous tissue which binds the ends of the fractured bones. How well the bone can heal depends on how well it is aligned and immobilized. The callous tissue is then gradually replaced with normal bone tissue as the break heals.

The Spine

The spine consists of 24 vertebrae, plus the sacrum and the coccyx. The spine supports the head on the top and carries most of the rest of the body, the shoulders, arms, ribs, hips and lower limbs.

Because it is segmented into vertebrae with joints in between, it allows flexibility – forwards, backwards, sideways and circular and twisting movement (see diagram page 11).

The spinal cord of the central nervous system runs through the spine.

Between the vertebrae are discs and strong ligaments. The discs have a strong, fibrous outer layer containing a spongey, elastic, pulp centre, which allows the movement of the vertebrae and cushions impact. Excessive strain can over-compress the vertebrae and push the disc tissue out into the spinal canal, putting pressure on the nerves. This is the infamous 'slipped disc' and causes severe pain (see diagram, page 213). The discs will also lose some of the spongey, elasticity with age, which will mean we are more susceptible to these kinds of strains and damage. Looking after our backs throughout our lives, good diet and correct exercises will help significantly to protect against injury, keep us supple and is the easiest way to ensure we experience best mobility and least pain.

The medical term for a slipped disc is a herniated disc, or a herniated nucleus pulposus.

The spine is curved in 4 distinct curves. The curves offer a far greater strength than a straight line and enable it to support the weight and load it carries which enables us to stand upright. When we are born the spine is one curve from head to coccyx and as we begin to sit and stand, the other balancing curves develop.

VERTEBRAL COLUMN
(simplified)

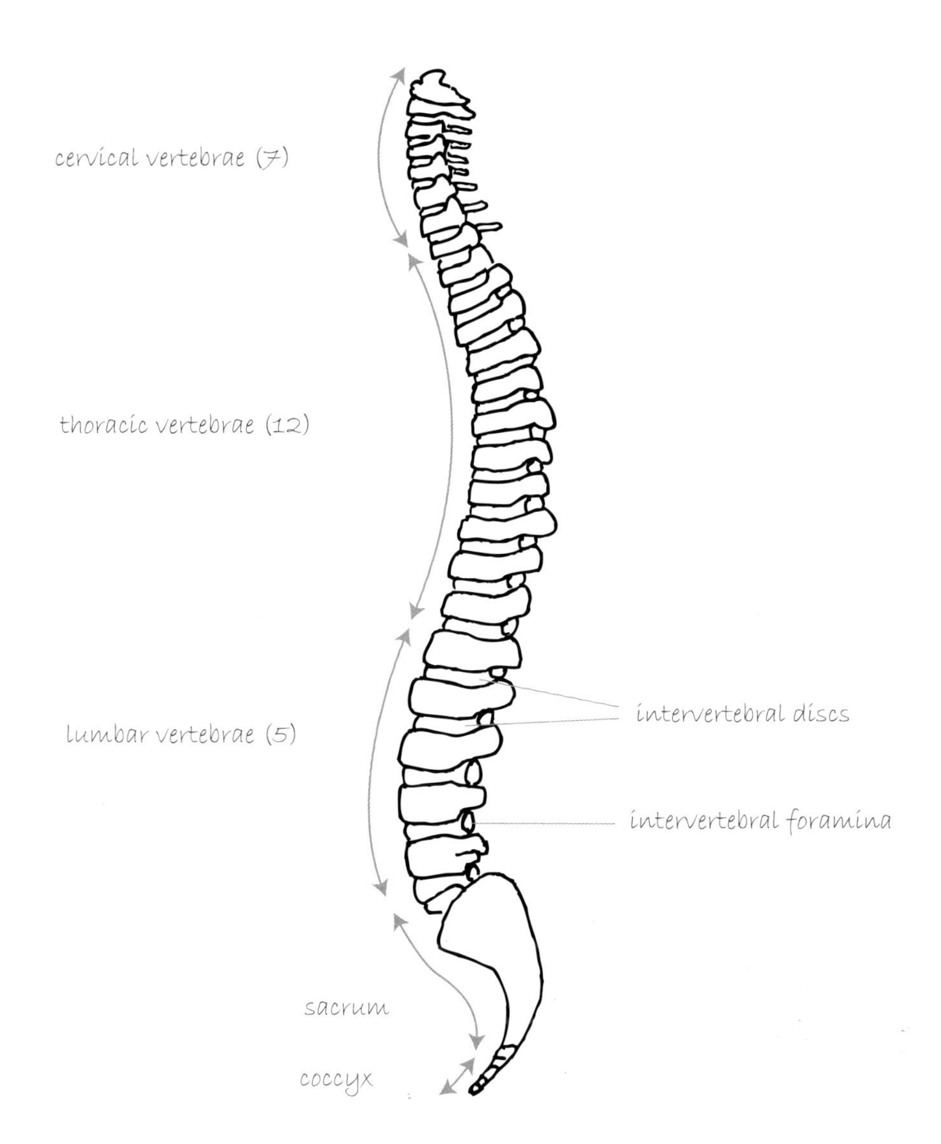

LOWER CERVICAL VERTEBRAE
SHOWING SPINAL CORD AND NERVES

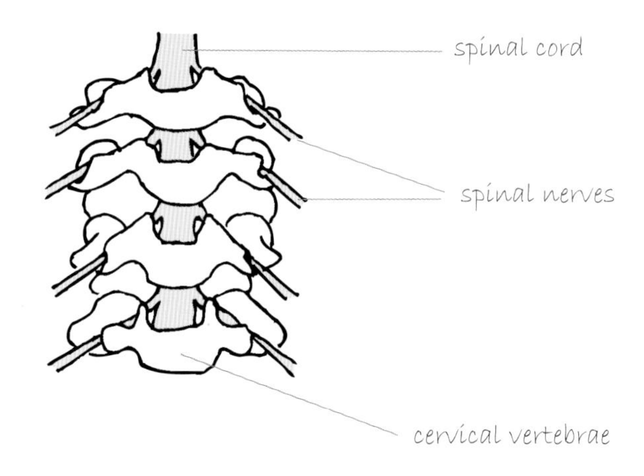

Whilst our bones are forming, when we are young, they are fairly resistant to toddler tumbles and the mechanical stresses of learning to walk. The bones then become harder and more dense and that density from adolescence to middle age gives great strength to allow hard work and carrying heavy loads. From middle age, loss of bone density leaves us more vulnerable to fracture. Loss of bone tissue can result in loss of height and can affect posture including the ability to stand tall. The loss of bone tissue can cause a compression or shrinkage which can be very different in different people. It may be very slight and barely noticeable, or if it occurs to a greater extent, it will be more noticeable and even disabling, causing stooping and bowed head and neck.

Our spine is such an important part of our body, taking care of it should be a really high priority.

Calcium and bone

Calcium is an alkaline element.

A modern, typical western diet tends to be quite acidic in digestion and in order to balance that, our body will draw on alkaline stores in the body. We can lose quite a lot of the body's calcium to neutralize acidity in the body. We need good nutrition to have the nutrients available to provide renewal and regeneration and calcium is an essential

PROLAPSED (SLIPPED) DISC

viewed from the side

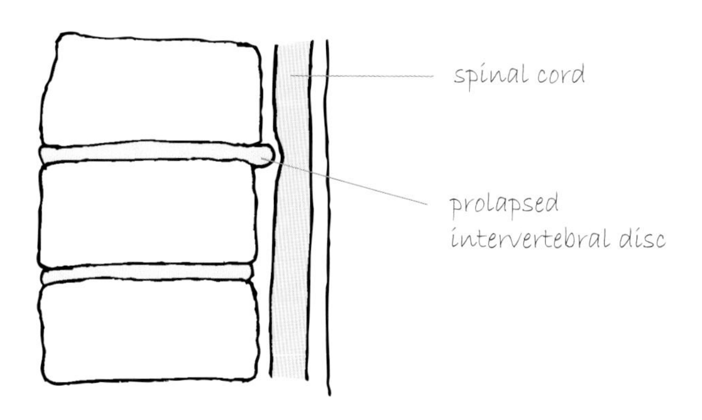

viewed from above

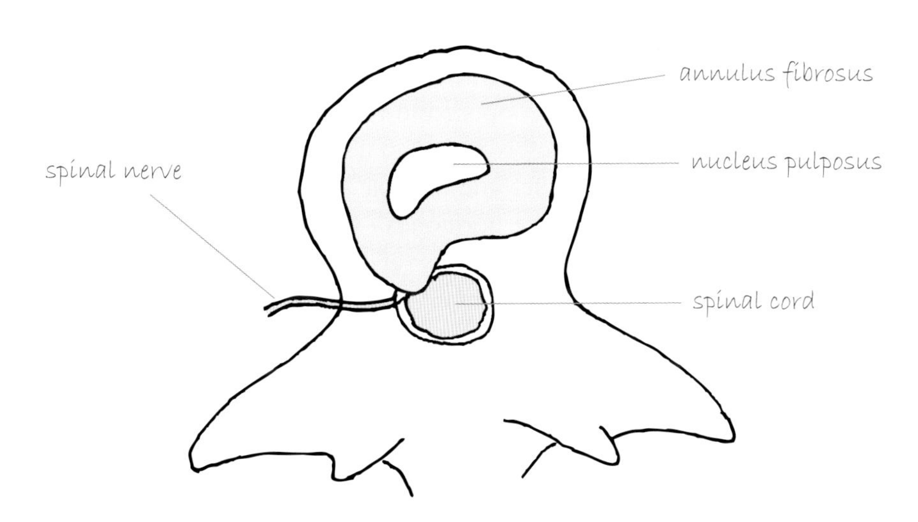

part of our diet in order to build a strong skeleton. Although we need calcium to form bones, you can't make your bones strong just by eating calcium. Use and activity is what builds a stronger skeleton. Exercise sends shock waves through the body and stimulates the osteoblasts in our bones to create tiny particles of calcium in the bone matrix. We need the calcium to be available but it is exercise that causes the signals and messages for bone formation. Lack of exercise with sufficient impact can reduce the messages that trigger the renewal and regeneration of strong bones and skeletal system. We have very cushioned shoes and carpets and floor coverings and try and cushion shock as much as we can – which is a long way from when we would have had to run on hard ground in bare feet. That general jolting and jostling is what the skeletal system needs to stimulate and promote repair and renewal. A good compromise is best – not to over-cushion impact all the time, in order to let the skeletal system function as it should and not to over expose the system to unnaturally prolonged, jarring activity on unnaturally hard surfaces. The bones and joints and tendons and ligaments and cartilage and muscles were all designed to do everything we needed to do and we need to work with that and with our level of fitness. Good fitness and personal trainers, physiotherapists, chiropractors, osteopaths, chiropodists and your GP can all advise on this. Also bear in mind what the body was designed for and what a relatively natural lifestyle would involve in terms of activity – and that will give a fairly good idea of what is good for us and what probably isn't.

An estimated 3 million people in the UK suffer from osteoporosis. 1 in 3 women and 1 in 12 men develop bone disease after the age of 50. In this country we have figures of 70,000 hip fractures and 50,000 wrist fractures a year. Every 3 minutes somebody breaks a bone due to bone disease, as opposed to breaking a healthy bone.

Although osteoporosis is believed to be genetic to a certain extent – we can definitely make a significant difference by our diet and lifestyle. Women are affected more than men because of the female reproductive hormones. Oestrogen slows the loss of bone tissue and progesterone builds bone density. If lower levels of oestrogen and/or progesterone have been produced due to times of missed periods, menopause, early menopause or hysterectomy, this can increase the risk of osteoporosis. (Missed periods can be due to malnutrition – including some dieting – or stress, or over-exercising, amongst other causes). Men with a low testosterone level can also have a greater risk.

Symptoms affecting men and women alike could be steroid medication, coeliac disease, Crohn's disease, ulcerative colitis, smoking, excessive alcohol, fizzy drinks and insufficient exercise.

Bone tissue is constantly being lost and renewed. It is estimated that a child's skeleton is replaced every 2 years. The rate will vary then to the skeleton being replaced approximately every 8 years. Anytime from our 30s onwards we may lose overall bone mass at a rate of approximately 1% a year but again the higher and lower rates will vary significantly from one person to another.

The best ways to make bones stronger is regular, weight-bearing exercise – walking, jogging, dancing, weight-lifting, weight-training. Cutting down on caffeine and salt and avoiding too much protein is also thought to help support the body's calcium levels. Japanese women whose diets are rich in plant proteins and traditionally no dairy produce have fewer incidences of osteoporosis than women with typical Western diets. One of the highest incidence of osteoporosis is found in the Inuit (Eskimo) population whose diet is typically extremely high in animal protein and very high in calcium.

Calcium doesn't work on its own. Like all the nutrients, elements, minerals and vitamins, it works in combination with many others. It works in partnership with magnesium, Vitamin D helps your body absorb calcium, Vitamin C is essential to help build collagen which strengthens the bone matrix – plus boron, zinc, copper, manganese and Vitamin K. All these will be present and sufficient in an all round, good diet. Taking a calcium supplement won't necessarily help increase calcium levels because it needs to be taken in balance with other nutrients, especially magnesium and Vitamin D. Too much calcium can in fact push the balance out to the point of causing a magnesium deficiency, which is not uncommon. If you need to supplement, or think you need to supplement, it is best to do so with qualified advice and products that contain the right ingredients in the right preparations and quantities.

High protein diets can be counter-productive and bad for bone health, including meat and dairy, protein-rich foods. Evidently dairy food is fiercely recommended by many as a source of calcium but too much protein, especially meat and dairy protein can end up using/depleting calcium reserves of more calcium than it provides. We are far more likely to eat too much protein than not enough and too much protein causes acidity in the body. Calcium reserves will then be stolen back from the bone, into the blood, to counteract and neutralize the blood acidity level. The more protein you eat, the more calcium you can lose. High dietary acid load is responsible, in studies of osteoporotic fractures, for more breaks than lack of calcium in the diet, menopause and inactive lifestyle.

It is important to have a balanced, complete, nutritious diet. We can't just load in calcium, especially animal calcium – and high protein diets are responsible for more than calcium loss. They cause additional stress to the kidneys and are linked to kidney disease and kidney stones, heart disease, cancers – particularly of the stomach and colon – and digestive disorders including appendicitis, colitis and diverticulitis. Plant proteins and plant calcium don't have the same overloading affect and are easily assimilated, metabolized or eliminated.

Vegetables, pulses, nuts, wholegrains and water provide good quantities of calcium and magnesium and would have been the sources we relied upon before the easy availability of meat and dairy produce from more intensive farming. Our body is designed and better able to process these foods and absorb the calcium from them.

With magnesium, calcium is also required for nerves and muscles to operate and assists in blood clotting.

Symptoms of insufficient calcium include muscle cramps, tremors or spasms, insomnia, nervousness, joint pain, osteoarthritis, tooth decay and high blood pressure.

It is easy to take bone health for granted. In the normal way, if nothing goes wrong – it won't be something we can see or feel. It is definitely something that can have a greater impact on our lives as we get older, beyond 35 and beyond 50 and at that stage the benefits we have given ourselves by good nutrition and exercise can make a significant difference. Making and keeping healthy bones is what we are supposed to do. It isn't something we can quickly put right later on, so the importance of looking after our bones really cannot be over-emphasized.

(There are many references for finding the calcium content in food – and often the amounts and figures and tables vary. 3 are included at the end of this chapter as examples, see pages 220-221.)

Posture, lifting, carrying and movement

As well as good diet and exercise, one of the most helpful ways to look after our back and our limbs is in our posture and movement.

Posture is all about balancing our body weight around our centre of gravity, our lower spine and pelvis, so's not to overstress or overload a particular area, limb or set of muscles. Our muscles generally work in pairs and the bones and muscles all counterbalance to keep us stable. The skeleton is the framework with our muscles acting like guy ropes, holding and supporting the frame – if something is out of line, some of those guy ropes will be straining.

Good posture helps avoid neck and back pain and many other aches and pains from stiff or overstrained muscles. There are many things that can contribute to bad posture, from simply slouching or standing and walking badly, to more serious conditions and muscular disorders. The key is to be aware of our posture and do what we can, develop good habits.

Standing – it is best to stand straight and try not to drop one hip. If you are standing for long periods of time or giving a presentation, standing with one foot slightly further forward than the other and changing sides now and again can help. Other than that, try and relax arms, shoulders and neck and change position from time to time.

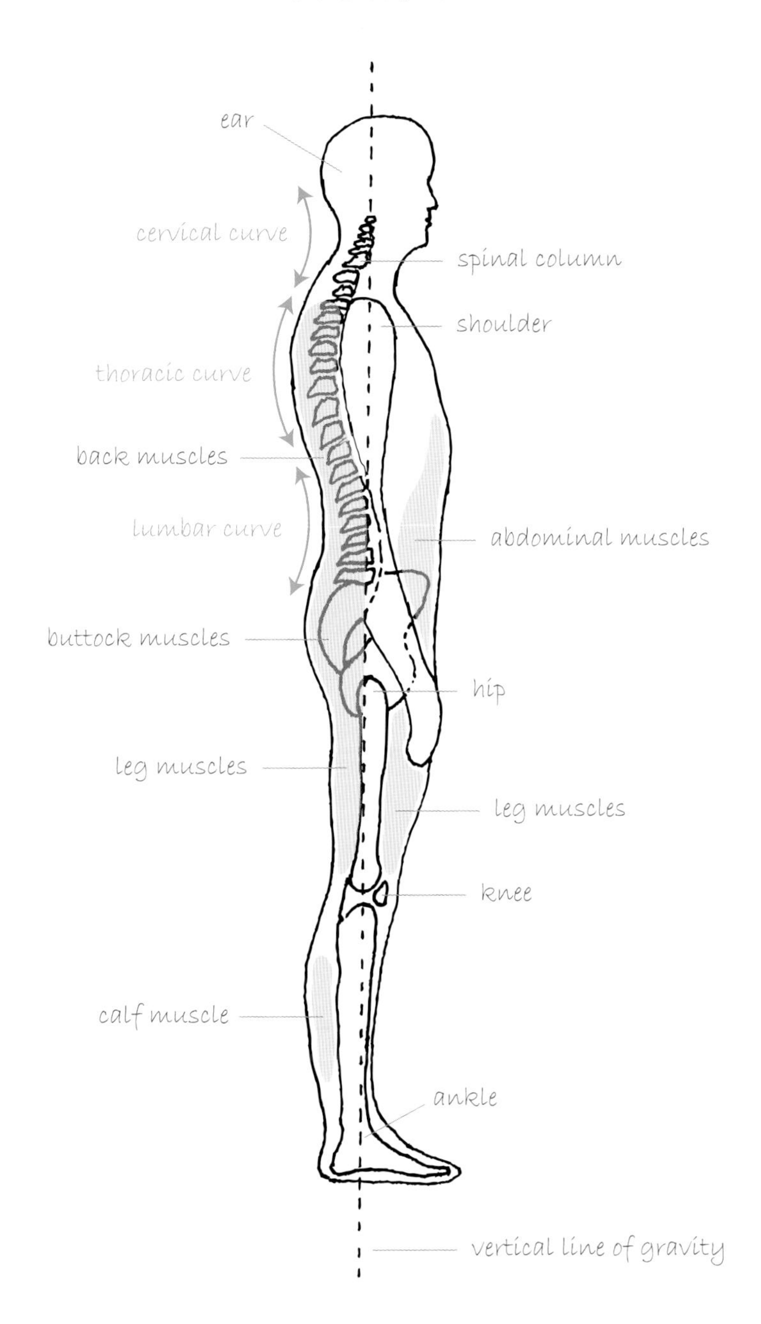
POSTURE
ear
cervical curve
spinal column
shoulder
thoracic curve
back muscles
lumbar curve
abdominal muscles
buttock muscles
hip
leg muscles
leg muscles
knee
calf muscle
ankle
vertical line of gravity

Sitting, at a table or desk, try and make sure you have a good chair, supportive to the back, especially lower back, adjusted to the right height, to have your head up and body upright, feet flat on the floor (or footrest), shoulders down and back and relaxed and keep your abdomen muscles firm to support your torso and spine and hold you in balance. All these things help to minimize strain on susceptible limbs and muscles. If you are using a computer screen and keyboard or anything similar, try and keep elbows close to your body and your wrists in line with your elbows. Check the height of the screen is eye level or just below - and try not to work in the same position for too long without taking a break or loosening your arms, shoulders and neck from time to time and doing some stretches. All these things make a big difference and there is a vast array of sources for good information. This is important for all of us to look after our own health, wherever we are - and in a workplace must also meet the current legal requirements. There is endless information available from independent osteopaths, chiropractors, physiotherapists and all the ergonomic workplace and health and safety advisers and consultancies have the best, up to date guidance.

The things to try and avoid are slouching, using a desk that is too high or too low, sitting with tense neck, shoulders or wrists and crossing legs. Crossing legs twists the spine, puts pressure on knees and hips and can compress the lower back. Making sure we are using the right kind of chair is important, a chair that is supportive, the right height and adjustable, if necessary - and a swivel chair if we are frequently turning for different things. Over time these things make a considerable difference and being in the wrong position, for long periods of time, or day after day, some muscles will compensate for the poor posture and can cause serious, long term problems which may be avoidable. Simply changing position frequently (say, every 30-40 minutes), getting up and walking around, stretching and varying or alternating what we are doing will all help avoid problems and tension.

We need to be especially careful carrying heavy bags, satchels, briefcases, rucksacks and suitcases. Even a handbag over the same shoulder, day after day can affect how we walk and take the spine out of line and that will pass on consequences, not only to the shoulders but to hips and even knees, legs, feet and ankles. For heavier bags, cases and shopping it is well worth using trolleys - but again, there are good and bad ways of using trolleys - so spare a thought for your limbs and your bones and your body and find out the best way to do things. There is plenty of information and advice, from qualified individuals, health publications and the internet.

Driving posture is important too. Again, make sure your lower back is supported. Many car seats don't allow for best posture but if you can, try and have your hips level with or slightly higher than your knees and your position close enough to the steering wheel not to round your shoulders. Keep your shoulders and neck loose and relaxed, physically moving and exercising them, especially on long journeys, in bad traffic, or tense and demanding conditions. You need enough headroom too so that you aren't bowing your head and straining your neck.

It is worth checking posture from time to time and having the benefit of an expert opinion. It is almost impossible to self-diagnose any imbalances and bad habits we may have spent a lifetime acquiring and there may be a few simple things we can do and changes we can make that will have significant long term benefits.

Getting rid of tension at the end of the day will help posture, muscles, nerves and limbs. Whenever you can just relax; if possible lying on the floor with knees slightly bent and relaxing lower back – and loosening arms, neck and shoulders. This isn't doing nothing, this is 'active resting' – a very important part of the executive schedule.

Needless to say, more demanding tasks like moving home or manual handling at work require real thought and planning. A couple of seconds' thought before some of these kinds of tasks can save us from ourselves. There are wrong and right ways to go about these sorts of manoeuvres but our own common sense can tell us to clear the area that we will be walking through before lifting and carrying heavy objects, making sure doors are open, asking someone to help, splitting large loads into smaller units. There is professional information available for all these things and there is also logic – just taking a couple of seconds to think things through and be kind to our bodies.

A balanced posture minimizes the stress on the nerves, joints and muscles. The nerves travel from your brain through your spine out into your body. An impinged nerve can cause localized pain or referred pain along the path of the affected nerve. So an impinged nerve in the neck may cause neck, head or arm pain and an impinged nerve in the lower back may cause lower back or leg pain.

Calcium content of Foods – examples

Recommended Daily Amount 800mg / Optimum Daily Amount 1,000mg

	mg per 100g
Swiss cheese	925
Cheddar cheese	750
Almonds	234
Brewer's yeast	210
Parsley	203
Corn tortillas	200
Globe artichokes	51
Prunes	51
Pumpkin seeds	51
Cooked dried beans	50
Cabbage	4
Winter wheat	46

(New Optimum Nutrition Bible: P Holford)

Calcium can be obtained from many different sources. The list below which is a modified version of a table available from the UCLA, gives the calcium content in commonly available foods.

Milk, non-fat, 1%, 2%, whole, 240 ml;	300 mg Calcium
Cheese, Cheddar, 25g;	204 mg Calcium
Salmon, Canned, with bones, 75g;	185 mg Calcium
Rhubarb, cooked, 240ml;	174 mg Calcium
Oatmeal, fortified 240ml;	163 mg Calcium
Spinach, frozen, cooked, 240ml;	138 mg Calcium
Tofu, firm, 240ml;	258 mg Calcium
Almonds, 240ml;	92 mg Calcium
Beans, boiled, baked or refried, 240ml;	50 mg Calcium
Mustard greens, cooked from fresh, 240ml;	52 mg Calcium
Orange, 1 medium;	52 mg Calcium
Halibut, baked, 75g;	51 mg Calcium
Kale, fresh, cooked, 240ml;	47 mg Calcium
Broccoli, cooked from fresh, 240ml;	36 mg Calcium (a good source of vitamin D)
Bread, wholewheat, slice;	32 mg Calcium

Calcium content of Food and Drink

	portion	calcium (mg)
Cereals and Bread		
All Bran	40g	136
Cheerios	30g	135
Ready Brek	40g	480
Swiss style muesli	50g	55
white or brown bread	1 slice	39
wholemeal	1 slice	19
Fruit		
Apricots – dried, ready to eat	1	29
Figs – dried, ready to eat	1	48
Orange juice	250ml	25
Oranges	1 (med)	75
Tropicana calcium enriched orange juice	250ml	305
Vegetables		
Broccoli, boiled	85g	34
Cabbage, Savoy	95g	35
Spring greens, cooked	95g	71
Fish and Eggs		
Pilchards, canned in sauce with edible bones	1 pilchard	138
Sardines, canned in sauce with edible bones	1 sardine	108
Prawns, cooked	10	33
Salmon, tinned	sandwich portion	145
Eggs	1	32
Beans, Nuts and Tofu		
Almonds	100g	240
Brazil nuts	100g	170
Peanuts	50g	30
Baked beans	2 tbsp	43
Baked beans	415g can	222
Red kidney beans	2 tbsp	42
Red kidney beans	420g can	300

	portion	calcium (mg)
Beans, Nuts and Tofu		
Chickpeas	2 tbsp	30
Lentils, cooked	3 tbsp	19
Lentil soup	av. portion	85
Sesame seeds	1 tbsp	80
Tahini (sesame seed spread)	1 heaped tspn	129
Tofu, cooked	100g	510
Dairy		
Skimmed milk	1 pint	705
Semi-skimmed milk	1 pint	702
Whole milk	1 pint	673
So!Good fresh soya milk	1 pint	840
Soya milk with added calcium	1 pint	795
Cheddar cheese	25g	180
Cheese spread	30g	126
Cottage cheese	small pot (200g)	82
Desserts		
Yogurts (various)	150g	210-240
Dairy ice cream	av. portion	134
Fromage frais	1 tbsp	40
Provamel Yofu	125g	100

Source of information from product labels and 5th edition of McCance and Widdowson's 'The Composition of Foods'.
Reference: www.diet-coaching.com/files/calciumtab

Inclusion of named foods and drinks is for information only and implies no endorsement

Joints

Joints – where 2 or more bones come together.

Some joints allow a lot of very flexible movement. Others allow very restrictive movement. Some of the joints of the skull are held rigidly in place, not allowing any movement. The joints of the spine hold the vertebrae firmly together and allow movement. Many other joints allow much freer movement – shoulders, elbows, hips, knees.

Joints can be made of fibrous tissues or cartilage or articulating disks, or ligaments or cushions of fluid, all designed according to their movement and function. A good book on anatomy and physiology will have pages and pages of descriptions and diagrams of all the different joints, how they are constructed and what they do. (I recommend one in the Reading section, page 308.)

Using them as they were designed to be used, within the appropriate range of movement, is the best exercise for the joints and using them helps to keep joints supple, mobile and strong. The exercise also keeps muscles, ligaments and tendons surrounding and supporting the joint strong. Over-use of joints or straining them, out of their designed range of motion or bearing too much load, stresses joints. Exercise and activity is good for our joints, we just have to take care that we are doing things in a joint-friendly way. If we develop habits of doing actions in a joint-unfriendly way, anything from walking to weight-lifting, typing or texting, there can be consequences for the joints, muscles and tissues. Dancing, cricket, football, golf, running, tennis are all good exercise but they could be hazardous for joints if we don't build in regimes to manage proportionate over-use of some joints, artificially repetitive actions, twists, sprains and straining muscles and joints. We will often, naturally use one side, right or left, more than the other. It is the same for various everyday tasks and work – vacuuming, lawn-mowing, kneeling, bending, driving, manual labour. Shoulders, hips and knees are common sufferers of pain and stiffness. Knee pads may not seem glamorous but if we are habitually doing work or hobbies that are tough on the knees, fitting a kitchen or bathroom, doing the garden, electrical re-wiring and repeated or prolonged kneeling is going to be involved, it may be a very practical precaution and knee pads in our 20s, 30s and 40s are more glamorous than permanently damaged knees later in life. Joints do heal from stresses and strains but they also tend to carry weaknesses once they have suffered any significant damage. Learning the best ways to do things and building in precautions to look after muscles and joints will make significant differences in avoiding or reducing pain and disability which we may be risking in the future. Any of the anatomy and physiology professions; doctors, chiropractors, osteopaths, physiotherapists and sports and fitness

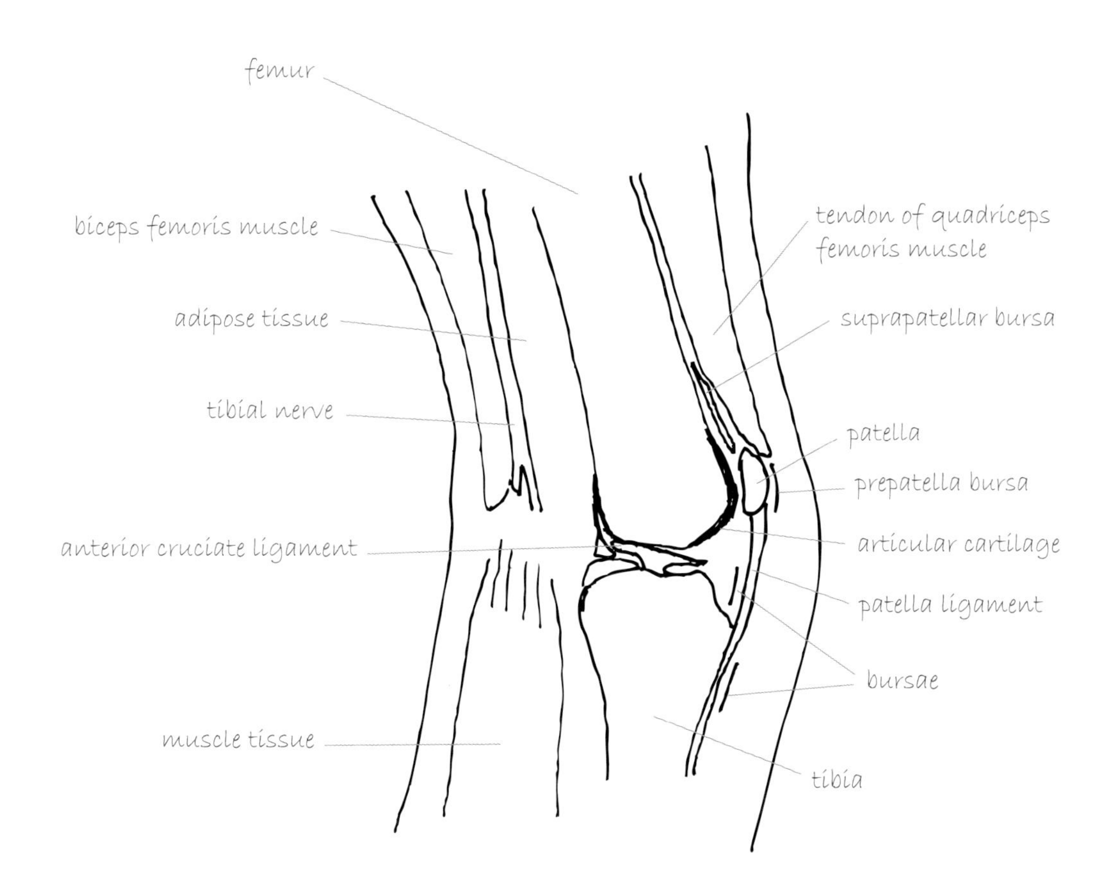
SECTION THROUGH KNEE JOINT
femur
biceps femoris muscle
adipose tissue
tibial nerve
anterior cruciate ligament
muscle tissue
tendon of quadriceps femoris muscle
suprapatellar bursa
patella
prepatella bursa
articular cartilage
patella ligament
bursae
tibia

trainers should be able to advise on good exercise regimes – and ways of compensating for imbalance, use and abuse. This isn't a weakness, our design and capabilities are extraordinary and good and strong. Looking after joints is just the simplest, most effective way of keeping them like that, a strategy for good, long term joint health.

Diet and nutrition is one of the best ways to protect and prolong joint health. Wear and tear can be responsible for the deterioration of joint health and so can diet. The synovial fluid that lubricates our joints depends on a good, mixed diet with adequate vitamins, minerals and anti-oxidants. It needs the nutrients to stay fluid and provide the lubricant properties. The same diet maintains the elasticity of the articulating disks, fibrous tissues, tendons and ligaments. Joints like the good, all-round nutritional diet that provides the nutrients and building blocks for all the component parts. If our diet is poor in providing the right nutrients, the joint tissues may be less flexible and less able to keep supple, renew and repair.

Diets high in refined sugar, or stimulants, fat or protein have been associated with aggravating arthritis and so have allergies and food sensitivities (which may be wheat or dairy or other common everyday foods) or pollutants – chemicals or exhaust fumes. They all challenge the immune system which is already having to deal with the inflammation and may be malfunctioning as a consequence of the disease.

Cartilage damage and sprains are amongst the most common problems. Cartilage damage is usually caused by stress and tearing, which may also cause internal bruising, bleeding, pain, lack of mobility and instability of the joint. Sprains usually affect ligaments – resulting from twisting or wrenching which can break blood vessels, and cause bruising and swelling, limiting movement.

The most common non-inflammatory joint disorder is osteoarthritis, characterized by deterioration of joint cartilage. The cartilage thins at points of frequent wear and impact, so there is less of a shock absorber and the space between the bones narrows. Bony spurs can form and ligaments harden, resulting is restricted movement and pain.

The inflammatory form of arthritis is rheumatoid arthritis. It is a chronic and systemic inflammatory disease of connective tissue and the cause is still not completely known. It usually affects small joints of the fingers, hands and wrists first but may then progress to affect larger joints. As well as the painful inflammation, this disease destroys cartilage and erodes bone, deforming and disabling joints with loss of mobility, aching and stiffness. It is an auto-immune disease, it triggers over activity of the immune system and can also affect organs of the body – blood vessels, lungs, heart and eyes.

Lifestyle and diet can directly improve the health of our joints even where there may be genetic conditions. Many conditions can be prevented or reduced. Sports people and dancers will generally have access to the professional advice they need, especially when training and performing to levels likely to affect joints in the short, medium and long term. For everyone else there is the straightforward knowledge that looking after joints is our best, long-term insurance policy. Omega 3 and fish oils are common anti-inflammatories and glucosamine and MSM are popular supplements to support joint health, for animals as well as humans. As with all the other references to supplements and special nutrition requirements, good, professional advice is really important. The wrong products taken in the wrong way can be ineffective or detrimental. Self-diagnosis and amateur treatments can be responsible for wasted time and money. Good nutrients, good hydration from drinking plenty of water, as low toxic load as we can manage and sensible exercise play a key role. So does avoiding accidents and injuries which is probably the most logical thing we can do to help ourselves. If we do have injuries, it's important to give joints and tissues the conditions and time to heal properly. Badly healed injuries can create scar tissue, which is less flexible and supple and poor healing may leave a weakness. Good posture also helps joints, especially hips and shoulders. Sitting square to a desk or table or when watching the TV, distributes our weight and balance evenly on both hips, to help avoid over-straining one. It also keeps the shoulders even and balanced. Carrying things, especially shoulder bags can distort shoulder joints, hunching one shoulder higher than the other. We need to try and balance any distortion, transferring weights from one side to the other and de-tense shoulders and relax them when we know we've been a bit hard on them. Finding out more needn't be expensive and may even be enjoyable. Dance classes, Pilates and all sorts of fitness training can be an introduction to another world of practical anatomy and physiology information and great physical exercise.

Muscles

Muscles work as co-ordinated teams of biological power centres, moving the different limbs and members of the flexible skeleton.

Muscles connect to bones by tendons and fibrous connective tissues which essentially make it one combined system – the skeleto-muscular system. They are not two separate systems.

Our muscles provide movement for us to physically and consciously move our bodies; walk, run, move our limbs and head, drive, eat, work, shop. They also provide movement for biological and metabolic processes; breathing, blood flow, digestion, elimination. The muscles maintain body position and posture. Muscles are the primary source of heat in the body – the heat is the by-product generated by muscles doing what they do, throughout the muscle mass, throughout the body.

As a baby we gradually learn to lift and hold our head, roll over, sit, stand and walk as development changes permit muscle co-ordination and control. Later in life, as we age, muscle cell volume starts to be replaced with non-functional connective tissues and we lose muscle strength. Most, if not all of this is due to disuse (atrophy) and so can be avoidable, or very greatly reduced.

Muscles are designed to work by contracting and relaxing and that action works like a pump, taking blood, nutrients and oxygen to the tissues and muscles and taking de-oxygenated blood and waste products away, including lactic acid. Using muscles properly keeps them healthy.

If we don't use our muscles enough, or we pull a muscle, have an injury or a disabling condition, such as arthritis – the pumping action will be lost by the lack of mobility/activity of the muscle. The muscle is then held in a sustained contraction without the flexing and stretching. Nutrients and oxygen still go to the muscle to maintain tissue health but some nutrients and metabolytes[1] may collect, instead of being pumped away, causing inflammation, pain and stiffness. This can also happen after exercise and the muscles seize up. It can also happen as a result of stress and tension. Muscles that tighten due to lack of use or abnormal use, stress, tension or arthritis, can be eased by massage, remedial soft tissue work, relaxation and gentle limbering up techniques. The right exercises and techniques can be a great help – and the wrong exercises and techniques can make things worse and cause more damage. It's important

[1] metabolytes: substances produced by the metabolic processes of the body

to work with qualified people who know what they are doing.

The skeleto-muscular system operates in conjunction with all the other systems. The nervous system senses the changes necessary to instruct movement, initiate movement and control movement by information and feedback loops – information from the brain or other sensory centres, to do something, to change that action and to stop doing something. The cardio-vascular system maintains blood flow for the muscles. The urinary system removes waste products from the muscles. The respiratory system brings in oxygen and removes waste products. The digestive system provides the nutrients the muscles need. The endocrine system produces hormones that assist the nervous system in regulating muscle contraction. The liver processes lactic acid produced by the muscles and converts it back to glucose. The immune system helps defend the muscles from infection and disease. The blood system delivers the nutrients and removes waste.

For many of us, the time when we are most aware of our muscles is when we have pulled or strained a muscle, or a muscle seizes up, or we experience pain. Good, balanced use of our muscles keeps them well and healthy. Warm-ups and warm-downs before concerted exercise or placing an extra demand on our muscles will always help to prevent damage – and it is a really important thing to do. If we do pull or strain muscles, they can also spasm – and hang onto stiffness and pain. Sometimes they can relax and recuperate on their own with rest and gentle reintroduction to activity – and sometimes we may need, or benefit from massage or manipulation. Muscles tend to work in pairs or groups and if we do strain or damage a muscle, the importance of correcting that is to prevent the knock-on effect on other muscles, joints and limbs. If a shoulder or leg muscle isn't working properly it can easily affect other parts of the body and cause further problems. A stiff shoulder can affect the neck, head, back, hips, legs and arms. A strained foot or ankle will affect the leg, hips, back and shoulder. Muscles are linked to ligaments, tendons and nerves and as well as keeping them in shape ourselves – it is critical to take exceptional care and consult only highly recommended, qualified therapists if we do need help. The body is a wonderful thing and usually mends very well. At times of injury or weakness it is essential to have the right knowledge to correct problems and not cause further damage.

An overview of what all our muscles are, where they are and summary of what they do, paints the best picture of their importance to our health, our function and performance and our mobility. Similarly to all the other organs covered in the chapters on Anatomy and Physiology, the muscles like being looked after, they need nutrition, blood supply and oxygen and they need to be used and kept in shape. The number of them and what they do for us makes their case. (There is a key to some of the terms at the end of the section.)

Muscles of the face

Occipitofrontalis	raises eyebrows, wrinkles forehead horizontally
Corrrugator supercilii	wrinkles forehead vertically
Orbicularis oculi	closes eye
Zygomaticus major	laughing, elevates angle of mouth
Orbicularis oris	draws lips together
Buccinator	permits smiling and blowing

Mastication muscles

Masseter	closes jaw
Temporalis	closes jaw
Pterygoids (lateral and medial)	grates teeth

Muscles of the head

Sternocleidomastoid	flexes head, rotates head
Semispinalis capitis	extends head, allows lateral bend
Splenius capitis	extends head, allows bend and rotation
Longissimus capitis	extends head, allows bend and rotation

Muscles of thorax

External intercostals	elevate ribs
Internal intercostals	depress ribs
Diaphragm	enlarges thorax, allowing inhalation

Muscles of the abdomen wall

External oblique	compresses abdomen, rotates trunk laterally, works pelvis, supports lumbar curve of spine
Internal oblique	as above
Transversus abdominis	as above
Rectus abdominis	as above, aids elimination, defecation, forced expiration, childbirth, flexes trunk
Quadratus lumborum	flexes vertebral column laterally, depresses last rib

An important function of all abdominal muscles is to pull up the front of the pelvis, flattening the lumbar curve of the spine, maintaining core strength and posture and supporting the back. Weak, untoned abdominal muscles / 'abs' can be the cause of many posture and back problems, affecting much of the body.

Muscles of the back	
Erector spinae group:	
Iliocostalis group	extends, laterally flexes vertebral column
Longissimus group	extends head, neck or vertebral column
Spinalis group	extends neck or vertebral column
Transversospinales group:	
Semispinalis group	extends neck or vertebral column
Multifidus group	extends, rotates vertebral column
Rotatores group	extends, rotates vertebral column
Splenius	rotates, extends neck and flexes neck laterally
Interspinales group	extends back and neck
Muscles of the pelvic floor	
Levator ani	with coccygeus muscles form floor of pelvic cavity and support pelvic organs
Ischiocavernosus	compress base of penis or clitoris
Bulbospongiosus (male)	constricts urethra and erects penis
Bulbospongiosus (female)	erects clitoris
Deep transverse perinei	support pelvic floor
Sphincter urethrae	constrict urethra
Sphincter externus anii	close anal canal
Muscles of the shoulder girdle	
Trapezius	raises or lowers shoulders and shrugs
Pectoralis minor	pulls shoulders down and forward
Serratus anterior	pulls shoulders down and forward, abducts and rotates shoulders forwards
Levator scapulae	elevates and retracts scapula and abducts neck
Rhomboid major	retracts, rotates, fixes scapula
Rhomboid minor	retracts, rotates, elevates and fixes scapula
Muscles that move the upper arm	
Pectoralis major	flexes upper arm, adducts upper arm anteriorly
Latissimus dorsi	extends upper arm, adducts upper arm posteriorly

Scapular:

Deltoid	abducts upper arm assists in flex and extension of upper arm
Coracobrachialis	assists in flex and medial rotation of arm, adduction
Supraspinatus	assists in abducting arm
Teres minor	rotates arm outwards
Teres major	assists in extension, adduction and medial rotation of arm
Infraspinatus	rotates arm outwards
Subscapularis	medial rotation

Muscles that move the forearm

Biceps brachii	flexes supinated forearm supinates forearm and hand
Brachialis	flexes pronated forearm
Brachioradialis	flexes semi-pronated or semi-supinated forearm, supinates forearm and hand
Triceps brachii	extends lower arm
Pronator teres	pronates and flexes forearm
Pronator quadratus	pronates forearm
Supinator	supinates forearm

Muscles that move the wrist, hand and fingers

Flexor carpi radialis	flexes hand, flexes forearm
Palmaris longus	flexes hand
Flexor carpi ulnaris	flexes hand, adducts hand
Extensor carpi radialis longus	extends hand, abducts hand
Extensor carpi radialis brevis	extends hand
Extensor carpi ulnaris	extends hand, adducts hand
Flexor digitorum profundus	flexes distal interphalangeal joints
Flexor digitorum superficialis	flexes fingers
Extensor digitorum	extends fingers

Opponens pollicis	opposes thumb to fingers
Abductor pollicis brevis	abducts thumb
Adductor pollicis	adducts thumb
Flexor pollicis brevis	flexes thumb
Abductor digiti minimi	abducts fifth finger, flexes fifth finger
Flexor digiti minimi brevis	flexes fifth finger
Opponens digiti minimi	opposes fifth finger slightly
Interosseous (palmar and dorsal)	adducts second, fourth, fifth fingers (palmar) abducts second, third, fourth fingers (dorsal)
Lumbricales	flexes proximal phalanges, 2-5 extends middle and distal phalanges, 2-5

Muscles that move the thigh

Iliopsoas	flexes thigh, flexes trunk
Rectus femoris	flexes thigh, extends lower leg
Gluteal group:	
Maximus	extends thigh – rotates outwards
Medius	abducts thigh – rotates outwards stabilizes pelvis on femur
Minimus	abducts thigh, stabilizes pelvis on femur rotates thigh medially
Tensor fasciae latae	abducts thigh tightens iliotibial tract
Adductor group:	
Brevis	adducts thigh
Longus	adducts thigh
Magnus	adducts thigh
Gracilis	adducts thigh, flexes and adducts leg

Muscles that move the lower leg

Quadriceps femoris group:	
Rectus femoris	flexes thigh, extends leg
Vastus lateralis	extends leg
Vastus medialis	extends leg
Vastus intermedius	extends leg
Sartorius	adducts and flexes leg permits crossing of legs
Hamstring group:	
Biceps femoris	flexes leg, extends thigh
Semitendinosus	extends thigh
Semimembranosus	extends thigh

Muscles that move the foot

Tibialis anterior	flexes foot, inverts foot
Gastrocnemius	extends foot, flexes lower leg
Soleus	extends foot
Peroneus longus	extends foot, everts foot
Peroneus brevis	everts foot, flexes foot
Peroneus tertius	flexes foot, everts foot
Extensor digitorum longus	dorsiflexion of foot, extension of toes
Lumbricales	flex proximal phalanges extend middle and distal phalanges
Flexor digiti minimi brevis	flexes fifth (little) toe
Flexor hallucis brevis	flexes first (big) toe
Flexor digitorum brevis	flexes toes 2-5
Abductor digiti minimi	abducts fifth (little) toe, flexes fifth toe
Abductor hallucis	abducts first (big) toe

Key:

abduction	–	moving away from the midline of the body
adduction	–	moving towards the midline of the body
anterior	–	front
anteriorly	–	towards the front of the body
posterior	–	back
posteriorly	–	towards the back of the body
medial	–	of or towards the middle (opposite of lateral)
medially	–	towards the middle of the body
lateral	–	of or towards the sides (opposite of medial)
laterally	–	towards the sides of the body
adduct	–	to draw inward toward the median axis of the body or toward an adjacent part or limb; toward the centre line of the body
abduct	–	to draw away from the midline of the body or from an adjacent part or limb; away from the centre line of the body
pronate	–	to turn or rotate the hand or forearm so that the palm faces down or back
supinate	–	to turn or rotate the hand or forearm so that the palm faces up or forward
distal	–	farthest; distal interphalangeal joints – furthest from wrist/body
palmar	–	palm side of the hand
dorsal	–	back; eg: back of the hand – back side of the hand
evert	–	to turn outward.

Teeth

Between the ages of 6 months – 2 years, we grow 20 baby teeth (deciduous teeth).

These are then replaced by 28 permanent teeth, usually between the ages of about 6 to 13 years old. We may then have 4 more molars or wisdom teeth appear, between approximately age 17 and 25, 1 at the back of each side, top and bottom. A grand total of 32.

We have to take good care of our permanent teeth – because these ones have to last, no more natural replacements. Any replacements from there are ones artificially made for us.

Unlike our bones and our skin and our blood and many parts of the body which are sustained and renew and regenerate from what we eat – our teeth are not renewed, we can't strengthen them as we go along from the nutrients in our food. We can damage them by food.

The general make-up of a tooth is (see diagram page 235):

- the crown – the exposed part of the tooth
- the neck – where the tooth emerges through the gum
- the root – below the gum.

The crown is covered in enamel – the hardest tissue in the body – and under the enamel there is a layer of dentin which makes up most of the tooth and contains the pulp cavity where the blood and lymph vessels and nerves are.

The neck joins the crown to the root and the root is where the tooth is secured into the jaw by fibrous tissue.

The best ways to look after our teeth are:

- to keep them clean
- to have a good diet
- to have regular appointments at the dentist.

Plaque

Plaque is a film that builds up on teeth. It is the coating of bacteria that naturally forms on our teeth all the time and is slightly sticky. Sugary, sweet foods and drinks will encourage a greater production and build-up of plaque in the mouth. High water content foods and fibrous foods that move the plaque over the surface of the teeth cause minimal plaque and build-up. In modern life, with a modern diet, our teeth can't keep themselves

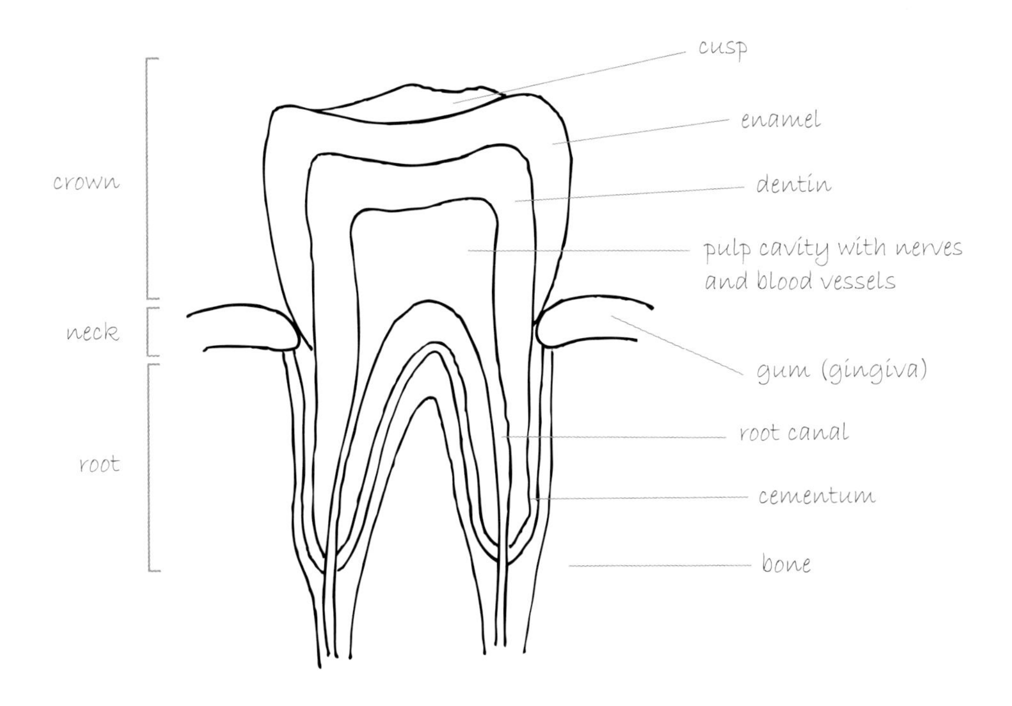
SECTION OF A TYPICAL TOOTH
cusp
enamel
dentin
pulp cavity with nerves and blood vessels
gum (gingiva)
root canal
cementum
bone
crown
neck
root

clean and it is necessary for us to clean our teeth to prevent build-up of plaque that will discolour teeth, contribute to bad breath and encourage tooth decay.

To check how clean teeth are, you can use disclosure tablets that are usually available from most dentists. Disclosure tablets contain a special stain which highlights areas of plaque to indicate where teeth and gums may need extra brushing. The stain is harmless and temporary.

Tooth Decay and Dental Erosion

When we eat or drink, a certain amount of acidity is created in the mouth. It takes about 40 minutes for the acid caused by eating and drinking to be neutralized in the mouth. So for that length of time the enamel coating of the teeth is under attack. Sugary things have a greater affect and tend to linger, take longer to clear. Long after we have swallowed our toast, or apple, or peanuts, or any of our meals, work is going on in the mouth to return to neutral. Nearly everything we eat and drink will affect the enamel to some extent which is why it is recommended not to brush teeth within an hour of eating. The enamel is slightly softened and vulnerable. Between food and drinks, the mouth tries to return to normal, neutral, 'clean' state. If we have a snack or sugary drink within an hour of the previous snack, meal or sugary drink, or are frequently sucking sweets – our teeth are under a constant attack and we are preventing our mouth re-establish the clean/neutral state it is always striving to achieve.

Acidic foods and drink can cause decay too. They can soften and breakdown the enamel, protective coating of the teeth and we need to give teeth the time to rebuild the mineral content after these kinds of food. Acidity is measured by pH, the lower the pH number, the more acidic the food or drink is. Some common guideline examples are:

vinegar	2.0		high
cola	2.5		
white wine	2.5-3.8		
red wine	2.9-3.9		
pickles	3.2		
grapefruit	3.5		
orange juice	3.8		
lager	4.4		
Cheddar cheese	5.9		
milk	6.9		
mineral water (still)	7.6	good/neutral	low

Having something acidic now and again won't normally cause a problem – but repeatedly exposing your teeth to substances that can affect and damage the enamel will eventually cause decay. The enamel isn't replaced and the softer dentin and the nerves are then open to inflammation, infection and disease.

Many commercially prepared drinks, including sports drinks, contain citric acid which can be erosive. If you do use any of these drinks, drinking them quickly, not holding them in the mouth and perhaps using a straw, will help your teeth.

Loss of enamel is called dental erosion and makes teeth sensitive and painful. If the enamel becomes worn it can expose the softer dentin underneath and the tooth can start to decay, forming holes or cavities which will need fillings and crowns. If the decay is not treated quickly enough, the nerve of the tooth can become infected and die, causing an abscess and possibly leading to root canal work being necessary.

Gum disease

Gum disease (gingivitis) is the most common cause of tooth loss in adults. It is caused by the build up of plaque and tartar (hardened plaque) around the teeth and gum line and the gums become red and are likely to bleed when brushed or flossed. The plaque releases toxins which inflame the gum and if the gum swells, drawing it away from the tooth the exposed area becomes infected. In very serious cases this can even lead to the bone being affected and the tooth becoming loose and either falling out or needing to be removed – which is when we may require dentures, bridges or implants.

Regular dentist inspections of your teeth and gums help protect against decay and erosion and gum disease by picking up any signs and symptoms early and the dentist and hygienist can clean areas that are difficult for us to reach or keep clean. Although regular, thorough brushing will usually remove plaque, it won't remove tartar. Once tartar has formed it will need to be removed by a dentist or hygienist.

Apart from the pain and expense of tooth decay and gum disease there is also the aesthetics to think about. Rotten teeth and gaps affect our appearance too.

Care of teeth

The professional advice is to brush your teeth properly twice a day and there is good information about how to clean your teeth on the British Dental Health Foundation web site www.dentalhelpline.org.uk and the British Dental Association web site www.bdasmile.org.uk

The emphasis here is on the word properly. If you don't get chance to brush your teeth properly at any stage – then you will need to give them an extra clean next time you can. To clean your teeth thoroughly will take 2 or 3 minutes plus flossing and interdental brushing and it's worth timing that now and again to gauge the time you spend. You need to know that you have got your teeth thoroughly clean, twice a day – so you need to make up for any rushed cleaning as soon as you can.

Generally, we need to:

- brush over the cutting surfaces of upper and lower teeth
- brush over the outside and inside surfaces of upper and lower teeth, brushing over the gum and away from the gum – or in small circular movements – and do this quite a few times for each tooth and the crevices between teeth
- also, brush over the tongue which helps remove residues and bacteria to help keep the mouth clean and freshen breath.

The amount of toothpaste is not the effective part of teeth cleaning, only a very small amount is needed – it is the brushing that is the key – and the state of the toothbrush. Your dentist can give you good advice on what kind of toothbrush will suit you best – generally, avoid the hard toothbrushes and use medium or soft toothbrushes – but replace them regularly, at least once every 3 months.

It is very important to clean teeth last thing at night because saliva production in the mouth, which is the natural cleansing agent for the teeth and mouth, reduces overnight and bacterial residues and sugars left in the mouth and on the teeth overnight have a greater chance of causing plaque build-up, damage and decay.

It is also better for your teeth not to eat sugary snacks and drinks between meals. As soon after brushing that you eat and drink sweet, sugary things, the bacteria and plaque build-up will start again and this includes tea and coffee. Periods of time between meals with a clean mouth, without food and drink will minimize plaque build-up and tooth decay. Water is fine! – still water and natural foods without added sugars, such as nuts, seeds and fruit are the best snacks if you need some.

As mentioned above, professional advice usually recommends not cleaning your teeth within 1 hour of eating. Eating and drinking does slightly soften the enamel coating of the tooth and you can cause damage by brushing if the enamel is softened. This includes apples and fruit and fruit juices. Fruit is very good, natural food and good for your teeth too – we just need to remember to wait after eating fruit before brushing our teeth. The important thing is to clean our teeth – not to use the timing of meals and snacks as an excuse not to.

Fruit Juices and Smoothies

In fruit juices and smoothies the sugars present in the fruit have been released in the pressing and blending and juicing process, they are no longer in their natural state, making them far stronger and more concentrated. Too many of these types of drinks may cause excessive damage to the enamel and gums.

The dental advice web sites (www.dentalhelpline.org.uk and www.bdasmile.org.uk) will also give a lot of information on:

Electric toothbrushes
Different toothpastes
Floss and interdental brushes
Bleeding gums
Dentures and Implants
Dental erosion
Wisdom teeth
Gum disease
Use of Mouthwash
Dental care products
Removal of Wisdom Teeth

Regular appointments with a dentist are the best way to check that you are managing to keep your teeth clean and prevent plaque build up and tooth decay. Your dentist can spot potential problems before they arise and identify other problems early to prevent them becoming serious. The benefit is having fewer problems and needing less treatment.

Bad breath

There can be various causes for bad breath. Most commonly bad breath is caused by odour given off as a gas from the bacteria around teeth and gums. Keeping teeth and gums clean and preventing the build up of plaque is a direct way to minimize and eliminate this problem. One of the most common symptoms of gum disease is having a bad taste in your mouth – which will also be being given off as bad breath. Any medical conditions or drugs which cause you to have a dry mouth may make bad breath more likely because they reduce the saliva in the mouth which is your body's natural way of cleaning the mouth. Breathing through the mouth instead of the nose can also increase the potential for bad breath.

4 possible tests or indicators for bad breath are:

- people pulling away when you speak, or turning their face if you are kissing hello, or goodbye
- asking a good, trustworthy friend, just to be honest and say
- licking your wrist and sniffing
- foul taste in the mouth

and it's unfortunate that all too often it can be the person with the bad breath who is unaware.

It may seem slightly excessive to make a dentist appointment simply to ask for an opinion on the freshness of your breath – but if you are worried, it is worth doing – and if there is a problem, at the dentist you are in the right place to make an immediate improvement. If the problem is plaque, tartar or gum disease, you will know straightaway and have the best advice to deal with the cause. The dentist will also be best placed to tell if it isn't a dental problem. Other causes could include; throat, nose or lung infections, sinusitis, bronchitis, diabetes, liver or kidney problems. If you get the all clear from the dentist, you need to check for other causes with the doctor. Bad breath is telling us something. It isn't pleasant for the other people who have to suffer it but the cause is a symptom of something and needs treating.

The affect of Dental and Oral Health on other Health Conditions

Studies and research have linked infections in the mouth with:

- Heart disease
- Strokes
- Diabetes
- Premature and low-birth-weight babies
- Respiratory (lung) disease

It really is worth looking after oral health. Infections in the mouth do affect our overall health.

There is further information on these associated conditions on the web sites.

Bacteria from the mouth can enter the blood stream. There they can attach to fatty deposits and can cause clots. Clots can reduce normal blood flow. Some studies have suggested that people with gum disease are twice as likely to have coronary heart disease. Again, according to information available from the British Dental Health

Foundation, studies have found a much higher incidence of people with gum disease suffering strokes, than those without. People with diabetes are more susceptible to infections and heal more slowly – so dental check-ups for people with diabetes, to treat any infections early, are especially important. Gum disease can also increase blood sugar. The research indicates that we are more likely to develop diabetes if we have gum disease.

Gum disease is also linked to premature births and low-weight babies. It is believed that this is due to gum disease raising the levels of fluids in the body that bring on labour. This risk will be higher for women whose gum disease worsens during pregnancy.

Respiratory diseases are thought to be caused by droplets inhaled from the mouth and throat. Bacterial infections can increase the risk of these conditions and make them worse.

Conversely, the studies show that people who are fit and healthy are 40% less likely to develop gum infections and disease.

Headaches can also be caused by jaw and teeth problems. If stress causes you to grind your teeth, during the day, or at night when you are asleep, the strain and tension of the jaw and facial muscles and nerves could easily cause a headache and damage your teeth.

Headaches can also be caused by occlusal problems – the way our jaw bites together. Our jaw should be comfortable and relaxed when resting (ie: not eating and speaking). If you are aware of your bite becoming uneven, or an otherwise unexplained increase in headaches or migraine, or clenching or grinding your teeth, or your jaw being stiff or tender in the morning – it is worth checking this with your dentist. It is possible for our bite to become out of balance and uneven. This is estimated to affect up to 1 in 4 people, male and female and sometimes the symptoms are linked to hormonal changes and menopause.

Tooth Whitening

There isn't a standard colour for teeth and the natural colour of our teeth will vary from person to person. Very few people have brilliant white teeth and teeth may discolour slightly with age. Teeth may also be surface stained by tea, coffee, red wine, smoking, etc.

Very few people need teeth whitening treatment – for most people it would be a purely cosmetic choice. Your dentist would be able to advise whether it was a good thing to do and teeth whitening should only be carried out under dentist supervision.

The process involves bleaching, usually with hydrogen peroxide or carbamide peroxide and it is essential that it is used properly and you have correct shields and mouthguards.

The treatment has typically taken up to 4 weeks, initially at the dentist and then with subsequent 30 min applications at home and the effects can last up to 3 years. Newer products available may work more quickly and there is also laser whitening. Teeth whitening can be quite expensive and there are some side effects – sensitive teeth and gums, sore throat – usually temporary, during or after treatments.

Suffice to say – this is something to be very careful about and shouldn't be undertaken without adequate consultation.

A dentist would be able to judge whether your teeth are suitable for the treatment. The bleaching agent in Home/DIY kits is considerably weaker than the products used professionally, because they are restricted by law, so they won't be as effective and may include other harmful acidic or abrasive products which could damage gums or cause ulcers.

Whitening toothpastes don't actually alter the colour of your teeth but may help reduce and remove staining. For these types of products it is worth checking that they have been approved or accredited by the British Dental Association.

Cosmetic and fashionable treatments for teeth can be very harmful. Your teeth really just want to be looked after and kept clean. If you consider any of these treatments, only do that with the professional supervision of your dentist. Correcting damaged teeth will be very expensive and may not always be possible.

Wisdom Teeth

The last 4 molars, at the back of the mouth, that usually appear between age 17 and 25, may come through without any problem and just sit happily behind our other teeth. It can also be quite common now that our jaw is too small for the last molars and there is not enough room for them. If that is the case the emerging wisdom tooth may get stuck or come through at an angle, causing pain and discomfort – they may even start to decay part way in and out of the jaw or gum. If they are going to cause problems, the dentist will recommend removing them. There is lots of further information available from the web sites and your dentist.

Diet

A good diet of adequate vitamins, minerals and fresh fruit and vegetables will support the health of our mouth and teeth, in the same way it supports our health generally. It will certainly help minimize tooth decay.

Mouthwash

There are several mouthwashes available on the market. Again, ask your dentist, hygienist or pharmacist which one is suitable for you and what it is needed for and there is a lot of information on the web sites.

A good home-made mouthwash for pain or inflammation is a teaspoon of salt dissolved in a glass of medium hot water. Slosh the mouthwash round your mouth to clean around the teeth and gums and hold the mouthwash in your mouth for a few minutes near painful or affected teeth and gums. Salt water is a mild antiseptic.

Number and name of teeth in the set of baby (deciduous) teeth and permanent teeth per jaw

	number of teeth per jaw	
Tooth	Deciduous teeth	Permanent teeth
central incisors	2	2
lateral incisors	2	2
canines	2	2
premolars	0	4
first molars	2	2
second molars	2	2
third molars	0	2
total – per jaw	10	16
total – per set	20	32

ADJUSTMENT OF LENS TO SEE OBJECTS DISTANT AND CLOSE

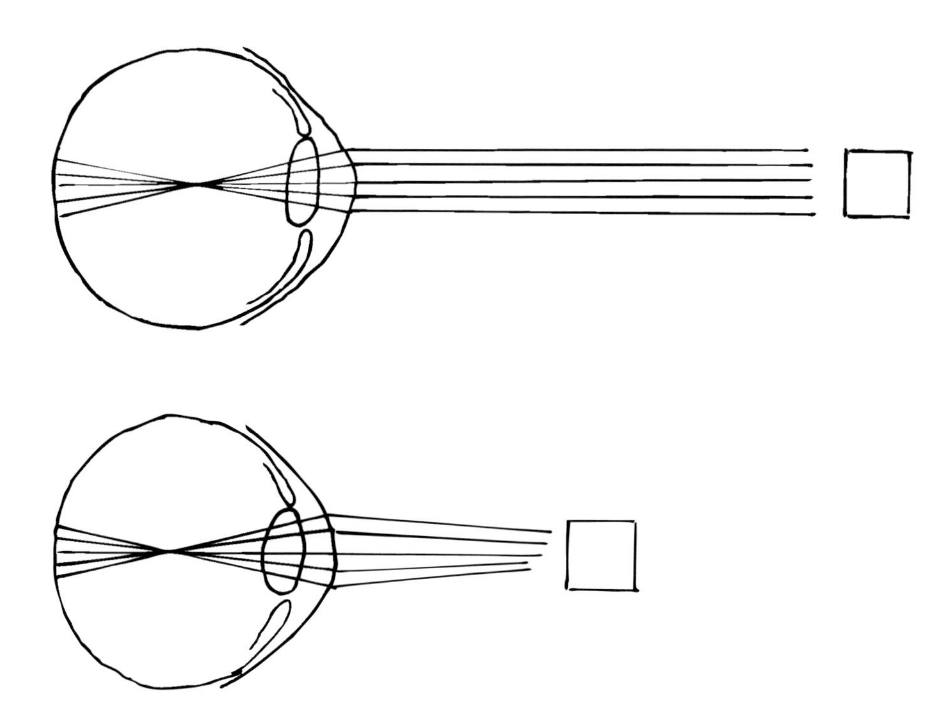

Distant image – to focus the image on the retina, the lens flattens (the ciliary muscle relaxes)

Close image – to focus the image on the retina, the lens becomes rounded (the ciliary muscle contracts)

Eyes

Most of our eye is inside the eye socket, protected by the bone of the eye socket. About one sixth of the eye is exposed beyond the bone socket and protected by the eyelids.

There are 3 main layers coating the eyeball. The outer layer is a transparent film and the visible part of this layer, the surface part of the eye is called the cornea. Immediately under that is the layer of white fibrous tissue which gives the white appearance to our eyes. Beneath the white fibrous tissues is the layer of the eyeball where many of the blood vessels are. These layers around the eyeball incorporate the muscles and ligaments which hold the lens, the pupil and the iris, which we see at the front of our eyes – and the retina, macula and fovea towards the back of the eye – and contain the vitreous gel within the eye.

When we see, what we see are the rays of light from what is around us. The light rays entering the eye are being focused on the retina and an image formed which stimulates receptors to send nerve impulses to the visual area of the brain. Vision/sight is the receipt and interpretation of rays of light. The rays meet the eye and are then deflected, bent and directed via the cornea, to the lens and pupil, to the retina.

To see things further away, the pupil has to relax and the curve of the lens flatten. Light rays from objects at 20 or more feet away from us are just about parallel when they meet the eye and don't need to pass through a more curved lens. They pass on through the cornea and the pupil to the retina.

To see things close to us, the muscles of the lens constrict, increasing the curve of the lens. Light rays from close objects diverge and are spread out when they reach the eye. The lens has to draw them back to parallel, adjust them to focus and they pass on to the retina.

The eyes are making these adjustments very, very quickly and all the time. The lubricated, vitreous nature of the tissues and the health of the muscles and ligaments, allow this to happen all day, everyday.

If our day consists of long periods of close work we can strain our eyes because of the long time the muscles are constricting. Looking at more distant scenes and objects as often as we can to relax the muscles, helps to balance that and keep the muscles working. As we get older and the muscles lose their elasticity we tend to become far-sighted. The muscles are less able to constrict on their own.

When the lens muscles constrict to see close objects, the pupil also constricts. The fibres of the iris surrounding the pupil tighten, reducing the pupil and this prevents rays straying out to the peripheral areas of the cornea and lens which would cause blurred vision. The pupil also reduces in bright light to prevent damage to the retina.

THE EYE

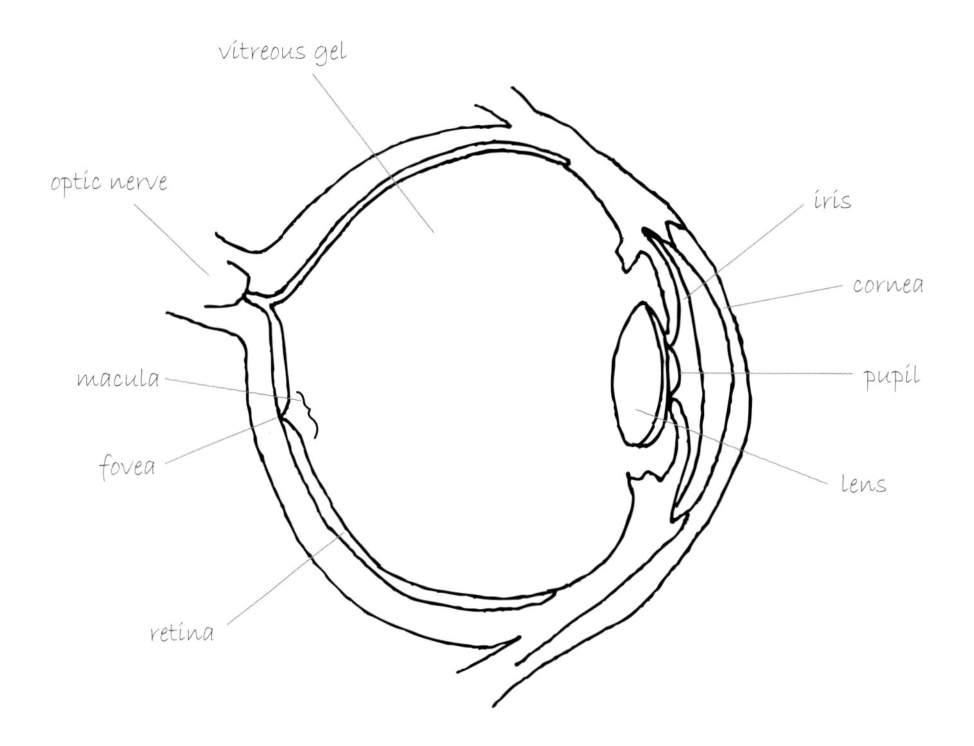
vitreous gel
optic nerve
iris
cornea
macula
pupil
fovea
lens
retina

The eye has three main parts: the cornea and lens, which focuses light at the front of the eye; the retina, the light focusing film at the back of the eye, including the macula and fovea; and the optic nerve which connects the eye and the brain.

The cornea is the outer layer or skin of the eye which focuses the light that reaches the eye, to pass through the pupil to the lens and then to the retina at the back of the eye. The muscle surrounding the pupil is the iris. At the back of the eye, tiny, light-sensitive receptors pass the signals to the optic nerves.

Different parts of the eye most commonly referred to are:

the cornea	–	the exposed surface film of the eye
the iris	–	the coloured circular muscle around the pupil.
the pupil	–	the dark, circular opening at the centre of the iris, through which light passes
the lens	–	in the middle of the eye behind the pupil, focuses the light rays received onto the retina
the vitreous gel	–	the colourless mass of the body of the eye
the retina	–	the inner film at the back of the eye which focuses the light
the macula	–	a small area of the most acute vision, on the retina
the fovea	–	the tiny area of clearest vision on the macula
the optic nerve	–	the nerve which carries the visual messages from the retina to the brain.

In normal room light, a healthy human pupil has a diameter of about 3-4 mm. In bright light, the pupil has a diameter of about 1.5 mm. In dim light the diameter is enlarged to about 8 mm. The narrowing of the pupil results in a greater focal range.

When bright light is shone on the eye, the pupil automatically decreases. This is the pupillary reflex, which is an important test of brainstem function. Conversely the pupil dilates if we see an object of interest.

Certain drugs cause constriction of the pupils, such as alcohol. Other drugs, such as psychedelics/hallucinogens, cause pupil dilation.

Caring for our eyes

Regular eye tests identify symptoms or problems and this could easily include things we are not aware of. Many eye conditions begin with no pain or visual affects, so we may not know about them for some time. Early detection of problems greatly affects the results that can be achieved to maintain and improve the health of our eyes and our sight.

Information and studies from medical organisations associated with eye health and the Royal National Institute of the Blind (www.rnib.org.uk) all emphasize several things that we can do to keep our eyes healthy and reduce and delay the onset of any problems:

- regular eye tests
- not smoking
- keeping fit
- reducing UV damage
- healthy diet and nutrition
- protecting eyes from dust, dirt and physical damage
- drinking sufficient water.

Eye tests are recommended every year for children up to age 16 and people over 60:
for people between 16 and 59, every two years;
for people with family history of glaucoma, every year;
for people with diagnosed diabetes, screening every year.

We shouldn't wait until we have symptoms before having an eye test, even if we have a healthy lifestyle. Some eye conditions are genetic and family history, ageing and other risks may affect our eyes, without us knowing. Early diagnosis and treatment make a significant difference. Optometrists can look at the retina at the back of the eye for early signs of macula degeneration and diabetic retinopathy and check the pressure in the eye for indications of glaucoma. They may also identify symptoms of diabetes or hypertension.

It can be easy to get used to deteriorating eyesight. If it happens gradually we can start to think of it as normal and put off doing anything about it – but in many cases corrective treatments will make a good difference and preserve our sight, so that we have the best quality of sight and for longer. Summed up at its briefest, an eye test can save your sight.

This is particularly worth bearing in mind for children. Symptoms and conditions can occur without us knowing and they can be treated. If any problems develop they can affect reading and schoolwork and learning – and mood, tiredness and concentration. (Details of eye tests and who is entitled to free eye tests are on the NHS Direct web site. At the moment, under 16s and 16, 17 and 18 year olds in full time education qualify for free eye tests, and so do over 60s, plus people registered with certain degrees of blindness, diabetes or glaucoma).

Smoking has become one of the major concerns affecting eye health. Smoking can cause reduced blood flow in the eye and altered blood vessels and toxins from tobacco smoke can accumulate in the lens. It has been demonstrably linked with age-related macula degeneration (AMD) and cataracts. Normal processes going on in the body all the time, produce free radicals and so do introduced substances from toxins and disease. Inhaling cigarette smoke is inhaling over 4,000 chemicals. Although we have natural protections against free radicals, where this protection is not enough, damage can occur, called oxidative stress. Oxidative stress damages cells and prevents them from regenerating as they should and smoking increases the production of free radicals and oxidative stress. The information and studies referred to also say that increased risk of developing eye disease can be reversed over time. Smokers are estimated to be between twice and four times as likely to develop AMD and possibly 10 years earlier than non-smokers.

Keeping fit, taking regular exercise and monitoring blood pressure and cholesterol levels will all help towards maintaining good eye health. Fitness reduces the risks to eye health from problems related to strokes, cardio-vascular conditions, overweight conditions, diabetes and high blood pressure. Fitness supports the immune system and cardio-vascular system to protect against disease and toxins and keep us healthy.

Sun and UV

UV rays are ultraviolet radiation from the sun. UVB rays can affect the surface of the eye and damage the cornea. UVA rays penetrate more deeply and can be the cause of eye conditions later in life. We are also at an increased risk of UV damage after cataract surgery (unless special lenses were inserted at the time of the surgery). Sunlight contains UVA and UVB rays. Normally throughout the year, exposure to UV in the UK is small. Most of the UV rays can be absorbed by the structure of the eye without causing damage but over exposure to UV rays has been related to some eye disease, cataracts in particular and also AMD. Although cataracts are a treatable condition, they are still a major cause of loss of sight in the UK. It is a good idea to provide extra eye protection from UV for people spending lots of time outside or spending time in sunnier countries. Many prescription specs and contact lenses now have UV filters built-in but it's always worth checking. Sunglasses can protect our eyes from UV rays. A CE mark indicates that they meet the approved European standard and BSEN 1836:1997 is the British standard mark. Surfaces that reflect sunlight, like glass and other surfaces, water and snow, intensify the rays.

(There are also UVC rays. UVC rays don't reach the earth's surface – so are not usually mentioned in sun and UV damage and protection advice).

There are several different types of sunglasses for different conditions, including wraparound frames which in conditions of strong sunlight can reduce the amount of UV rays by up to 35% compared to standard frames. A wide-brimmed hat can also block up to 50% of UV rays from the eyes. Children are at an increased risk and opticians and optometrists can advise on best protection for adults and children and for different conditions.

Try and avoid facing directly into strong, bright sunlight, adjust blinds to prevent unwanted light and glare. Try and avoid glare or bright reflections from screens and the TV, windows, water and shiny surfaces.

Healthy diet and nutrition play a significant part in maintaining healthy eyes and delaying and reducing eye and sight problems. Our diet provides the nutrients for the repair and renewal of cells, including the tissues and muscles of the eye. It also provides the anti-oxidants which provide our natural defence against the free radicals which cause cellular damage, including AMD. There is lots of information available covering studies on anti-oxidants and eye health. Good anti-oxidants, vitamins A, C and E are fruit and vegetables, nuts and seeds (oranges, kiwi fruit, grapefruit, dried apricots, tomatoes, peppers, raw carrots, peas, green beans, Brussel sprouts, kale, spinach, broccoli, lettuce – excluding iceberg lettuce). Adequate polyunsaturated fats and omega 3 oils reduce the risk of developing AMD and the severity and progression of the disease. It is possible to include some of these nutrients as supplements but, as covered in the section on nutrition, this should only be done with expert advice. It is easy to take supplements in the wrong proportions and all nutrients need to be taken in the right combinations and forms – so a good all round diet is the best basis, with additional, professional help, if necessary. One important component of macula health, is macula pigment which is derived completely from our diet, in the same foods as the anti-oxidants (fresh fruits and dark, leafy, green vegetables). Level of macular pigment is an indicator of overall eye health.

People with diabetes are at risk of a particular condition called diabetic retinopathy – when the tiny blood vessels of the retina are affected by becoming blocked or breaking, which can lead to loss of sight. This is very successfully treated by early diagnosis, laser treatment or surgery – with sight loss avoided in up to 90% of cases. The risks of this condition increase the longer someone has had diabetes and it is more likely to occur if diabetes has been left undiagnosed or uncontrolled. In one study showing between 1.8 and 2 million people diagnosed with diabetes in the UK it was also estimated there could be up to another 1 million people having the condition without diagnosis. Annual eye health screening is recommended and available for people with diabetes. (Further information at www.diabetes.org)

Being overweight has been linked to the risks of AMD, diabetic retinopathy, glaucoma and cataracts as well as other eye conditions associated with high blood pressure and raised cholesterol. Cardio-vascular disease and high blood pressure can result in hardening and narrowing of the blood vessels, including hypertensive retinopathy. High cholesterol can also result in a thickening and hardening of arteries near the retina, causing pressure on veins and possible blockages.

Protecting eyes from dust, dirt and risks from activities, including sport and DIY is also important. This comes generally into the category of common sense. We need to do whatever it takes to keep damaging objects and chemicals away from our eyes, including the fumes from strong substances and chemicals, or getting chemicals on our hands and putting hands and fingers to our eyes. Using things safely helps protect us plus wearing safety glasses or goggles. It's a question of remembering and then taking that minute to do the right thing – eyes and sight are so precious. Around the home and garden most things we use have instructions, advice and warnings on them – and if there is something that may flip or fly into your eye, wear protective glasses – getting things down out of the loft or trimming the hedge, we know what the hazards are and it's quicker to put some glasses on than having a sore or irritated eye for the next 12 or 24 hours or causing serious damage. Cycling or motorcycling seem to be activities when you discover just how many air borne assaults there can be to your eyes – and when it's also quite important to see. Once it starts to get technical, there are goggles and glasses that protect against dry hazards, like dust and different goggles to protect against wet, fluid chemical and substance splashes. There isn't one overall item of eye protection, having the right protection for the job is important.

In the workplace there are guidelines, procedures and regulations governing conditions and what we should and shouldn't do. Be sure to know what the correct advice is and who is responsible for what you are doing and the regulations to be complied with.

The potential risks are many and varied and they are common, possibly everyday encounters: glass, sawdust, grass and hedge trimmings, wood chippings, house dust, road dust, grit, sand, medicines, lotions and potions, chemicals, sharp corners of furniture, protruding fixtures and fittings – indoors and outside, belts and buckles, squash balls, golf balls, fish hooks, flies and bugs, aerosols, nails – there are lots of web sites with lots of information on the best way to take effective, simple precautions – and protect your eyes. People who wear lenses need to be particularly careful as dust and fragments can become lodged between the lens and the eye. Out and about we also need to be careful of animal and bird droppings that may carry contaminants. It is surprising how often we put our hands to our face, hair and eyes. If hands may have come into contact with a contaminant, it is very easy to transfer those contaminants that can irritate and infect the eyes.

Drinking sufficient water can be a simple way to help tired, dry and itchy eyes. There are a multitude of different eye washes, eye baths and eye drops to soothe and lubricate tired eyes. They are often called 'false tears'. In the normal way the fluid produced naturally by our eyes and secreted from the tear ducts can keep our eyes lubricated and comfortable. If we are dehydrated, it does affect every part of us and drinking sufficient water will often solve frequently recurring dry and itchy eyes. It is one of the signs of being generally dehydrated.

Eye Washes, Eye Baths and Eye Drops

If you do need to use eye washes, eye baths and eye drops they are very effective and have useful labelling and information. Most of them have strict information on how long they should be used after being opened to avoid contamination and infections. There are also various ointments for eye conditions, such as styes and inflammation. These products also have information and labelling and pharmacy staff can advise which ones are best for which circumstances. A good home made eye wash for certain conditions, including styes, is warm/hot salt water, as salt water has mild antiseptic properties. (A teaspoon of salt in a cup of water, using boiling water if possible and allowing it to cool a little, until a comfortable temperature to use).

Adequate light

The light needed to do things depends on who we are and what we are doing.

The light required by someone in their 70s may be 3 x as much as a teenager, to do a similar activity, eg: reading, hobbies and crafts, because as we age our pupils get smaller and our eyes become less transparent. Different activities require different amounts of light. Needing to distinguish colours requires more light than activities that don't. Contrast makes things easier to see in less light, whereas things of similar shades and tones are more difficult to see without good light.

For work and activities where colour is important, there are different types of light because not only does sufficient light make a difference but also having light of a broad enough spectrum.

We don't hurt our eyes by trying to do things in insufficient light, we simply can't see to do them. You don't hurt your eyes by trying to read under the bed covers by torchlight – but if it isn't sufficient light, you won't be able to read.

Sufficient light, is the light you need to be able to see what you are doing. You may not hurt your eyes if the light is too poor but you may well get a headache.

We were designed to do things requiring sight in the daylight, before the invention of artificial light, sight is the interpretation of light rays. What we are doing, for how long, age and other factors will affect light requirements – opticians or optometrists will have best advice and answers to specific questions.

20/20 Vision

One of our most common eye tests is to identify letters or objects, usually decreasing in size, from a chart or light box.

We sit or stand 20 feet from the chart and that defines the first '20', the distance in feet we are from the object. The second figure is determined by what we can see clearly/identify compared to 'normal'. A pre-set standard of 'normal' is what someone with normal vision would be able to see and identify at a distance of 20 feet.

If our result is 20/20 we have 'normal' vision.

If our result is 20/100, it means we can see at 20 feet, what someone with normal vision would see at 100 feet.

Our eyes are wonderful things. 90% of us say that sight is the sense we most fear losing. They are designed to look after themselves and for many of us days, weeks and months go by with us hardly having to think about them. The best thing we can do is simply to remember to take care of them.

There is 24 hour help and advice available on NHS Direct
tel: 0845 46 47 www.patient.co.uk

Information from the RNIB and others will also cover much more, including specific conditions:

Conjunctivitis
Cataracts
Macula degeneration
Glaucoma
Trachoma
Diabetic retinopathy
Detached retina

Ears

The ear is an exceptionally intricate and delicate mechanism to enable us to hear and to balance. The sequence of spaces and shapes and bones and hair and fluid all act to convey and process the sound waves and convert the vibrations to electrical impulses and pass them along the auditory nerve to the brain.

In anatomy and biology the ear is generally referred to as the outer ear, middle ear and inner ear. Sounds travel through the air in sound waves and as they reach us, the part of the ear which we can see, called the pinna, channels the sound waves towards the ear canal. The shape of the pinna also acts as a mild amplifier. Sounds vary in pitch from very low to very high, which is determined by the frequency of the sound waves. As the sound passes towards the ear canal it is filtered and this filtering process particularly enhances sound in the usual frequency range of the human voice.

As the sound waves hit the eardrum at the end of the ear canal, it vibrates and these vibrations are passed on into the middle ear.

Beyond the eardrum are three tiny bones of the ear, the anvil, the hammer and the stirrup. The vibrations of the ear drum move these little bones, which are suspended on delicate membranes and ligaments. The vibration of the stirrup bone converts the sound waves into hydraulic pressure waves which pass through to the cochlea. The cochlea is lined with over 2 million hair cells which are sensitive to the movement of the cochlea fluid and membrane and convert the signals into electrical impulses. The electrical impulses are then passed to the brain along the auditory nerve.

The pressure of the inner ear needs to be kept equal to the pressure outside the ear and below the cochlea there is a tube (called the Eustachian tube) which acts to balance air and drain fluid to equalize the pressure. This is what we are aware of when we yawn or swallow or on a flight, usually the descent, or diving in water.

It is all a very fine sequence of reactions and balances.

Our balance is determined by the level of fluid (endolymph) in complex tubing in the inner ear, called the labyrinth – made up of the vestibule, cochlea and semi-circular canals.

This sensory system, called the vestibular system, provides information to the brain about our movement and our orientation. Our movements consist of rotational and linear translations and the system sends signals to the nerves that control our eye movements and the muscles that control our posture, to keep us upright.

When our sense of balance is interrupted we may have dizziness, disorientation or nausea. This can be caused by ear infections, colds and a number of medical conditions, including Meniere's disease. We can also temporarily disrupt our sense of balance by

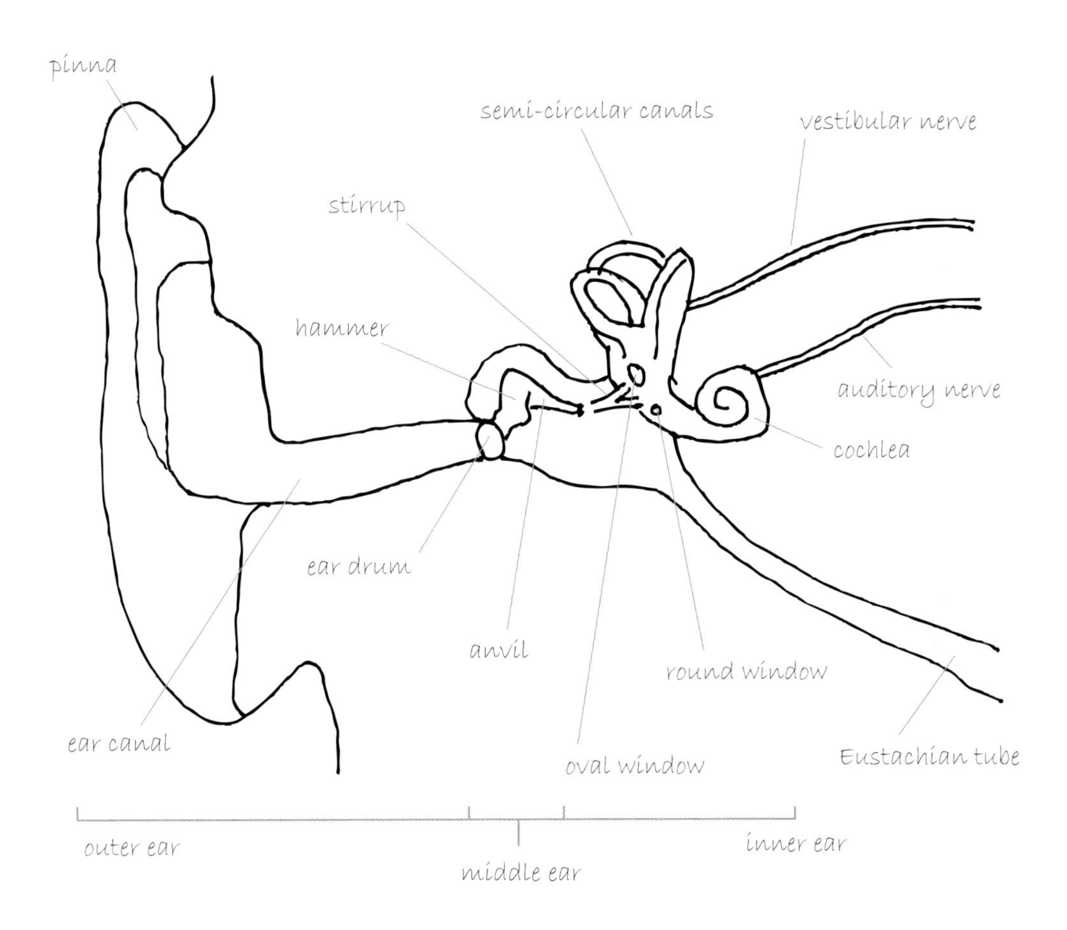
THE EAR
pinna
semi-circular canals
vestibular nerve
stirrup
hammer
auditory nerve
cochlea
ear drum
anvil
round window
ear canal
oval window
Eustachian tube
outer ear
middle ear
inner ear

rapid, vigorous movements – being shaken, circling quickly or getting up quickly, being swung round, sliding down a helter-skelter or riding on a merry-go-round.

Hearing loss tends to be common in older age but varies enormously. The hair cells in the inner ear die off naturally. This is different and far more subtle to hearing loss caused by damage and distortion caused by noise.

To look after our ears we need to keep all those working parts healthy and cause as little damage as we can.

We need to try and prevent water entering the ear.

Most important is not to put anything in our ears. We can keep the outer part of our ears clean with normal washing but the ear has its own self-cleaning mechanism from the inner ear, working outwards. Pushing things in our ear, weather a soft flannel or a cotton bud or a finger, can not only damage the delicate, sensitive tissues of the ear but can also push wax backwards into the ear canal, which can cause blocked ears and/or infection.

Anyone who has spoken to someone who has caused some damage to their ear will know it is a very difficult thing to live with. Whilst the ear heals we can be partially deaf, have pain and a constant background noise – and it can take quite some time to get back to normal.

If you need extra help keeping ears clean and/or suffer from a build-up of wax, or any hearing problems, consult the GP or nurse. They can clean ears safely and hopefully diagnose why the problem is occurring and help with advice. Seeking advice early is important.

Protect your ears from loud noise.

Earplugs are more attractive than damaged hearing.

Noise legislation

Research has shown that 'noise' at 55dB to 60dB creates annoyance, at 60dB to 65dB increases annoyance considerably and above 65-85dB causes serious damage to hearing.

No single agency has overall responsibility for legal noise control and for all aspects of environmental noise policy and legislation. So there's no one single piece of legislation that makes clear what noise levels are allowed. There are more than 100 different noise-related laws controlling different types of noise in different places, all of which may contribute to background noise. The UK Noise Act 1996, for example, only covers noise emitted from dwellings at night, while a number of EU directives control noise from transport sources, such as vehicles, trains and planes, outdoor machinery and industry.

The World Health Organization has suggested a standard guideline value for average outdoor noise levels of 55dB, applied during normal daytime to prevent significant interference with the normal activities of local communities (also 50dB for indoors, 30dB for bedrooms, and more specific limits such as a 100dB for a four-hour period for concert halls).

In the work place there will be specific legislation and regulations for health and safety.

Prolonged and/or frequent exposure to noise above 85 decibels can cause damage to hearing. Above 130 decibels is very damaging and on the pain threshold.

140	rock concerts
	big fireworks
	jet take-off
120	loud stereo
	night clubs
	chain saw
	pneumatic drill at 1 meter
100	pneumatic drill at 5 meters
90	lawnmower
	motorbike
	crying child
80	town traffic
	ringing telephone
70	vacuum cleaner
60	normal conversation
40	refrigerator
	bird song
20	whisper
10	quiet countryside
0	threshold of hearing

I'M OFFICIALLY GETTING OLD SO I DON'T NEED DRUGS ANYMORE. I CAN GET THE SAME EFFCT JUST BY STANDING UP REALLY FAST.

Jonathan Katz

Feet

The feet provide the body with support, balance and mobility.

The complex combination of all the intricate components of our feet act as a shock absorber and a mechanism to propel us in motion.

The foot and ankle contain:

- over 100 muscles
- 26 individual bones (25% of the number of bones in the body)
- 33 joints
- ligaments, tendons, blood vessels, skin and tissue
- over 125,000 sweat glands in each foot – producing anything from an egg-cup to half a pint of moisture a day
- the skin of the feet has over 7,000 nerve endings.

The bones of the foot are arranged in a way that they form 2 strong arches, one along the length of the foot and one across the foot. This is an excellent architectural structure for supporting weight. Arches are one of the strongest, if not the strongest, supporting shapes in any weight-bearing structure. This double arch provides a very stable and very strong base. The arches are held in position by strong ligaments and muscle tendons. Our feet support our full body weight all the time we are standing, all the time we are walking and multiples of our body weight if we run or jump. When we run, the equivalent of approximately 3 times our body weight is transmitted through each foot as it hits the floor. The structure of the foot is similar to the hand but the functions define their differences. The hand is for manipulation and there is more flexibility in the fingers, thumb and wrist – and the foot is for support and stability.

Looking after our feet includes:

- good hygiene
- cutting toe-nails well
- keeping feet warm
- exercise
- treatment for pain, cuts, burns, unusual changes in colour or temperature
- wearing good footwear – and the right footwear for the relevant activity.

Today's lifestyle for most populations means we have to wash. We don't live in a

THE FOOT

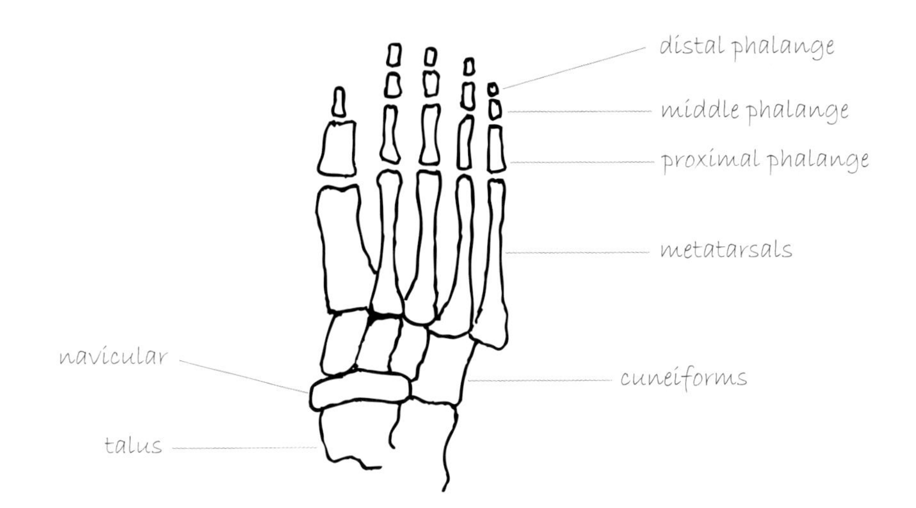

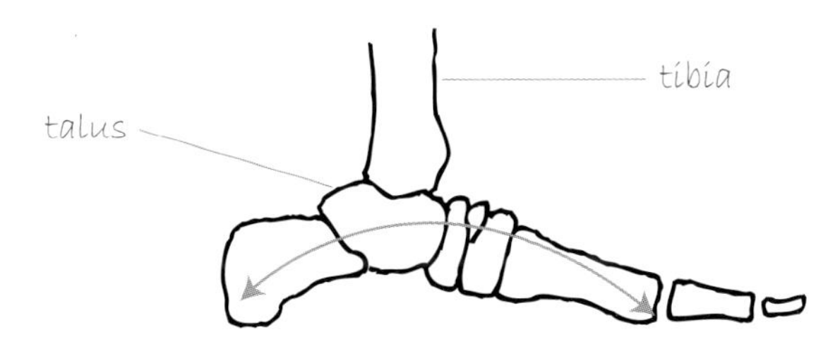

longitudinal arch

completely natural environment and we wear clothes, including shoes and socks, which trap moisture and particles given off through the skin. To wash our feet it is best in water that isn't too hot and not to soak them for too long which may remove the natural oils and dry the skin. Having got them wet and washed them, it's important to dry them thoroughly. If your feet are prone to dry skin, although we really need to nourish the skin from inside, from the diet - good moisturising creams, oils and lotions for the feet will help keep the skin supple and comfortable. Using a pumice stone helps prevent the build up of hard skin. If there is difficult build-up of dry or hard skin it is best to see a chiropodist - the comfort after an appointment will persuade you.

Cutting toe-nails is easier when they are slightly softened after a bath - and to prevent ingrowing toe-nails it is recommended to cut them as straight as possible across the top, not too short and not to shape them down at the corners - and definitely not to cut them down the sides. Use good quality toe-nail clippers and scissors. Again, an expert job done by the chiropodist from time to time is sheer luxury.

Keeping feet warm helps circulation which keeps our feet healthy - and warm feet also help us to keep our body warm.

Exercise helps stimulate circulation and keeps the feet muscles, tendons and ligaments healthy and strengthens the arches in our feet. We were designed to walk and run and be active and that is the best way to maintain the overall health, strength and mobility of our feet and ankles. A good work out for them from time to time is excellent - rotating and flexing the feet - and a good massage of the muscles and arches and toes. Another reason to exercise is that being overweight or unfit will put added stress on the feet.

Our feet work hard and it's important to treat cuts or blisters or other conditions promptly. Particularly seek professional advice for any changes in colour or temperature, especially for anyone with diabetes. There is a range of common foot problems (listed at the end of this chapter) and a range of advice and treatments from the chiropodist or podiatrist, GP and pharmacist and lots of information available.

To make an appointment with a chiropodist or podiatrist, choose those registered with the HPC - Health Professionals Council. Members of the Society of Chiropodists and Podiatrists will be HPC registered and will have qualified from a 3 year degree course (DPodM and BSc or BSc(Hons) Podiatry). Other practitioners may call themselves chiropodists or podiatrists - although those terms are now protected - and may even use the word 'registered' but may have had very little training or qualification. Feet and lower limbs are a specialist area. www.feetforlife.org gives lots of information on various foot conditions and how to find qualified chiropodists and podiatrists.

Basic hygiene and nail cutting will be all many people need to maintain strong, healthy feet. Problems can arise from illnesses, hereditary weaknesses, age-related conditions or from injuries or ill-fitting footwear. Correct treatment keeps us mobile, relieves pain and manages any risk of infection.

As we get older, usually around age 60 onwards, it becomes more necessary to check and look after our feet. Joints tend to stiffen, our feet can become more prone to the cold and the skin becomes thinner and more delicate. It also becomes more difficult to reach and see our feet. Using a hand mirror can help and having a professional check-up, approximately every 6 months, just makes sure and gets your toe-nails cut into the bargain.

Shoes and Footwear

It's usually a good idea to buy shoes in the afternoon because our feet swell during the day.

Shoes and socks need to be of material that will breathe to allow sweat and moisture to escape and keep the skin healthy. Shoes and socks that don't allow the feet to breathe can have the affect of making feet feel tired and ache.

The bones in our feet aren't fully set until approximately age 18, so good, well-fitting shoes for children and whilst we are growing are very important to long term foot health.

Poor-fitting footwear is an extremely common cause of foot problems for adults. Ideally the heel of our shoes should be solid, the width of the shoe and only up to 4 cms in height. The fit of the shoe around the heel and ankle is important not only for comfort but also to provide support and stability and hold the foot in place. Shoes need to have sufficient room in them but fit snugly so that the foot isn't moving and sliding in them – and shoes need to be foot shaped! A guide to size is to measure the length of the foot by drawing round it on paper or card, then cut a lengthwise strip from the longest point of the shape. The strip of paper or card should fit inside a shoe, along the sole, with 1 cm to spare. When your shoe is on you can test for adequate room in the shoe by pressing your thumb down in front of your toes. If the foot is too tight up against the front of the shoe, over time it can cause crumpled toes, corns, ingrowing toe-nails or even blackened and loss of toe-nails. Width is gauged from the width of your foot.

There is a lot of advice and assistance available to help with finding and checking well-fitting shoes, especially for children. A double-check is to look at children's bare feet just after taking shoes and socks off, to make sure that there aren't any red or irritated areas. Additionally, correct fitting shoes can help avoid children developing standing and walking with toes pointing inwards or outwards – by changing the shape of the shoe or using special insoles – but it is essential to do this with properly qualified advice.

There are many and various supports and fittings that can help us have comfy shoes, comfy feet and prevent problems developing.

For people on their feet a lot, the most comfortable shoes or boots for feet, legs, back and hips are likely to be ones made of a material that lets your foot breathe, with thick, flexible soles and adjustable fastenings, like lace-ups, to hold the foot firm in the shoe and stop it sliding and enough room and flexibility at the toe to be able to slightly wriggle your toes. Seams or stitching on the inside or any rough surfaces can irritate or rub the skin.

For shoes to let the feet breathe, socks also need to be of natural, breathable materials. Socks need to fit properly and not be too small or tight to cramp toes. Good socks will help to absorb moisture and provide additional cushioning.

Making sure that the heel of the foot is held firm in the shoe or boot and doesn't move up and down against the shoe – and that the toes and ball of the foot are held in place and don't slide and rub against the sole or shoe – provides comfort, reduces strain and tiredness and avoids blisters.

Sports Shoes

Modern shoes and hi-tech materials have become a multi-million pound industry with extensive research on performance and minimising risk and injury. Different sports and activities require different shoes. There isn't a super-trainer that suits everything. Running shoes are designed to be light and flexible and for running in, with mainly forward movement and not too much stopping and starting and changing direction. Shoes for racquet sports involving sharp stops and starts and turns and sideways movement at speed will have more support around the foot and the ankle. Aerobics shoes combine flexibility and support. There are big differences in the design, construction and support of these shoes and having the right shoes for the activity will safeguard feet and ankles from strains and injuries and protect the muscles and soft tissue in the feet and legs from strain, over-work and fatigue. If the muscles and tissues are over-working to compensate, referred problems can develop including back, knee and hip pain, inflamed tendons and toe trauma. The shoes are designed to provide varying degrees of cushioning to absorb impact. The right shoes will provide comfort and support, help improve performance and reduce fatigue and injury. Again, there is a lot of advice available to help buy the right shoes.

Football puts a lot of stress on the feet, especially on harder surfaces. If football boots are putting too much pressure on the feet, corns, calluses and ingrowing toe-nails can develop. Good, well-fitting boots shouldn't leave any signs of pressure after playing or training.

Running, walking, dancing, football, tennis, squash, basketball, netball, fencing, aerobics and all the sports and activities have extensive ranges of footwear and good retailers should be able to advise – but there is also a lot of independent and professional information and advice. For any sport or activity, footwear is one of the most important pieces of equipment to consider.

All that being said, don't let footwear discourage you from taking exercise. A good pair of shoes is usually sufficient for most normal walking and cross trainers are OK for a range of activities if you aren't going to become an enthusiast at any particular one.

For hiking and hill-walking good walking boots are necessary. When wearing heavier footwear, typically walking boots, it often adds to comfort and helps avoid pressure points and blisters to wear 2 or 3 layers of socks, which can reduce friction.

Working Feet and Working Shoes

Feet do work hard and anywhere that particular care or footwear is advised it will help towards comfort and safety. Different jobs and workplaces may specify particular footwear such as safety shoes and hard toe caps to guard against injury – it is important to comply with current, relevant health and safety regulations and protect your feet. It's also important to keep feet warm and dry to guard against chilblains or athlete's foot.

High Heels

Wearing high heels throws our weight in our footstep onto the ball of the foot, instead of being distributed through the heel and the arch and the ball and toes. It tilts us forward a little which makes the spine bend slightly to compensate. As the heel is elevated it is also more unstable which requires muscles to work harder to balance but leaves us more prone to twisting or spraining an ankle. The calf muscle is also shortened and tightened. Wearing high heels for short periods, now and again – probably won't do too much lasting damage. Prolonged wearing of high heels can cause calluses and bunions and corns, it can cause toes to become bent and cross-over, back problems and can lead to a continually shortened calf muscle causing the arch of the foot to lower and affect the knee and hip. Varying the shoes we wear and the height of the heels will help prevent serious problems developing. For long periods of time, a heel height of up to 4cms is recommended. Relaxing the foot after wearing high heels and some stretching exercises for the calf muscles will help to reduce side-effects. For people who love high heels it is always going to be difficult to resist the temptation but restricting them to special occasions and minimising the length of time to wear them will do very real favours for your feet and back.

Flip Flops

Flip flops are always likely to be popular, especially on hot, sunny days. The thing to remember is that they don't provide support for the feet and are as flat as you can get, so can lead to problems from strained arches and scrunched toes. They may cause aches and pains, especially for people who often wear high heels that may have encouraged tight calf muscles and restricted ankle movement because the contrast in position and movement can cause damage to the soft tissues in the foot. Flip flops are excellent for wearing in changing rooms, hotel bathrooms and around swimming pools to help avoid picking up infections. They are positively discouraged for driving when they could be a real hazard. Worn over long periods, flip flops also let your feet spread which may mean other shoes will then feel tight and that new shoes may need to be slightly larger than before. They are nice, relaxed footwear for certain times but it's worth being aware of the drawbacks.

Slip-ons, Crocs and Clogs

The guidance here is on the fit. Slip-ons, Crocs and clogs are looser fitting shoes because they don't fasten round our feet. A lot depends on how hard our feet have to work to keep the shoes on and stay firm in them. Looser fitting shoes can build up hard skin on the soles of our feet and heels and encourage our toes to scrunch. Some of the more expensive designs tend to have a structured shape and a rim around the heel to hold the foot more firmly. The test is in the wearing. If your foot is sliding around, or your toes are clinging for dear life or you are getting tired or achey feet and legs, or a build-up of hard skin, or dry, cracked heels - then these are the best sort of indications that it's down to these type of shoes. Crocs are very light and easy to wear but they do have synthetic soles which may not suit some feet.

High Arches and Flat Arches

There are different types of feet and that will affect how the foot works and moves. We are all a bit different and slightly out of synch or misaligned somewhere and our bodies adapt to compensate. Often we won't be aware of these adaptations and compensations. Flat or low arches (pronation) can lead to aches and pains as the arch isn't being as supportive as a higher arch and this can be helped by shoes that support the inner side of the foot. High arches (supination) mean feet are slightly less flexible and this can be alleviated by more cushioned shoes to help absorb and reduce the impact from the more rigid joints. Exercises that work on the strengths and weaknesses of your feet and ankles will reduce aches, pains and injuries and optimize strength, mobility and posture.

Diabetes and feet

Anyone diagnosed with diabetes will be advised to take particular care of their feet. High glucose levels can cause damage to nerve endings and loss of feeling which can mean that minor cuts or skin conditions aren't felt or noticed and become vulnerable to infection or ulcers. Visually check feet everyday or every few days and use a hand mirror if it helps – checking for any damage or change in colour or temperature.

Some common foot conditions: (see www.feetforlife.org)

athlete's foot
bunions
calluses
chilblains
corns
diabetic conditions
gout
ingrowing toe-nails
osteoarthritis
sweaty feet
verrucae

Like the rest of our body, our feet respond very well to good, tender, loving care and can go happily on for years and miles.

WHEN OUR FEET HURT, WE HURT ALL OVER

Socrates

A GOOD LAUGH AND A LONG SLEEP
ARE THE BEST CURES IN THE DOCTOR'S BOOK.

Irish Proverb

AND IF TONIGHT MY SOUL MAY FIND HER PEACE IN SLEEP,
AND SINK IN GOOD OBLIVION,
AND IN THE MORNING WAKE LIKE A NEW-OPENED FLOWER
THEN I HAVE BEEN DIPPED AGAIN IN GOD,
AND NEW-CREATED.

D H Lawrence

IF A MAN HAD AS MANY IDEAS DURING THE DAY
AS HE DOES WHEN HE HAS INSOMNIA,
HE'D MAKE A FORTUNE.

Griff Niblack

I'M NOT ASLEEP. . .
BUT THAT DOESN'T MEAN I'M AWAKE.

Anon

Sleep

Sleep plays a major role in our physical energy, mental performance and overall ability and stability – our wellbeing.

During the day, activity in the body is geared to providing energy and breaking down molecules for use (catabolic processes). This leads to waste by-products and an acid environment for cells which needs to be cleared. During the night, during sleep, the body is geared to detoxing, resting, repairing and re-building (anabolic processes). This clears acidity and restores the mildly alkaline state of tissues which keeps things working properly. Whilst we are asleep our bodies are still performing vital functions for our health. If we restrict our hours of rest and sleep, we are restricting the chance our body has to perform these functions. These functions require the body to be inactive and many require darkness.

This is why, when we are short on sleep, we can feel almost hung-over, irritable and tired. Our bodies haven't cleared. It is important for the body to be able to clear toxicity and metabolic waste – not doing so can be the cause of various chronic diseases as well as headaches and pain.

If we are particularly busy and/or stressed we may require more sleep – it is ironical that often it is at the times we need more sleep that our sleep patterns are disturbed and we may have insomnia.

A good night's sleep can increase resistance to infections. Sufficient sleep enhances relationships at work and socially and affects our performance and productivity.

If you sleep well and don't have sleep problems – value that, it is a wonderful thing.

If you do have sleep problems there are lots of simple, practical things which can help. We aren't all the same and how much sleep we need will vary – but we all need enough.

Sleep can be disrupted by:

chemical sensitivities
depression
eating late at night
emotional stress
food allergies
high animal protein diets
high blood histamine levels
hormone imbalances
imbalance of calcium and magnesium
pain, physical injury or illness
physical inactivity
poor blood glucose control
shift work
sugar and alcohol
too many or few B vitamins
too much caffeine, nicotine and other stimulants

Things which can help a good night's sleep

Sleep problems may be: not being able to fall asleep, waking up too often, not feeling well rested when it's time to wake up in the morning or simply wanting to improve the quality and quantity of our sleep. These tips and techniques have been found to be helpful.

- Avoid before-bed snacks, particularly grains and sugars, they will raise blood sugar and inhibit sleep. Later, when blood sugar drops too low, you may wake up and not be able to fall back to sleep.

- Sleep in complete darkness, or as close as possible. If there is even the tiniest bit of light in the room it can disrupt your circadian rhythm and the pineal gland's production of melatonin and serotonin. There should also be as little light on a landing or in the bathroom as possible. If you get up in the night, from a sleep point of view - don't put lights on to go to the bathroom. If you can't do that safely, then you have to judge that - but as soon as you turn a light on, that light will, for you, that night, cease all production of the important sleep aid melatonin. This doesn't mean you can't go back to sleep - but may make it more difficult.

- Listen to white noise or relaxation CDs, on a low volume. The sound of white noise or nature sounds, such as the sea, can be soothing and sleep-inducing.

- Don't watch TV right up to going to bed and don't have a TV in the bedroom. It is very stimulating to the brain and can make it take longer to fall asleep. It is also disruptive to the pineal gland, for the same reason. The same applies to computers.

- Go to bed as early as possible. Our systems, especially the adrenals, do the majority of their recharging or recovering during the hours of 11pm and 1am. Also, your gall-bladder dumps toxins during this period. During sleep the body processes that waste. If we have kept the body awake, we compromise that process and the extra toxins can back-up affecting our system as a whole and cause disruption to health. Before the widespread use of electricity, we would go to bed shortly after sundown or dusk, as most animals do and which nature intended for us as well.

- Have the temperature in the bedroom no higher than 70ºF/21ºC.

- Eat a high-protein snack several hours before going to bed. This can provide the

L-tryptophan needed to produce melatonin and serotonin.

- Eat a small piece of fruit, either half an hour before the snack, or an hour afterwards. This can help the tryptophan cross the blood-brain barrier.

- Avoid caffeine. In some people, caffeine is not metabolized efficiently and therefore can lead to side-effects quite a long time after it is consumed. An afternoon cup of coffee, or tea, will keep some people from falling asleep even several hours later. Some medications, particularly diet pills and cold remedies may also contain caffeine.

- Avoid alcohol. Although alcohol can make us drowsy, the effect is short-lived and people will often wake up a few hours later, unable to fall back to sleep. Alcohol will also keep you from falling into the deeper stages of sleep, where the body does most of its healing, mending and repairing.

- Avoid foods that you may be sensitive to. This is particularly true for dairy and wheat products, as they may affect sleep, eg: causing apnoea, excess congestion, gastro-intestinal upset and gas, among others.

- Limit fluid intake for a couple of hours before going to bed – simply to reduce the likelihood of needing to get up in the night, or minimize the frequency.

- Have a hot bath, shower or sauna before bed. When body temperature is raised in the late evening, it will fall at bedtime, facilitating sleep. (Baths are less stimulating than showers – so see what suits you).

- If you are menopausal or peri-menopausal the hormonal changes at this time can cause sleep problems. Lots of advice on naturally managing these changes will include helping good sleep patterns.

- Keep your bedtime and getting-up-time as consistent as possible. Going to bed and getting up at similar times each day will significantly help you to have good sleep – even at weekends or when you have had to have a late night or particularly early start. Keeping to a regular pattern helps your body maintain a sleep rhythm, making it easier to fall asleep and get up.

- Don't worry about lack of sleep. Worrying about lack of sleep is a very effective cause of insomnia! Lots of people, all over the world, miss sleep for all sorts of reasons. If you miss some sleep, just try and do what you can to have some good sleep the next time you can – your body is very good at catching up – do what you can to help. Relax, breathe, lie down and rest – worrying won't help.

- If you do wake in the night, try not to get up, and not to make a cup of tea or do things. Try to lie still, relax, focus on the fact that you are horizontal and resting, warm, comfortable – the next best thing to sleep. If you can focus on that calm, comfortable state, you are still resting your limbs and resting your body physically and probably giving yourself the best chances of dozing off again. Very low volume radio or music may help. If we get up when we wake in the night and make drinks and do things, we are training ourselves not to sleep/to have the wrong reaction.

High stress levels

Repeated or prolonged stress leads to increased levels of stress hormones, adrenalin and cortisol. When stress is continuous and prolonged it can result in under-production of these hormones. High and low levels of cortisol mean stress. Cortisol is produced in the body on a circadian rhythm. It is highest in the morning and lowest at night. Raised cortisol at night is associated with difficulty in going to sleep. Depressed early morning cortisol is associated with difficulty waking up and getting going. Stressors include; unresolved problems, caffeine, nicotine, food allergies, chemical sensitivities, pain, physical injury, illness, poor blood glucose control, hormone imbalances, shift work and physical inactivity.

Nutrient imbalances

For a small percentage of people, supplementing B vitamins can cause agitation and insomnia. Being deficient in B vitamins can also cause insomnia.

Magnesium is a relaxant and calcium causes contraction. Modern diets tend to provide more calcium than magnesium. Magnesium rich foods are: nuts, seeds and dark green leafy vegetables. These foods supply a good balance of calcium and magnesium.

High blood histamine levels

A high blood histamine level is associated with allergy. Managing allergies can reduce histamine levels and improve sleep. Some individuals naturally produce more histamine. They are genetically more prone to allergies, insomnia and depression. There is a lot of nutritional advice on managing and eliminating allergies, particularly: 'New Optimum Nutrition Bible', by Patrick Holford (see pages 308 and 311).

Balancing the diet

Ideally we should have our last meal no later than 7.00pm. The body is not designed to digest food as we sleep. We are designed to detoxify overnight. The gradual build-up of toxins in the system can affect our sleep pattern. Too much animal protein can inhibit the sleep-inducing amino acid tryptophan from reaching the brain. Eating a moderate amount of animal protein foods, soy products, nuts, bananas, papaya or figs for an evening meal can provide good levels of tryptophan in the brain and help improve sleep.

Relaxation

Should be natural and is definitely the key – but this is something more people are having to re-learn. Watching a horror film, or reading an over-stimulating book in the evening before going to bed, not winding-down after work, or doing something too exciting, will have the effect of preventing us reaching low levels of cortisol and we wake up in the morning not feeling as though we have had a good night's sleep, not feeling refreshed. How we are in the evening is important to affect a good night's sleep. If you've been to a good party in the evening and you're feeling up, even though it is late, when you come back it can still take a while to come down. This unwinding is where we just sit and do nothing and allow our cortisol levels to come down. Having your own relaxation routine will make a significant difference.

Why it is important to go to bed early

A good night's sleep is an important key to stay healthy.

Naturally, once upon a time, ideally, a person would have slept during the hours of darkness and woken up naturally with the sun rise. The further you move into the Northern Hemisphere, the more difficult that is.

There have been many studies completed that show that sleeping before midnight is very important. Sleep during the hours before midnight is said to be twice as important as in the hours after midnight – due to the synchronising of the various organs and systems of the body.

Sleeping less than 6-8 hours a day can create problems with our insulin levels – but we are all different. It is important to try to sleep in complete darkness, as light will disrupt or affect the quality of our sleep.

Too little sleep may accelerate ageing

Regularly catching only a few hours of sleep can hinder metabolism and hormone production in a way that is similar to the effects of ageing and the early stages of diabetes. Chronic sleep loss may speed the onset, or increase the severity, of age-related conditions such as type 2 diabetes, high blood pressure, obesity and memory loss. Sleep research has shown that just one week of sleep deprivation altered the subjects' hormone levels and their capacity to metabolize carbohydrates. People who trade sleep for work or play may get used to it and feel less fatigued. Some people will 'get away with it' but they are still preventing their body carrying out all the detoxing and revitalising it would normally be doing.

During sleep deprivation, the researchers found that men's blood sugar levels took 40% longer to drop following a high-carbohydrate meal, than during a normal sleep-recovery period. Their ability to secrete and respond to the hormone insulin, which helps regulate blood sugar, dropped by 30%. These changes reflect the effects of insulin resistance, a precursor to type 2 diabetes. In addition, the sleep-deprived men had higher night time concentrations of the hormone cortisol, which also helps regulate blood sugar and lower levels of thyroid-stimulating hormone. These raised cortisol levels are like the levels often seen in older people and may be involved in age-related insulin resistance and memory loss.

Sleep debts resemble stress. Most sleep deprivation research has focused on what it does to the brain but it is likely that sleep has many functions. In the study, subjects' blood sugar and hormone concentrations were restored after the sleep-recovery period. Earlier research has shown that in developed countries, the average night's sleep has become shorter since the beginning of the century, from 9 hours to 7.5 hours. Many people give up sleep to make room for work and leisure. An adequate amount of sleep is as important as an adequate amount of exercise. Sleeping is not a sin.

Rational thinking will help with sleep

Insomnia is often caused by our thoughts and behaviours, habits and routines. In addition to looking at our sleep routines and habits we also need to look at our thoughts and beliefs about sleep. If our thoughts keep us awake they can also help us to sleep. People with insomnia will often have negative thoughts about sleep, such as 'I didn't sleep a wink last night', 'I dread going to bed', 'I must have eight hours sleep or I am damaging my health'. These thoughts are unlikely to help anyone to sleep better as they increase stress and worry. When we think more rationally about insomnia and avoid distortions and exaggerations then, the mind and body are more calm, relaxed and ready for sleep. We can talk and think ourselves into looking forward to lying down, relaxing, switching-off for a while, being warm, being comfortable. Rest is good and from there it is one beautiful, small step to sleep.

Mental Health

At some stage it must have been convenient to distinguish between physical and mental health and it's still easy to go along with this differentiation. There seems to be some sort of implied understanding as to which is which. Some symptoms and conditions fit conveniently into physical health and some into mental health. Fortunately we now also appreciate that both have everything to do with each other. How we think and how we feel affects how our body functions and what we can do – and how we are and what we are doing affects how we think and how we feel. What we do can change our chemistry and what we think can change our chemistry. Just looking at a list of symptoms or conditions easily demonstrates that there are no boundaries between physical and mental health: fatigue, anxiety, mood swings, panic attacks, ADHD, autism, neurological disorders, depression, eating disorders, obesity, self-harming, paranoia, psychoses, schizophrenia, inferiority, superiority or dominant complexes, concentration, performance, addictions, dementia, cardio-vascular disease, immune deficiencies, diabetes, cancer, arthritis, sleep problems, pain. Very few conditions are purely physical or mental – most are both.

In this chapter I've discussed a few of the everyday aspects of and influences on mental health. We can be very easily affected by many things. How we cope will depend on how we are, how much support we have, what the problems and threats are – and knowing what we can do about them.

In mental health as in physical health, some of us will be pre-disposed to some symptoms and conditions and some to others. Physically, health challenges can manifest themselves as allergies and sensitivities, heart, cardio-vascular, skin, liver, stomach conditions, muscles or joint disease, inflammation and so on – and mental health challenges may be stress, depression, eating disorders, anxiety, panic attacks, mental or nervous breakdown, psychoses, mood swings, dominance, vulnerability or inferiority.

Our health, mental and physical, depends on nutrients, chemical balances and energy. Circumstances impose some conditions on us and others develop from how we are. We can change our make-up. We can make it less likely to have some of these problems – and we can make ourselves more susceptible to them. We can protect against things. This will either make it less likely for conditions to arise or develop – or easier to cope and resolve them when they do. We can also increase our understanding and awareness to look after ourselves and others, preventing serious illness – as well as the care and treatment for it.

Things that affect our physical health, affect our mental health: coffee, alcohol, drugs, glucose, stress, music, exercise. Life affects how we are and how we feel – it affects the environment we provide for the brain and the body. What we do and our physical, emotional and mental health are influenced by just about everything that we encounter and experience.

Slow pace of life can send some people round the bend, a fast pace of life will do the same for others. Challenges and threats motivate some people who immediately want to rise to them and succeed – other people will feel intimidated and overwhelmed and want to withdraw. Both are perfectly good and rational responses but will be helpful and appropriate in different situations. In between is the wonderful world of indecision and 'I don't know what to do'. Balance and coping and adjustment are critical – the fine-tuning mechanisms that constantly need to identify, manage and rebalance – everything.

That we do manage and can make these adaptations is in itself quite marvellous. It isn't that surprising that sometimes there'll be different or peculiar reactions.

In the same way that many aspects of life have changed dramatically in the last 50-100 years, a very short span in the scheme of things, the experiences of modern life have changed in extreme ways. We have completely transformed how we live, what we do and all the general apparatus and equipment of our days and weeks. New things have developed at a very rapid pace and gone from being new and extraordinary to being everyday, ordinary, accepted parts of our lives; lighting, heating, cars, 'phones, televisions, computers, endless technology, inventions, discoveries, machines, gadgets, possibilities and aspirations. Our places of work and leisure, business practice, management models and techniques, politics, economics, population, housing and transport have all seen extraordinary change and development and take up a greater part of our lives. Very few lives can be free from bewildering administration, finance, insurance, tax, rules and regulations, legislation and legal matters – all requiring us to learn systems and procedures – all with aspects beyond our control. We have to take part in a vast puzzle with an awful lot of rule books. No one is in charge, there is no one point of reference – but it's not optional, we have to play whether we want to or not.

Many people now live in fast-moving, changing, transient neighbourhoods and communities. Communication has broken countless boundaries. We have, and are assumed to be comfortable with, artificially lengthened days, extensive travel, mobile 'phones, e-mail, instant and 24 hour news and information. We have a lot to deal with, a lot is expected of us. Whatever we think our day may hold at the start, can change numerous times. That may be exciting and stimulating and it may be bewildering and overwhelming. Some of us can keep up, some of us can't. We may keep up for a while then start to struggle. Some can keep up with some things but not everything. Some things make sense and we can understand, others don't. Some things suit us, others don't. Whilst we cope and adapt to everything we need to do, things are fine – but if we hit snags, it will have different consequences for different people, in different ways. This is always likely to be the case because we aren't all the same. We have different reactions, different natures and characteristics and different circumstances. Our coping ability will also differ from one day to another. Depending on recent events, general mood, weather and a host of conditions, how we feel and how well we cope can vary enormously. Something that wouldn't cause a problem one day can affect us quite seriously another. Sometimes we'll know why and sometimes we won't. Some people adore going out, they adore the buzz and the stimulus – unfazed by challenges, competition and diverse expectations. It's also true that for many people, the thing they want and long for most when they wake in the morning – is the end of the day – when it's all over and when they are in and safe – when the onslaught subsides, just for a while.

Most of the easily accessible information on mental health starts by emphasizing how normal and commonplace several conditions are. These are various pieces of work published for various reasons. There aren't neat, comparative statistics across ages, genders and countries – but there are endless examples to show that many mental health conditions affect a lot of people.

According to the World Health Organisation, 1 in 10 people suffer from a mental health problem at any one time and 1 in 4 people will suffer mental health problems at some time in their life.

1 in 6 children in the UK has special educational needs; 1 in 3 has behaviour, attention or learning problems; 1 in 86 has autism.

In the UK depression affects 1 in 5 of us. Apparently 1 in 10 women in the US is on anti-depressants and 1 in 4 in Spain.

In a year, 3 out of 10 employees in the UK can typically have mental health problems, the most common being depression – and depression is cited as the cause of 70% of recorded suicides. Depression is estimated at costing England and Wales £8m a year in lost productivity.

350,000 elderly people a year are diagnosed with cognitive impairment and 185,000 with dementia – that's 500 people a day – in the UK.

Each year we prescribe 532 million tranquilizers, 463 million sleeping pills, 823 million anti-depressants and a myriad other drugs for mental health treatment and management.

A lot of health care has evolved focusing on the treatment and care needed for many of the symptoms and conditions – but the treatment and care is only half the story. The same focus needs to be given to the prevention of these conditions. We can slow the rate at which these symptoms and many degenerative diseases occur and develop. Looking after health and mental health is something we can do.

The benefits are good levels for mood, motivation, memory, concentration and IQ – and greatly reduced risks and implications of depression, stress, autism, psychoses and other conditions.

Memory is a good example of how nutrition, anatomy and physiology, lifestyle and personal behaviour all come together and how our brains work. It is also a subject frequently referred to by people concerned about their mental health and often one of the things we notice playing up if tired or stressed or anxious – or growing older.

Memories are stored over a network of brain cells. They aren't all in one large, super brain cell or cluster. We don't have a one-stop memory bank. The memory isn't stored as one chunk but in lots of different pieces, like a jig-saw – that has to be reassembled. To access and recall those memories the system has to work. Different cells of the brain have to co-operate in a joint effort. The best way to keep the system working well is good exercise and stimulation: informative reading and listening, quizzes, research, conversation and debate, planning, thinking things through, creative skills, learning new things, new challenges, original ideas, humour. With good use, the brain cell connections stay healthy and we grow new connections. In benign conditions lots of little, happy connections are made and our brain can build the information we need – we remember the right words to use, we remember how we have done things before, we remember who people are and their names, where things are that we need and what we're supposed to be doing. We remember that if we get flustered the best thing to do is calm down or take practical, logical action. If we inflict adverse conditions of tiredness or stress, the opposite happens. The connections don't work properly. The brain can either just seem to seize up and not want to work at all, hit a blank; or work poorly and slowly and make mistakes; or create some sort of improvised chaos. In stress conditions the excess cortisol can literally cause the connections to shrivel. We can force the brain to keep going, to keep on thinking and that may be successful – but this will normally only be for the short to medium term and probably happening over less connections, what is, in affect, a reducing capacity. We'll be trying to process the same or more workload over a decreasing network.

Homocysteine (see page 117) and other chemicals we introduce or create in different circumstances, will also cause damage and destroy cells in the brain.

Memories have features, associations, the most common being what we saw, heard or how we felt/acted – visual, auditory and kinaesthetic. There is also taste and smell – our memories are linked to our senses. These are the pathways by which the memory enters the brain cells and part of the reason why different parts of a memory go to different places. The stronger those associations are and the more of them there are – helps to make it easier to recall them and reuse that information. The more pathways that are used, the more brain cells there are collaborating to restore and recreate the memory. Quite often when we are trying to remember something, we might say something to the effect of, 'Oh, I can just see it now . . . ' – so a part of the memory is flickering into life and we just need the rest of the pieces to fall into place.

If a memory is linked to something we saw written down and we also say it out loud, or sing it, make a rhyme or a song about it, tell it to someone else and we copy it by writing it out or making a picture of it – we are increasing the chances of recall. We are increasing the number of links. We have seen it, heard it and done something with it – we have increased the associations and the sensory pathways connected to it. When we want to remember a conversation, we often think of where we were and when and any other clues associated with that conversation. We all have different styles and preferences for this kind of learning and memory. Some people are particularly strong visually, so the words, or numbers, or sights that they saw will have most influence. Some people are particularly strong on auditory signals and will be most influenced by what they heard, what they were listening to. Some people are particularly strong kinaesthetically and will remember their involvement, the part they played in something and what they felt like. And there is every mixture and combination of those three, plus the other senses. This is why we all learn differently as well. Some of us will want to read about things, others will want pictures and diagrams, others will want to listen to lectures or recorded media material, others will want to do experiments, scribble on flipcharts and whiteboards – feel our way through whatever it is. It's why we teach children numbers by speech and rhymes and by drawing the numbers and writing out the sums and having counters, beans or shells to touch and move to demonstrate as well.

And it's why our memories are prompted by different things, a particular landscape or picture, voice, piece of music, aroma of baking bread, the smell of the sea, a familiar perfume. Some of those associations rebuild a memory without us even thinking about it – without us even trying to remember. We see that image, hear that noise or smell that smell and immediately a particular memory will spring to mind. Sometimes we have difficulty getting the memory to work – and other times it just happens without any conscious thought at all. This is a simple demonstration of how easy it can be for the brain to work, for the connections to be made and the signals sent or how even minor things can disrupt those processes – given certain conditions.

Stage plays and concerts are wonderful examples of storing and processing information whether we remember the play or the concert because of the stage and the scene and the costumes; the speeches, voices and music; or the event – the getting ready to go out, the anticipation, the meeting people, the atmosphere, the experience, what happened. It will depend on us and how we are as individuals, which of those associations are strongest and the extremely powerful combination of all of them together.

Acetylcholine is the key memory neuro-transmitter. Our memories exist, they are there but to access and retrieve them we need happy, healthy neuro-transmitters. It's believed that one of the problems of Alzheimer's is the hippocampus of the brain being unable to file memories. People with Alzheimer's typically have low acetylcholine. A deficiency in acetylcholine stops us being able to connect the different pieces of a memory together to form the whole memory, including remembering words we have used most of our lives and faces we have known for years.

For our thought processes and the memory to work well the brain needs its nutrients, it needs us to keep calm, for us to breathe to supply oxygen and it needs the mental exercise to keep the system working.

To help the brain generally, to help in times of stress or depression and to help struggling memories, we can exercise the brain cells by making and re-learning patterns – doing things we know, things we know we will get right. It feels good because we did it and got it right. It makes a pattern and imprints that pattern. Brains like patterns and repetition. We can do something easy, get it right, feel good – and do it again and feel good again. The feeling good bit is important – the brain likes that bit. The brain is like a muscle and if it is exercised and not abused, it will usually work well; if it is tensed or stunned or bombarded it can't think straight. It likes praise and recognition. Tell it how clever and wonderful it is. Then do it again. Doing simple, straightforward things we are likely to get right, is a fairly close parallel to the 'displacement activity' in Stress (page 158). When we are over-faced by difficult things, or anything and everything, it is very tempting to do something really simple, something easy that we know we can do – rearranging the CDs, playing with the paperclips, shuffling papers, chatting to someone on the 'phone or going out for a drive for no other reason, even some washing up or vacuuming or cleaning the kitchen cupboards. We may have crushing, urgent priorities or a hideously long list of things that need doing and instead of doing them, we'll find almost anything else to do instead. The brain is just preferring to operate in an alternative mode or automatic pilot rather than do some more thinking, working and reasoning. At that point we also have to manage the choices and the balance. Do we let that natural tendency dictate what happens, or do we step back in and impose some structure? Are we going to be passive to some mental down time, or do we need to be active and guide the thought process and activity back on track? and how do we know which choice to make? We probably do know but the healthy decision may not be the same as the life-situation decision – and anyway, all this means that there is another decision to be taken. It's easy to understand why the brain can reach a point of confusion, non-co-operation, or chaos. We need to keep a sort of balance sheet in our lives, clocking up when and why we've tasked the brain to keep going when it wanted a rest and then paying back with the rest next time we can. If we borrow brain time and keep going – and then think we feel fine so there is no need to pay back – we can just rack up a large mental debt. At some stage, that debt can be called in and may be with interest. The rest or reprieve doesn't have to be lying down in a darkened room. Changing activity, giving one set of brain cells a rest and using some others, is often all it takes. This is definitely where physical exercise can play a valuable role, completely changing the focus from study, or paperwork, or intellectual challenges to activity, different stimulus and change in environment – so long as we are mindful of energy levels. Changing the push from mental activity to physical activity, if we are tired or exhausted, won't pay back the debt – we are borrowing from the same pot. Then, a stroll, or some undemanding company and conversation, or complete relaxation is going to give a better chance of recharging the battery.

The use of going out for a drive as a coping mechanism is interesting and it seems to be a popular reaction. Lots of people use driving as a sort of mental buffer – perhaps there is something about covering distance physically that gives some more space mentally. Walking we can usually choose whether we are escaping or thinking about things. With driving we can't afford to switch off, we have to concentrate – so we are either switching focus, escaping from whatever it is, to the driving, which will achieve some respite – or we are daydreaming, or pre-occupied which clearly has serious dangers of its own. It's really important to be aware of our mental state – the problem being that the more affected we are – the less we may know it or be prepared to acknowledge it.

A lot of our mental health is influenced by voices, including our own. We need those voices to be positive and constructive. If we have critical voices in our head which tell us how daft, or useless we are – we need to replace them with nice voices telling us how gorgeous and clever we are and run that message a few times. It makes the brain feel good – it relaxes and soothes and then funnily enough it's more able to work properly and think straight. There's a world of difference between; 'You stupid individual, now what have you done?' and 'Now, come on gorgeous, I love you to bits and you know we can do this'. One can lock and disable the brain – the other can relax it and enable it. We have to be aware of these conditions in looking after ourselves and looking after other people. Anyone can need help. It may be us and it may be someone else.

Impatience, intolerance, frustration and anxiety do tend to work in spirals and once we start getting cross, instead of solving it at stage 1, we can easily manifest things into something debilitating. This will compromise all our mental faculties, not just memory. A spike of acute stress to respond to something urgently will normally bring increased clarity of thinking – but sustained stress, tiredness or depression will blur and obstruct thoughts and mental acuity.

Higher cortisol can result in worse memory – and worse memory will cause increased frustration, anger and impatience.

Stress impairs the memory because of the raised cortisol levels and the areas of the brain responsible for learning and memory can actually reduce in size. A deliberate ambition to work like crazy to achieve an early retirement or early career change, if under increased stress levels, may achieve your aims but you may end up with less of the brain you started with. The good news is that the connections, the brain cells and dendrites and synapses do grow back and recover when the cortisol levels are reduced – although that will be dependent on the amount of damage and the circumstances of recovery – relaxation, help and support.

Stress also disrupts blood sugar balance which can blunt memory and alertness and lead to brain damage.

Cortisol levels are usually found to be high in Alzheimer's patients and the levels reflect the severity of the condition.

Alcohol can be a significant threat to mental health, clarity, memory, mood and ability. The liver will detoxify the initial amounts of alcohol detected in the body but once it has detoxified what it can, any more alcohol absorbed will reach the brain and disrupt the normal communication signals. That's why many people like and desire that feeling – it unhinges memory and blunts some senses, feelings and emotions so that worries can be dimmed or forgotten and we can escape reality. It can also create havoc and heighten other senses and emotions, so that sense, logic and reason are dimmed and anger and emotion and bravado artificially boosted. The constant mechanisms we take for granted, balance and co-ordination are disabled – the connections can't connect. The excess alcohol will also dissolve the fatty acids which form the most part of the brain and the fatty tissue which coats all the cells and nerves, it will block the conversion and production of those fats and destroy the essential vitamins.

There are all sorts of other stimulants that can interfere with brain function – tea, coffee, sugar, cigarettes, drugs and performance products.

Intake of sugar, in its common refined form, either as spoons of sugar or in sweets, biscuits, cakes, puddings and numerous food products, immediately affects blood sugar levels. Each time we have to rely on our insulin to come to the rescue and restore safe levels (pages 62 and 135). After the intake of the glucose raises the levels abnormally high, the correction will then typically drop the levels abnormally low. The disruption of random high and low blood sugar can cause fatigue, irritability, increased perspiration, poor concentration, forgetfulness – depression, emotional episodes and crying, digestive problems and dizziness. The digestion of the glucose also requires B vitamins, which can leave us deficient in B vitamins, which are needed for good mental performance. Sugar consumption is linked to aggression, anxiety, hyperactivity, attention deficit, eating disorders, learning difficulties, depression and fatigue.

There is no set of tables for who can eat what – we are all affected but some more than others and our tolerance levels will be changed by time, health and what else is happening.

Blood sugar affects behaviour and mental processes. Studies have shown direct links to blood sugar balance and habitual offenders. Juvenile offenders who took part in a reduced sugar experiment showed a 44% reduction in anti-social behaviour. Higher levels of refined carbohydrates are also linked to low IQ.

The high levels of blood glucose associated with diabetes can cause nerve, eye and brain damage. High blood glucose levels can damage nerve cells and stop them working properly and slow communication. Depression is prevalent in people with diabetes.

The brain likes constant, steady, stable levels of blood sugar. After eating something sugary and the level rising too high and the correction often taking the sugar level too low, we can have a roller-coaster effect going on. When the level falls too low, we can bring it back up again either by another sugar fix, or by releasing our own adrenalin and cortisol, which could be from a stress reaction, some anxiety – or from a stimulant, tea, coffee, chocolate, a cigarette, alcohol, etc. This can easily create a sugar, stimulant, stress circle, which can, in turn, become a stress, tiredness and depression loop. Artificially raised blood sugar does give for abnormal lows which we can experience as flat moods or low energy, often first thing in the morning but at any time during the day. At that point we can reach for something as a jump start, which might be coffee or sugar – or it may be adrenalin triggered by the worry (sudden panic) about lateness, or workload, or lack of performance. There are quite marked comparisons between stable, sustained blood sugar, energy and mood and the highs and lows of the roller-coaster which is more difficult to manage, tiring and fertile ground for mistakes and confusion.

The usual tips on nutrition apply to manage blood sugar: wholegrains, soya yogurts, fruit, seeds, nuts, pulses and beans – and avoiding processed, low-nutrient food, additives, high sugar, salt and fats – and it isn't good to go too long without food and skip meals. Regular meals help maintain blood sugar – and vitamins and minerals help maintain blood sugar and appetite.

Coffee/caffeine is addictive, even in quite small amounts which is why we like it so much. Having a coffee appeals because we like the taste and/or it makes us feel better. Not having a coffee may mean drowsiness, headache, low mood or fatigue. Strictly, these aren't how we feel if we don't have coffee – but they are coffee withdrawal symptoms – so if we have another coffee, they go away. The drowsiness, headache, low mood and fatigue aren't so much health deficiency as coffee management syndrome. Having regular or frequent coffees, we are giving our brain and our body a fairly strong stimulant, beginning to experience the withdrawal symptoms and having another shot. That's quite a lot of chemistry going on, all of which involves more effort and energy expenditure.

Caffeine blocks receptors in the brain that naturally control adrenalin and dopamine. With that control blocked, the levels rise and we feel more alert, about 30 minutes after the coffee. The more we do that, the more we depend on it but we are consequently forcing the body to produce more adrenalin and dopamine, which leads to adrenal exhaustion. Adrenalin and dopamine are our natural stimulants for motivation and communication, so we are not only depending on artificial stimulants, we are exhausting and damaging our own. We can experience this as apathy, depression, exhaustion and inability to cope.

We may often not be having a coffee because we want one, because we like the effect of coffee – but because we are managing coffee dependency symptoms. The feel-good experience we like and associate with coffee is how we'd feel if we didn't use coffee. A coffee fix lasts 30-60 minutes; being non-coffee-dependent lasts all day – and the next one – and the next one.

To test the affects coffee has on us – if you give up caffeine for 3 or 4 months and then have a large, strong, real coffee – you will probably get the shakes, a slight fluttery feeling, even palpitations. That is the impact coffee has. It is a strong stimulant. When we are used to it, we don't notice that to the same extent – but that is still what is happening.

Caffeine is in several drinks and products. Our first line of therapy for many things is a tea or a coffee and it's very nice and it's sociable – but we need to try to balance this with tea and coffee/stimulant-free times – experience reality. Let the body sort its chemistry out, get back on an even keel – let the natural mechanisms operate and maintain good working order. If we keep interfering with how the body functions, we can cause short and long term disruption. If we are dependent on caffeine and we reduce or remove it, energy level and performance can be a bit wobbly for a week and we may even be physically shakey, a fairly clear message in itself – but after that time energy levels and performance should recover and to higher than they were – and the shakes go away. We have to remember that the caffeine is also in cola and energy drinks, along with sugar, colourings, additives and stimulants. (See example caffeine table on page 130).

The plus side of reducing or almost eliminating coffee and tea, is that they then become luxurious indulgences rather than things we regularly depend on - and they become really special. We tend to take coffee and tea for granted - there are a lot of part-drunk or wasted cups of tea and coffee in the world. We literally don't think about it. We are making and drinking tea and coffee by sub-conscious reflex. Chocolate cravings also reduce after about a month if we cut down or remove it from regular intake - and again, it becomes a treat, something special, rather than downgrading it to everyday predictability.

The brain loves lovely, refreshing, clear water. It is 85% water and constantly uses lots of water. Alcohol, tea and coffee, medicines, many additives and other foodstuffs are diuretics and can easily cause dehydration.

Another hormone linked to stress is DHEA (dehydroepiandrosterone). When it's working well it's nick-named the anti-ageing hormone. It maintains mineral balance; manages building lean body mass, reducing fat tissue; manages the production of sex hormones; aids memory; controls stress and guards against depression. Our DHEA levels decline naturally after age 20 but this reduction is exaggerated in states of prolonged stress. DHEA is used as a supplement and can be effective to help improve memory and reduce depression. As with most supplementation it works in combination with other hormones, vitamins and minerals. It isn't an easy, miracle cure in a bottle and only part of a bigger picture so would form part of a professional diagnosis and treatment with qualified advisers and practitioners.

There are several pollutants in our everyday lives. In our foods and homes and communities we meet aluminium, lead, cadmium, mercury, copper, tartrazine and cocktails of chemicals, detergents, fertilizers and pesticides. The best defence is to try and keep intake and absorption as low as possible and to take lots of nutrients, good vitamins and minerals and water on board. Many of the things we come into contact with the most, are assured to be at safe levels but we are the only people who know about our own cumulative effect, the cocktail. It is quite easy to consume or absorb a gallon of chemicals a year just sprayed onto our food. If we know levels of some hazards are high, we can try and avoid others to compensate. A lot of health care is a contract with ourselves - being aware of the positives and negatives and doing deals, managing them.

If we've spent time in a busy place with above average traffic or pollution - have a day in the fresh air. If we've had a day with not the most balanced diet, heavy on some of the foods it's normally best to avoid - make a point of having a few days without them, treat ourselves to the good, clean, fresh stuff. If we've had a day with a little too much alcohol – have a few days without. If we've been overdoing it, try and take some time out, rest, relax, recoup.

As the activity and ability of the brain depends so crucially on the nutrients and environment provided for it – what we eat and our lifestyle have everything to do with our mental health. What we consume and how we live have a direct affect on intelligence, mental acuity, memory, concentration, emotional balance, stress, depression, happiness – fatigue, anxiety, sleeping problems, mood swings, psychoses, schizophrenia, suicide or addictions.

Maintaining a healthy, stable environment for our brain and our body directly affects our mental health. We can prevent disorders by looking after our health and we can also treat and overcome disorders.

Patrick Holford's book 'New Optimum Nutrition for the Mind' covers this in careful, clear, detail and is firmly endorsed by André Tylee, Professor of Primary Care Mental Health at the Institute of Psychiatry, King's College, London; Professor David Smith, Division of Medical Services, University of Oxford; and Hyla Cass, Professor of Psychiatry, UCLA School of Medicine. There are comprehensive chapters on improving IQ, memory, mood and digestion – and detailed information on hormone imbalances, mood swings, stress, sleep problems, energy levels, depression, mental health of the young and old, addiction and a great deal more (430+ informative, thoroughly researched pages).

Our environment, our circumstances and our food all affect our chemistry.

Eating good food has been proved to affect IQ, mood, emotional stability and memory.

The body and brain are made entirely of molecules from food so we cannot help but be affected by what we consume and its ingredients. Our thoughts and our mental energy operate across brain cells which depend on the right supply of vital nutrients. They can't exist and can't work properly without them. When we experience problems, we can try to correct them with intervention of medicines on top of the existing chemical cocktail – or we can provide what we need to be at our best and re-adjust the environment to reduce the agents that obstruct and compromise function. Poor nutrition equals chemical imbalances and most physiological and mental illnesses are caused by chemical imbalance. Psychologically we can provide support and help and bring about changes, which will affect and improve the chemical status but we have to eat EFAs and minerals and vitamins. We can't take them in in conversation. It's quite possible that there are many people who operate below their potential or experience more problems than they need to – and nutrients and lifestyle can improve or solve this, often without drugs and without their side-effects. If further treatments are still necessary, they can then be based on knowing that the best balance and environment has been established – which will clarify what the problems may be and simplify what may be needed, plus making the treatment more effective and possibly more successful.

Crucially we need to provide 5 brain foods in our diet. Glucose, the fuel; EFAs that keep the brain lubricated; phospholipids, known as the memory facilitator and which coat the neurons, the brain cells, allowing the transmission of all the signals; amino acids, the messengers; and the fine-tuning nutrients, the vitamins and minerals.

Our thoughts and all our instructions are ripples across the network of intricate nerve tissue and nerve-endings, eg: serotonin to keep us happy, or help mental and physical performance, or adrenalin and dopamine to keep us motivated. The signals, the neuro-transmitters, made of amino acids, hop from one neuron to another, over the gaps, the synapses. For the amino acids to become neuro-transmitters they require enzymes, again dependent on nutrients. Neuro-transmitters are what programme us to be happy, depressed, motivated, disinterested, have energy or lack energy. They are released from one neuron and cross the synapse to take the message to the next neuron, electrical impulses that are released and then reabsorbed and used again or broken down and destroyed. Millions of these tiny connections and explosions are going on all the time – the communication system beyond anything we can imagine – every fraction of every thought built, sent and dispersed – rather like millions of relay races all going on at once, in different directions and our lovely brain cells trying very hard not to drop the batons.

The digestive system contains 100 million neurons and produces as many neuro-transmitters as the brain. Two thirds of our serotonin is produced in the gut. Our digestive system and brain are in constant communication.

Eating a good breakfast can give you a great start and set you up for the day. This helps children to be able to concentrate at school, behave well and enjoy themselves. For adults it will help with concentration, mood, energy and performance. A general guide for best brain fuel would be low glycaemic-load (slow-release) carbohydrates and good amino acids – typically: wholegrains of rice, oats, millet – fresh fruit, nuts, seeds, beans, pulses and vegetables. This ensures good nutrients for the brain and avoids things that obstruct the nutrients, eg: sugar, alcohol, stimulants and oxidants – trans-fats and pollution. It is important to include the good fats and minimize or eliminate the bad fats. The brain tissue is more than half fat and the fat we eat directly affects the fat tissues of the brain.

Serotonin and melatonin, amongst others, are made from tryptophan – from nuts, seeds, bananas, soya, eggs, fish, chicken and turkey. All the amino acids are from protein sources; grains, pulses, beans, nuts, seeds, fish, eggs and meat.

Two thirds of a typical western diet can be fat, sugar and refined flour, especially from processed foods and snacks. If these foods make up so much of a daily food intake, it is impossible, in the rest of our food, to take on board the nutrients we need. The sort of foods we need are referred to as vital, life-giving – and the others as non-vital. Whole foods are vital food sources, they haven't had too much done to them and are full of goodness. Refined and processed foods are largely non-vital. They have been through so much, they don't/can't offer the same nutrition – they haven't got any or much vitality left.

We have also invented 10 million new chemicals – they are all around us, in and on our food, detergents and preparations we use in the house and garden, hygiene products and cosmetics, the water we drink and the air we breathe. In addition to what we eat there are several ways that we can affect the intricate balance of our chemical make-up.

As well as the meals we may immediately think of, we also consume, per week, 1.5 billion caffeinated drinks in tea, coffee and colas; 6 million kilos of sugar; 2 million kilos of chocolate; 1.5 billion cigarettes, 120 million alcoholic drinks; 10 million cannabis joints: plus the 532 million tranquilizers, 463 million sleeping pills and 823 million anti-depressants prescribed per year. That's an awful lot of chemistry.

On top of the physiological symptoms and difficulties from mental health conditions – there is one characteristic that comes into a class of its own – stigma. However widespread and normal these conditions are – they have accrued the most almighty stigma. Many mental conditions are perfectly explicable and rational reactions to different threats and circumstances – but we have categorized them as abnormal. Despite how common they are, we have to hide them and deny them or risk severe misunderstanding, prejudice, discrimination, condescension and patronisation. As various conditions become better understood and the extent of the reality becomes known, this is something that is improving. It has received valuable help from well known, respected people speaking about personal experiences, sharing views and supporting what needs to be in place to help understanding.

One example of this is that 'Time to Change' led by Mind and evaluated by the Institute of Psychiatry, King's College, London, has been set up specifically to deal with ending the discrimination surrounding mental health.

In 2006 Stephen Fry made a documentary called 'The Secret Life of the Manic Depressive' talking openly about bi-polar disorder and its affects on his life. He graphically described the implications and almost impossible conditions that come with it, including low self-worth and suicidal thoughts and intentions. This was a rare opportunity to hear and see the experiences of someone talking about a condition lived with since school days and culminating in a very dramatic and public event in 1995, 20-30 years later.

Towards the end of 2008 Alastair Campbell also made a documentary, called 'Cracking Up'. He gave a very real and vivid insight into breakdown and all that goes with it. In 1986 Alastair Campbell, in his own words, 'cracked up' as a result of months, if not years, of intensive stress, alcohol and all the associated complexities of public, political, media, working and family life. He made and screened this documentary, 22 years later.

Whatever our personal or political views, both these people clearly come into the category of exceptional achievement. Mental health conditions can occur for anyone, anytime, they don't discriminate. They can affect clever, capable, successful people and less able and vulnerable people. They can also be treated and overcome. The correct understanding of the condition and circumstances, the right treatment and crucially support, are the key elements of successful recovery and/or management. Some conditions won't necessarily go away completely and may recur or we may be prone to them but being aware of symptoms, early warning signs, parameters and having strategies in place, means we can live and make the most of life – especially knowing that it is a human condition, not some kind of dreadful curse that means we have to be locked away in a tower.

For many of us, it will be true that we don't have to have many of these conditions or, if we do, can overcome them more easily than we may think.

Numerous geniuses in the worlds of art, science, music, invention, writing and humour, people from all walks of life and world leaders are known to have, or have had, different forms of depression, breakdown and madness: van Gough, Einstein, Spike Milligan, Peter Sellers, Buzz Aldrin, Beethoven, Tchaikovsky, Mozart, Winston Churchill, Eric Clapton, Patricia Cornwell, Vivien Leigh, Frances Ford Coppola, Michelangelo, Picasso, Nelson, Napoleon, Christopher Columbus, Mao Tse-Tung, Robert Burns, Oscar Wilde, Peter Cook, Isaac Newton, Charles Darwin. We all have our moments.

We can also be affected by lack of daylight, now called Seasonal Affective Disorder (SAD). The weather is another good demonstration of how we are all different. Although there is a fairly strong consensus about enjoying warmth and sunshine, there are different preferences for all sorts of weather; cool, hot, breezes, calm, windy, rain and storms. SAD is thought to be the limited daylight disrupting the circadian rhythm. This would be particularly noticeable in the months of the year when we get up and go out in the dark and make our journey home in the dark, often spending a lot of the day out of the daylight as well.

Good diet, nutrients and vitamins, exercise and including daylight where possible, help to reduce the depression. Exercise, including walking and gardening, releases the hormones and neuro-transmitters that help lift the mood, reduce stress and improve our sense of purpose and self-esteem. Company and interaction also usually alleviate these conditions and conversely isolation can amplify them.

It can be difficult coming out of strong, limiting moods and psychological states. It is very frequently time when we want to be alone. It may be important to be alone, it may be important to switch off but keeping people away is typically a symptom rather than a reaction and one that can worsen and deepen the problem, rather than help. All too often it is nearest and dearest that are shunned or given a hard time – and they are just the people we are likely to need. It is another of life's ironies that when we need people and we need help – we reject them and turn away. When we need help, we shut people out. When we are cold we don't want to move around which will help us get warm, we sit and shudder. When we aren't supposed to scratch a scar, it itches like hell. Just when everything starts to fall apart and we need help – we can go into states of denial, refuse help offered to us, or are simply unable to ask for help or know what we need. We can deliberately, consciously say and do things we know will make the situation worse. It's part of the madness. We may shout at people, walk out, be dramatic, self-harm, not eat, binge, take drugs or alcohol. It may be loss of control, it may be seeking attention, it may be cries for help – it could be all manner of things, just a way of dealing with the situation, there and then – telling someone we desperately need, to get lost.

Whether we ever expect to need it or not, it's important to identify our support network; friends, family, colleagues, professionals – so that we know who is there. Companionship and support are invaluable throughout life and safeguard our physical and mental health. Isolation often leaves us more vulnerable to mental health problems and can make them more exaggerated when they do happen and more difficult to overcome. If for whatever reason you don't think you have a personal support network, you can build one. There are groups and organisations which will act as first points of contact and from where you can gradually put things in place. For many people that will be the GP, who should also have access to a range of different treatments, therapies and referrals – but sometimes anonymity will be important or we just aren't ready or brave enough to go to the GP. We need to find a way of knowing what to do and how. That is where conversations with trusted friends or professionally run helplines can establish the first few steps. The initial acknowledgement of what is happening and deciding to do something about it are the all-important key.

We are all subjects of our psychological environment – who we are, who we're with, what we do. In the last 50 years our experience of time and space has fundamentally changed.

As well as technological advance there is complete cultural change. Our culture and our life is exposed to a vast array of other cultures and lives and vice versa. Small, protected, known environments have evolved into completely open, merged, diverse environments with new and strange experiences, extended opportunities, attractions, bewilderment, threats and risks. With so much new to cope with, strong and fragile individuals and communities can struggle to survive. We need a combination of physical health, nutrition and psychological support.

A good, healthy, psychological environment also includes a base, a home, a safe place and respect - respect from others - but very importantly our respect for ourselves.

Counselling and help is a very individual thing and highly dependent on who we work with. The wrong help or counsellor can make things worse and the right help and counselling can be wonderful. The difficulty is that when we are stressed or experiencing difficulty, we are often less able to take the right decisions for ourselves, judgement can be affected and we can be very vulnerable. Just at a time we need to make important assessments and arrangements for ourselves - we may be least able to do that. Friends, family and good, reliable referrals and recommendations will often be the best safeguards - but we also have to know for ourselves whether something is working and helpful, or not. There are lots of people more than happy to take our money. It's hard to be clear-thinking and have your wits about you when you don't know what day it is. There are a range of organisations that can advise and can provide crucial support and treatment to restore health and a more stable psychological environment. We can be lucky and find the right solutions quickly and easily and it can also be a maze. It's not easy to be strong and keep making our way through when very debilitated to start with - but the organisations that can help are impartial, used to nearly every condition we are battling with and trying to describe - and exist to provide the benefit of experience. No one is ever completely alone - there is a helpline out there for all of us - it's just finding the right one. The importance of personal support really cannot be overestimated.

Ideally the personal support network will be made up of people who can understand - plus others who will need to know and if they don't understand are prepared to try - and this will typically include those very closest to us. For a partner, family member or friend to understand what someone is going through will involve patience and information. We need people to understand. Finding pieces of work which have been produced - books, fact sheets, articles, pamphlets - on stress, depression, eating disorders, panic attacks or breakdowns, things that give good, researched, objective descriptions, can be a way of letting other people know, giving them information and helping them live with the symptoms and treatment too. There is a book 'Living with a BLACK DOG' by Matthew and Ainsley Johnstone, which is a great example of this. Many partners and close friends may find it difficult to appreciate all the different aspects of what someone is experiencing and how it affects them, or not know what they can do – or think that they do know what to do and get it completely wrong. Third party accounts, written to help others understand, give a safe point of reference for everyone.

Many states of anxiety, stress, chaos or depression are accompanied by something that I call the death-wish – either knowingly or unknowingly we do things that can only make the situation worse. It's also fairly common to expect people around us to notice that something is wrong, even what it is and what to do about it. We expect a magnificent level of telepathy – possibly from people who have never demonstrated these extraordinary powers of telepathy before. If we are given more and more to do when our workload is impossible – we think someone will notice and rescue us. If we keep turning down invitations and stay in and become tired, nervous or withdrawn – we think someone will notice and help. Sometimes they may – but for the most part – no, they won't. If people do something that upsets us or shows a complete lack of understanding, perhaps over and over again, they may be being hurtful, or it may be that they just don't have a clue. This is a sure sign of the madness – when we know what is wrong and let it get worse and think it is everyone else's fault because they haven't realized.

How we live our lives does change our chemistry.

We also have a lot of innate intelligence and information. We have information systems running throughout the body. When they are working well they know what we need and how to look after us – but modern life has a tendency to overrule them, blur them, mask them or shut them out. There is quite a lot of guidance going on inside as to who we should spend time with, whether it is a good idea to do something, whether we are wary, frightened, feeling good, tired, in the right job, ignoring things that are important to us or need to make changes. Our bodies are often trying to tell us things. Habit and conditioning and lack of time to think can cancel out all that personal, bespoke wisdom. Taking time to listen and access that inner wisdom makes a difference. Many successful people just naturally have great access to that intuition or have developed ways to build it into their lives.

Howard Gardner's[1] work in the '70s and '80s identified 7 (or 11) different intelligences. Following that line of thinking we will have these intelligences to varying degrees. Not only do we have them but we need to look after them. He talked and wrote about: linguistic intelligence, logical-mathematical intelligence, musical intelligence, bodily-kinaesthetic intelligence, spatial intelligence, interpersonal intelligence and intrapersonal intelligence; plus naturalist intelligence, spiritual intelligence, moral intelligence and

[1] Howard Gardner. BA summa cum laude in Social Relations, Harvard College, 1965; PhD Psychology, Harvard University 1971; author of over 400 research papers and 20 books.

existential intelligence. These influence our skills and natural attributes - why we are better at some things than others. The brain and the mind have these different abilities and to be well we need to respect them. If we have in-built strengths that are being restricted, or not used, that could cause underlying discontent. If we have things we aren't so good at, that make some things a struggle, make some aspects of life hard work, we could work on those, so we are aware of them and perhaps make life a bit easier. 'Know thyself' is an anonymous inscription on the temple of Apollo at Delphi, that Plato ascribed to the Seven Wise Men. Being something we are not, will usually be stressful. Some people can perfect that art but it will usually take a toll, in some form, physically or mentally. Knowing who we are and how to live with that, plays a very important part in our health.

A life and/or a job that allows us to express who we are, finding and allowing room for our strengths and managing what we are not so good at, is good for our mental health. It's very easy to disappoint or depress ourselves if we try to be something we're not. It's highly unlikely we can devise the perfect life but it is also remarkable what we can cope with - how well we can manage - if we do have enough opportunity, in amongst everything else, to acknowledge our strengths, to enjoy things that do suit us and to relax. Then all the other stuff isn't quite so daunting. We can put up with the hassles and things we don't like, or aren't good for us because there's a little chink of light somewhere - there is a reprieve.

The most debilitating circumstances are when there is wall to wall oppression, loss of control, nothing we can do about things. To come back from that means re-finding the room for the chink of light, the good stuff. Not going there is even better.

Looking after mental health will include, nutrition, lifestyle, exercise, friendships and support and, should we need it, professional advice, 'talking therapies', helplines and groups. Many instances will be short and easily overcome - they are natural reactions to a range of circumstances.

The basics are very simple. We need to try and have a varied diet from a wide range of foods and natural, refreshing drinks and lots of water. Ensure a good balance of physical and mental exercise and rest and relaxation. Look after your brain. Take notice of early warning signs. Seek help early if you need to. Like so many things, biological and medical symptoms respond much more quickly and are easier to deal with, the earlier we act. Never underestimate the support network. Mental health depends on physical health and physical health depends on mental health.

The summary is:

Acknowledge what is going on.
Identify the support network.
Do whatever you can about nutrition, exercise and lifestyle.
Remember it's all chemistry.
You are in very good, revered company.
Act early if you think something needs doing.
Look after your brain - provide for its strengths and weaknesses - your strengths and weaknesses - your brain has needs, don't neglect them.
Know thyself - praise the good stuff, work on the other stuff

. . . and there is so much help and information available.

The following websites offer all kinds of information, advice and resources, including helplines and support groups.

www.mind.org.uk
www.rethink.org
www.mindout.clarity.uk.net
www.time-to-change.org,uk
www.mdf.org.uk
www.depressionalliance.org

Patrick Holford and Professor Andre Tylee, Professor of Primary Care Metal Health at the Institute of Psychiatry, King's College, London founded the Food for the Brain Foundation: www.foodforthebrain.org

I'D HATE TO ADVOCATE DRUGS, ALCOHOL
OR INSANITY TO ANYONE,
BUT THEY'VE ALWAYS WORKED FOR ME

Hunter S Thompson

Longevity

It is really difficult to get good, comparable figures for life expectancy. There are many available - but by the time you take into consideration whether they are national or international, for males and/or females, include or exclude childbirth mortality - and take into account regional differences, increase in population and the changing make-up of the population - it is almost impossible to be left with anything meaningful to compare life expectancy between today and other times. Many different influences affect these figures.

Generally, from the Office of National Statistics data, between 1992 and 2006 average life expectancy rose from 73.4 years to 77.3 years for males and from 78.9 years to 81.5 years for women. The increase was greater in England and Wales and less in Scotland and Northern Ireland. The figure is higher for males and females in the south of England and lower in the north and Scotland - and there are lots of other regional variations. In 2006 the local area with the highest figures was Kensington and Chelsea with 83.7 for males and 87.8 for females - and the lowest figures were in Glasgow, 70.8 for males and 77.1 for females.

Life expectancy figures for comparison with today are often taken from the year 1900, the turn of the century, as a nice, easy, convenient start point. Life expectancy of new born children in 1901 was 45 years for males and 49 years for females. This obviously shows a distinct improvement in life expectancy figures between 1900 and the early 2000s. If we compare current figures to just 50 years prior to that, ie: the mid-Victorian era - we have a completely different picture.

The Victorian era (1837-1901) is often portrayed as a hard time, with poor, hungry people living on dirty streets, for all but the wealthier, higher classes. There is extensive evidence that the urban mid-Victorian population (1850s, 60s and 70s), including working classes, ate a noticeably good diet, including significant amounts of fruit and vegetables, and life expectancy matched ours today.

Mid-Victorian working class men and women consumed between 50% and 100% more calories than we do, also burning many more calories than we do - to work and survive. Consequently they had a very high nutrient intake. Their diet was high in vegetables and fruits, equating to what we would probably consider to be about 8-10 portions a day. They ate considerably more nuts, legumes[1], whole grains and omega 3

[1] legumes – generally peas, beans and pulses; there is a page on legumes at the end of the chapter.

fatty acids. A lot of their meat consumption was offal, higher in micronutrients than most of the muscle meat we eat in a modern diet. Margarine was not introduced until the later Victorian years, so intake of trans-fatty acids was very low. There were few processed foods, so hardly any hidden salt and very little salt was added to meals in cooking. At the table, if used, salt was put at the side of the plate, rather than shaken over the meal, making it easier to control how much was taken and it was used sparingly. The ingredients of the mid-Victorian diet had a lower calorie content and higher nutrient content, was higher in fibre and had a lower salt/potassium ratio – this is in line with many of the health recommendations to us today. They were typically very fit, strong and healthy and had very strong immune systems – and this despite the conditions many of them would have lived in.

The simple, basic guidance we use for a natural, healthy diet is usually attributed to paleolithic/stone age times[1] – but our mid-Victorian ancestors were following many of the same principles – the main difference for us is that from the Victorians there is extensive documentary evidence. The mid-Victorian working classes were closely following the current health advice we see and hear today – a good, broad variety of good food. They had very few processed foods. Their diet was closer to the high-plant-based Mediterranean diet or Paleolithic diet than it is to our modern, western diet and they suffered from far less degenerative diseases. High levels of physical fitness are also borne out by high levels of physical performance, activity and strength. The main influences of individual experience and variance would be subject to region, seasonal availability of food and economic status – financial stability or instability.

After the well known misery and suffering of the 'hungry forties' (1840s) there was a rapid improvement in provision of vegetables and fruit, especially to the urban poor. By 1850 the working class diet and affordability of food had improved significantly. (It was to begin to decline again in the later 1870s with the introduction of processed foods).

In 1840 the average lifespan in the Whitechapel district of London was 45 years for upper class men, 27 for tradesmen and 22 years for labourers and servants – but from the mid-Victorian era (1850/1860) once infant mortality is removed from the data, life expectancy at age 5 was 75 for men and 73 for women – whilst ours today is 77 for men and 81 for women – and for today's working class, 72 for men and 76 for women[2].

[1] Paleolithic times – 300,000-30,000 years ago representing by far the greatest part of human history, spanning more than 2 million years to a time only a few thousand years ago

[2] Infant mortality increased in the economic depression of the late 1920s and during the Second World War. With economic prosperity and the establishment of the National Health Service, larger fluctuations in the number of infant deaths no longer occurred and infant mortality steadily declined.

These figures are striking because of the many environmental disadvantages of that era and the provision of medical care today - modern drugs, screening programmes and surgical techniques - with cleaner, more sanitary conditions. Mid-Victorians had relatively good health in old age, many working to within a few days of death, even in the workhouses. Current figures for the first few years of the 21st century show males may spend 7.7 years of their lives in a state of increasing medical dependency and women 10 years.

We frequently hear the theory that current increased life expectancy is linked to modern health care. If we compare figures from 1850, as well as from 1900, or 1920 then there have to be other, additional explanations.

From the 1880s to 1900 there had been a decline in nutritional standards, adversely affecting health and life expectancy. Prior to 1850 poor health and nutrition were affected by ineffective food distribution, lack of transport systems and the high prices connected to the Corn Laws.

Causes of death in mid-Victorian times were typically infection, peri-natal mortality and accidents at work or at home. Non-communicable, degenerative diseases, the highest causes of mortaility today (heart attacks, cardio-vascular disease, COPD - chronic obstructive pulmonary disease, cancer, dementia) were relatively insignificant. In 1869, the Physician to Charing Cross Hospital described lung cancer as 'one of the rarer forms of a rare disease. You may probably pass the rest of your student life without seeing another example of it'.

Records of that era indicate that breast cancer was a lot less common and less rapidly progressive than today. This is understood to be attributable to significantly higher intakes of a range of micro and phyto nutrients creating an internal constitution less conducive to cancer growth - our own natural equivalent to chemo-therapy without the harmful side-effects. Cancer cells are a natural occurrence - but the cells should be naturally detected quickly and instinctively and zapped, eliminated and removed. What has changed in recent times is their ability to beat the system, their opportunity to beat the system - if we are down-grading the defences we rely on to protect ourselves. The odds should be stacked against them - their survival and proliferation should be immensely difficult in an internal environment, intricately designed to overpower them. Our part is to do what we can to maintain that healthy environment so that it can act early and successfully - our most effective defence against disease. Our immune system and prevention and maintenance is how we are designed to deal with these threats. We are following a pattern of becoming increasingly dependent on remedial treatment which can be highly successful but which may also cause stress to internal systems and organs or have side-effects - asking more of our own, natural defences. Whether we follow prevention or cure – we will still need to rely on our own underlying health and strength to see us through. Health and prevention will almost inevitably offer the best route – by supplying the body with what it needs to look after itself.

The mid-Victorian diet contained higher levels of vaso-protective flavanoids, omega 3 polyunsaturated fatty acids, B vitamins and anti-oxidant vitamins and minerals. Although the carbohydrate, sugar and glycaemic content was higher, due to large amounts of potatoes, bread and baked foods, this was offset by very much higher levels of physical activity. There was a much higher proportion of plant-derived foods, similar to the Mediterranean diet, which is known to reduce the risk of heart disease and Type 2 diabetes. Heart disease was much less common and Type 2 diabetes very uncommon. Better blood sugar control, vaso-protection from higher nutrients and a lower sodium intake also lowered the risk of cognitive impairment, including symptoms of Alzheimer's disease, age-related cognitive decline and dementia. Allergies and sensitivities were also far less common.

Despite the medical knowledge and practice, diagnostic tools, drugs, contraception and surgery of the time – the life expectancy figures of the mid-Victorian era and now, are not that different.

The most obvious and crucial development was the success of early antibiotics – being able to fight infection and bringing infectious diseases under control. That was then the major cause of death. 50% of all infant deaths of all classes were due to infectious diseases. Their nutrition and lifestyle had prevented susceptibility to the long term, degenerative diseases which we experience so much more today. In general we have a less active lifestyle, lower calorie intake and/or nutritionally poorer diet. Many of us wouldn't be here if it wasn't for antibiotics. Most of us have had a course of antibiotics in our very early years, teens or adulthood. Such a very short time ago, we managed to live through infections and diseases without them and it is very difficult to say that we would now. There are still many populations that manage to stay healthy without them and the most likely reasons will be diet and lifestyle.

The extraordinary advancement of medical science and pharmaceuticals has brought phenomenal breakthroughs – but shifting towards reliance on medical and pharmaceutical intervention is suppressing our understanding and appreciation of the basis of strong nutrition – of all the vital constituents, vitamins, minerals, fatty acids, anti-oxidants, flavanoids, phenols, carotenoids, salicylates, xanthophylls – providing all the anabolic (building) and anti-catabolic (declining/ageing) ingredients we need to be well and strong. Many of the diseases prevalent today are not new, including heart disease and cancer – but what has changed is our ability to resist or overcome them. These diseases can be avoided through better understanding of lifestyle and nutrition and treated through lifestyle and nutrition. We have very rapidly turned away from the nutritional wisdom we had accumulated over generations and ages of man. Our earliest medicine was based on food and nutrition. It almost disappeared from medical training very, very suddenly during the 1900s but still many our most potent medicines are plant based and we need food and nutrition to reclaim their obvious place in our healthcare.

We know that populations suffering from hunger and deprivation in poor or war-torn countries need nutritional support – but we don't apply the same logic to ourselves because food is in plentiful supply. We have more food than we need and our wastage of food is higher than ever – but a lot of it just isn't the right sort of food. Because we have more food than we need, we don't think to assess ourselves as malnourished. We need to re-engineer our nutrition and lifestyle to provide the natural basics that our body is designed for – that keep us well. Much of the natural food we would have eaten contains the natural ingredients that guard us against many modern diseases. Eating a good, varied diet – we didn't even have to think about it and work it out. If we ate what was available, berries, fruit, green leafy vegetables, oily fish we were wonderfully dosing ourselves with many of the chemical properties now administered by drugs or being discovered as critical to fight against the conditions we suffer from. That is why the mid-Victorians were so effectively protected from the non-communicable, degenerative diseases which should be avoidable today.

The rise of serious and long-term medical conditions and dependence on medication is extraordinary. Each of us would find it difficult to think of anyone who hasn't taken some kind of medication or treatment. We barely even think about some of the basics we rely on. Our expenditure on medical science and pharmaceuticals is astonishing. Not long ago, substantial proportions of the population survived without medical interventions and degenerative disease was scarce. Whatever happened? Despite modern advances, pharmaceuticals and incredible expenditure we may not have achieved quite the extended life expectancy we like to think and degenerative diseases have become more and more common. We mustn't throw away nutritional wisdom which we had previously, experientially accumulated over hundreds of years and generations.

We can eat and exercise ourselves to health and fitness.

Most of the mid-Victorian population was working class and manual – the people who built the industrial landscape. The average British navvy – standing in a trench – shovelling dirt from the ground near his feet to above his head – could shift 20 tons a day. A British labourer today would struggle to shift 1 ton.

A navvy would be given 2lbs of beef, 2lbs bread, 2-3lbs of veg, 1 gallon beer per day: high in calories, high in phyto-nutrients.

Beer was the most commonly consumed alcohol but generally with a significantly lower alcohol content than today's beers, probably 1-2% and 2-3%, often weakened as it was watered down. It also had a far higher yeast content as beers and wines were not subjected to the ultra-filtration of modern production. Although many people now have to avoid yeast in their diet and others think they should – it was and is a natural probiotic and stimulus for the immune system. Brewer's yeast tablets are still used in this way but have also been superseded by the effective ingredient in a yeast-free immune primer Beta Glucans 1-3 and 1-6. The new preparation concentrates the effectiveness in 1 tablet of approximately 6 of the original yeast tablets.

Fruit and vegetables were produced without additional chemicals. Produce and the food chain generally were far less sterile than we are used to, continually exposing consumers to yeasts and low-level immunological challenges and micro-organisms – constantly priming and enhancing the activity of the immune system – including natural killer cells. Despite the extreme difference in production and hygiene, even food-poisoning was relatively rare.

Cooking methods, usually slow oven cooking and boiling, would also have produced less carcinogens. Frying and grilling were little used and would have been at a lower temperature due to cooking styles and the cost of fuel – unlike the high temperature grilling and frying we use and is so common in fast/convenience foods.

In the late Victorian era, we imported large quantities of processed, low grade foods, eg: margarine and fatty corned beef, cheap sugar and by the end of the century there was industrial scale cigarette production and health took a nose-dive and worsened until the end of the Victorian era.

Given the right nutrition and lifestyle our bodies have amazing powers of healing and regeneration. Some people age faster and some slower than others. As covered in the chapters on Anabolic and Catabolic Stages (page 302), during the first 20 years of our lives our bodies generate and build tissue faster than it is broken down, we grow. Between roughly age 20 and 50 there is a period of balanced wear and repair and over 50 wear starts to overtake repair. Arteries start to fur up, bones become weaker, cartilage becomes thinner, brain and other cells can start to malfunction, symptoms of degenerative disease can begin to appear and we begin to age – which may be gradually or rapidly. If we want to there is a lot we can do about that.

The most commonly known diseases that risk our health and longevity are heart and cardio-vascular disease, cancer, dementia and hypertension – and the risk of those is increased if we have diabetes – plus pneumonia and flu, viruses and infections. Many of these diseases share 4 common underlying causes – free radical damage, inflammation, immune system failure and excessive insulin stress:

- free radical damage – ageing, tissue/organ damage and deterioration, cancer, Alzheimer's; free radical damage is caused by excess free radicals (see page 112) damaging body cells

- inflammation – arthritis, heart disease, bowel and colon cancer, asthma and Alzheimer's; caused by irritation, injury or infection and collection or pooling of toxins

- immune system failure – infections and cancers; caused by weakened immune system, and health threats from poor nutrition, stress, insufficient rest or sleep, drug use, alcohol, obesity, auto-immunity, immune dysfunction or immune system hypersensitivity

- excessive insulin stress – type 2 diabetes, raising risk of heart disease, stroke, blindness, kidney failure and dementia: caused by diet high in starchy foods and sweet foods and high blood sugar leading to insulin resistance.

How we are also affects the next generation. Being well means we leave a better inheritance to our offspring. Inherited health does make a difference but so does what we do through our own lifetime. If we don't eat well or exercise well and nor does our next generation, the effects are cumulative. We are likely to become less well, less strong, less active and more sickly. Some conditions are becoming much more common, noticeably obesity, diabetes and cancer. How well we look after ourselves may be our legacy to our children and grandchildren.

Are we living longer? and are we well if we do?
Good nutrition, exercise, sufficient sleep and avoiding/reducing stress contribute enormously to longer, healthier lives – and the earlier we start the better. We must re-adopt the strategy of prevention as well as cure.

In better words than mine . . .

Food and nutrients, at the right levels and in the right combinations, together with regular exercise, adequate sleep and reduced stress, can extend the period during which wear and tear are in balance. Achieving that outcome should cut the risk of disease and slow the ageing process.

Dr Paul Clayton

Legumes

There are so many legumes, easily 50+ commonly used. Some of the most familiar are:

aduki beans
black-eyed peas
broad beans
cannellini beans
chickpeas
chili beans
fava beans
French green beans
green beans
kidney beans
lentils
lima beans
marrowfat peas
mung beans
peas
pinto beans
red kidney beans
runner beans
sugar snap peas
soy beans or soya beans
white kidney beans

Legumes are low in fat, high in fibre and are an excellent source of protein. One serving, approximately 3 tablespoons, can actually provide about half the folate we need for a day. They're also high in vitamin B and rich in anti-oxidants. Beans and grains are considered legumes and so are seed pods. Legumes are edible seeds that come in two types: immature, which we eat straight from the garden, like green beans and peas – and mature, such as dried, tinned or fresh beans.

The term 'legume' refers to a plant from the Leguminosae (or Fabaceae) family, the third largest flowering family in the world and the fruits of the plants are also called legumes. They form in a pod that splits along the seam when it's ripe. The pod contains seeds attached to one side of the wall. Peanuts are also legumes but we rarely buy or eat them in their natural form. Roasted and salted peanuts don't have quite the same nutritional benefits.

Legumes are nutritionally valuable foods. Mature legume pods contain 20% protein and plant protein (unlike animal derived protein), contain no cholesterol and are low in fat. Compared to grains, legumes contain about twice as much protein. Legumes are:

high in protein
high in iron
high in folate
high in potassium
high in magnesium
high in fibre
low in fat
a source of B vitamins.

An unsuitable and degraded diet?
Paul Clayton, Judith Rowbotham
Part one: public health lessons from the mid-Victorian working class diet
Journal of the Royal Society of Medicine (2008: 101: 282-289 DOI 10.1258/jrsm.2008.080112)
http://jrsm.rsmjournals.com/cgi/content/citation/101/6/282
Part two: realities of the mid-Victorian diet
Journal of the Royal Society of Medicine (2008: 101: 350-357 DOI 10.1258/jrsm.2008.080113)
http://www.jrsm.rsmjournals.com/cgi/content/citation/101/7/350
Part three: Victorian consumption patterns and their health benefits
Journal of the Royal Society of Medicine (2008: 101: 454-462 DOI 10.1258/jrsm.2008.080114)
http://jrsm.rsmjournals.com/cgi/content/citation/101/9/454

AGE IS NOTHING BUT EXPERIENCE –
AND SOME OF US ARE MORE EXPERIENCED
THAN OTHERS.

Andy Rooney

Anabolic and Catabolic Stages

As mentioned at the end of the second chapter, Health and Wellbeing - Why It's Important, and the chapter on The Cell, our bodies are in a constant state of wear and repair. The process of tissue growth and re-growth is called anabolic and the process of wearing out and deterioration is called catabolic.

During anabolic stages, new cells replace old ones, growth and development or renewal takes place. During catabolic stages, cells become worn out and break down, they die.

For the first approximately 20 years of our life we would typically be in a state of distinct anabolism. We would then have a few years of more gradual growth until around about our late 20s. From that stage we would generally have 20 or so years where growth or renewal and wear and tear are about equal and then anytime between 50 and 60 start a gradual decline where wear and tear and ageing of tissues becomes greater than the renewal and replenishment. From late 60s and 70s that decline would again, typically, become more noticeable. This affects our bones, muscles, joints, arteries, eyes, skin - all of us and cells can start to malfunction. Although we may inherit different aspects of our health in our genes that will affect and influence these stages - the most everyday, common, obvious things that will extend and support anabolism and delay or reduce catabolism are nutrition, exercise and lifestyle. With good nutrition and exercise we can remain healthier for longer. We are mortal, we can't live forever but we can make a considerable difference to how well we are and for how long. We can be as well as we can, for as long as we can - if we want to.

We may not be able to live forever - we may not want to! - but we may as well be as well as we can whilst we're here. Two of the main benefits are reduced pain and increased mobility, which become increasingly valuable as we get older. Catabolic dominance takes its toll as we age because we can become more depleted in micro-nutrients. Eating well, years before our older years and into our older years will ensure an adequate supply and the best range of those vital nutrients. Nutrition, what we eat, will help support us against a wide range of symptoms and disease. We benefit from eating the good things and we benefit by not eating the not-so-good things.

STAGES OF ANABOLISM AND CATABOLISM

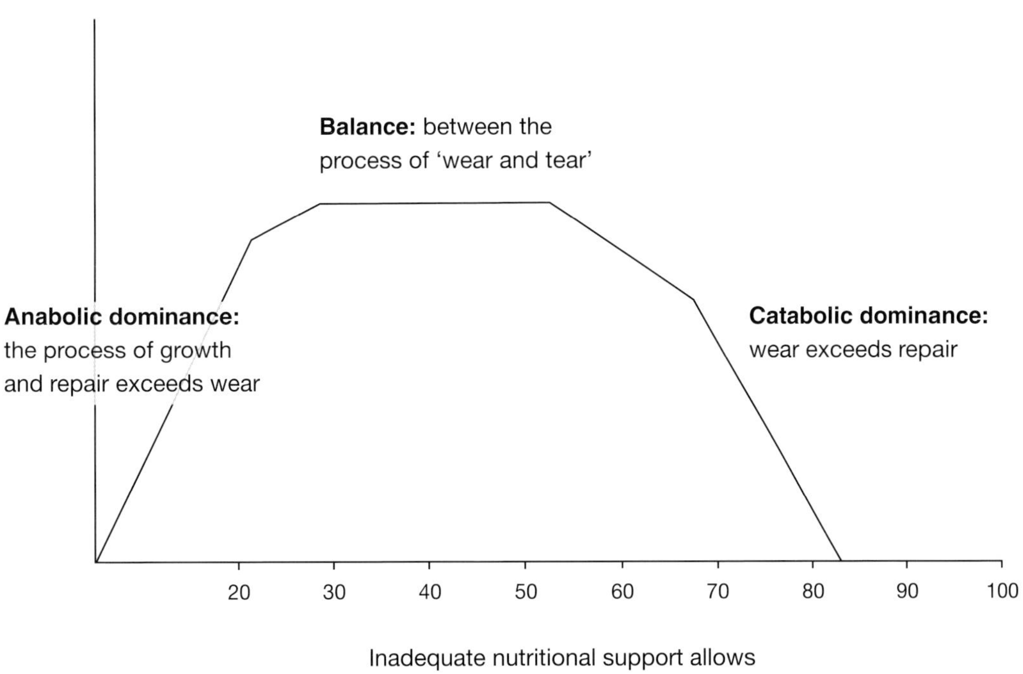

Inadequate nutritional support allows catabolism to begin to dominate

Facts and figures

- 164 million days lost to the UK economy during 2005 attributed to ill health
- costing the UK economy £13 billion a year
- similar figures were reported for 2007 costing £13.2 billion; 2008 slightly up, 2009 slightly down
- the most significant causes of absence, for manual and non-manual workers, are back pain and musculo-skeletal injuries
- smoking causes half of all premature deaths
- excessive alcohol consumption causes 33,000 premature deaths a year
- 1 in 2 adults are overweight and 1 in 5 are obese
- obese men are 33% more likely to die of cancer
- obese women are at 50% greater risk of getting breast cancer
- 1 in 4 of us dies prematurely of cancer and 2 in 4 of heart disease but these diseases are 75% lifestyle related and therefore possibly preventable
- half a million people each year experience stress at a level that will make them ill

A diet rich in saturated fats and processed foods, smoking, stress, alcohol and lack of exercise are all contributory factors to these statistics.

Work-related stats from employer surveys during 2006, 2007, 2008 and 2009

- average level of employee absence was 3.5% of working time lost in 2006
  3.7% of working time lost in 2007
  back to 3.5% in 2008 and 3.9% in 2009

- average cost of employee absence per employee was £598 in 2006, £659 in 2007, £666 in 2008 and £694 in 2009

- days lost per employee pa were 8 in 2006, 8.4 days in 2007
  8 days in 2008 and 7.4 days in 2009

- absence levels for public services employees were 4.3% in 2006
  4.5% (10.3 days pa) in 2007, 9.8 days in 2008 and 9.7 days in 2009

- absence levels for private sector employees were 3% in 2006
  3.2% (7.2 days pa) in 2007, 7.2 days in 2008 and 6.4 days in 2009

- absence levels for non-profit sector employees were 3.6% in 2006
  4.2% (9.6 days pa) in 2007, 8.5 days in 2008 and 9.4 days in 2009

- absence levels for manufacturing and production employees were 3.5% in 2006
  3.3% (7.6 days pa) in 2007, 7.2 days in 2008 and 6.5 days in 2009

- on average employer respondents predict approx 16% of absence may not be genuine

- 50% of respondents identify Statutory Sick Pay as a significant or very significant cost to the employer

- approx 40% of respondents rate strategy and provision on employee well-being as poor and wish to work on improvement in future years

Surveys based on 819 UK-based HR responses, of 1.6m employees: average size of organisation – public sector 5,606 employees; private sector 1,412; non-profit 403; manufacturing and production 531.

Another survey reported that in 2007 the average direct cost of absence was £517 per employee (3.1% of payroll) which included lost production and the expense of covering absence with temporary staff or overtime. It was also estimated that indirect costs, such as lower customer satisfaction or reduced morale and efficiency could add another £263 per employee per year. Adding these indirect costs to the direct cost would take the loss to the UK economy to £19.9bn in 2007.

ref:

CIPD - Eighth, Ninth and Tenth National Survey of Absence (2007, 2008, 2009)
CBI - Confederation of British Industry
ONS - Office of National Statistics
WHO - World Health Organisation
Cancer Research UK
HSE - Managing sickness absence

Summary

So

- we are wonderful, complicated, clever, sophisticated beings
- we have hearts, lungs, livers, kidneys, intestines, brains
- we have a skeletal system, a muscular system, a nervous system, an endocrine system, a cardio-vascular system, a respiratory system, a lymphatic system, an immune system, a digestive system, and a urinary system
- it all works on hormones and enzymes and neuro-transmitters
- the body and brain are made entirely of molecules from our food
- it is all completely inter-dependent
- and it all relies on homeostasis
- and we, consciously, are in charge of providing that safe, healthy environment
- it is all working, all the time, whatever we do, 100% committed to keeping us well. It has no choice – it is pre-programmed for survival – meet yourself halfway – or hopefully better than that
- eat well – enjoy good food
- keep fit
- learn more and be involved in who you are and how you are

Reading and Reference

Anatomy and Physiology: Gary A Thibodeau and Kevin T Patton

Health Defence: Dr Paul Clayton

Healing Foods Cook Book: Jane Sen
More Healing Foods: Jane Sen

Survival of the Fittest: Mike Stroud

Your Life in Your Hands: Jane Plant

New Optimum Nutrition Bible: Patrick Holford
New Optimum Nutrition for the Mind: Patrick Holford
Optimum Nutrition for Your Child: Patrick Holford and Deborah Colson
Optimum Nutrition for Your Child's Mind: Patrick Holford and Deborah Colson
The Low-GL Diet Bible: Patrick Holford
The Holford Low-GL Diet Cook Book: Patrick Holford
(many, many titles by Patrick Holford on all aspects of nutrition, and different health conditions: asthma, cancer, arthritis, skin problems, digestion, pregnancy, allergies, heart disease, hormones, stress and fatigue)

Your Body's Many Cries for Water: Fereydoon Batmanghelidj

Fit for Life: Harvey and Marilyn Diamond

The Greatest Story Ever Told: Bernard Jensen

The Endorphin Effect: William Bloom

Shape Your Self: Martina Navratilova

Candida Albicans: Leon Chaitow

Passage to Power: Lesley Kenton

Eating Without: Barbara Cousins

What Do You Eat?: Liz Cook

Living with a BLACK DOG: Matthew and Ainsley Johnstone

www.centreofthecell.org
Centre of the Cell
Queen Mary University of London, and Barts and The London School of Medicine and Dentistry

www.feetforlife.org
Society for Chiropodists and Podiatrists

www.dentalhelpline.org.uk
British Dental Health Foundation

www.bdasmile.org.uk
British Dental Association

www.rnib.org.uk
Royal National Institute of Blind People

www.lizcookcharts.co.uk
nutrition, vitamins and minerals charts and information, plus lots more

www.thefoodcalculator.com
diet analysis

www.mendprogramme.org
MEND – Mind, Exercise, Nutrition... Do it! a social enterprise dedicated to reducing global overweight and obesity levels, helping children and families become fitter, healthier and happier, offering free healthy living programmes in the local community. Set up in 2004 by Great Ormond Street Hospital for children and the University College London Institute of Child Health.

All these sites have excellent information on mental health and helplines:
www.mind.org.uk
www.rethink.org
www.mindout.clarity.uk.net
www.time-to-change.org,uk
www.mdf.org.uk
www.depressionalliance.org

www.foodforthebrain.org
Patrick Holford and Professor André Tylee, Professor of Primary Care Metal Health at the Institute of Psychiatry, King's College, London founded the Food for the Brain Foundation.

An unsuitable and degraded diet?
Paul Clayton, Judith Rowbotham
Part one: public health lessons from the mid-Victorian working class diet
Journal of the Royal Society of Medicine (2008: 101: 282-289 DOI 10.1258/jrsm.2008.080112)
http://jrsm.rsmjournals.com/cgi/content/citation/101/6/282
Part two: realities of the mid-Victorian diet
Journal of the Royal Society of Medicine (2008: 101: 350-357 DOI 10.1258/jrsm.2008.080113)
http://www.jrsm.rsmjournals.com/cgi/content/citation/101/7/350
Part three: Victorian consumption patterns and their health benefits
Journal of the Royal Society of Medicine (2008: 101: 454-462 DOI 10.1258/jrsm.2008.080114)
http://jrsm.rsmjournals.com/cgi/content/citation/101/9/454

A Century of Change: Trends in UK statistics since 1900
http://www.parliament.uk/commons/lib/research/rp99/rp99-111.pdf

CIPD - Chartered Institute of Personnel and Development
National Survey of Absence (2007) (2008) (2009)
CBI - Confederation of British Industry
ONS - Office of National Statistics
WHO - World Health Organisation
Cancer Research UK
HSE - Managing sickness absence

http://www.dh.gov.uk/en/Publicationsandstatistics/Publications/PublicationsPolicyAndGuidance/DH_4080994

Professor Jane Plant is one of the world's leading geochemists and chief scientist of the British Geological Survey from 2000 to 2005, as well as Professor of Geochemistry at Imperial College, London. She graduated with a Class 1 Honours degree in geology at Liverpool University in 1967, gaining her PhD in Geochemistry at Leicester University ten years later. Jane has worked at the British Geological Survey for her whole professional career and took a leading role significantly (and at first unexpectedly) in the new field of environmental health. During the 1970s it was Jane Plant's team which identified links between deficiency diseases in livestock and the geochemistry of the land on which they lived.

Patrick Holford researched the role of nutrition in mental health and illness, whilst completing his bachelor degree in Experimental Psychology at the University of York. He is a leading pioneer in new approaches to health and nutrition and is widely regarded as Britain's leading spokesman on nutrition and mental health issues. He is author of over 30 health books, translated into over 20 languages and selling over a million copies worldwide. In 1984 he founded the Institute for Optimum Nutrition (ION). Patrick retired as Director of ION in 1997 to focus on writing, teaching and researching. He is an Honorary Fellow of BANT (the British Association of Nutritional Therapists).

Jane Sen is an accomplished chef and has worked with chefs throughout the world. She is dietary adviser to Bristol Cancer Help Centre, a nutritional expert and a popular lecturer to health professionals and interest groups throughout the world.

Index

Some of the hormones and what they do

Hypothalamus

Hormone	Function
growth hormone releasing hormone (GRH)	stimulates secretion of growth hormone
growth hormone inhibiting hormone (GIH)	inhibits secretion of growth hormone
corticotrophin releasing hormone (CRH)	stimulates release of adrenocorticotropic hormone (ACTH)
thyrotropin releasing hormone (TRH)	stimulates release of thyroid stimulating hormone (TSH)
gonadotropin releasing hormone (GNRH)	stimulates release of gonadotropins (FSH and LH)
prolactin releasing hormone (PRH)	stimulates secretion of prolactin
prolactin inhibiting hormone (PIH)	inhibits secretion of prolactin

Pituitary

Hormone	Function
growth hormone (GH)	promotes growth by stimulating protein anabolism and fat mobilization
prolactin (PRL)	promotes milk secretion
thyroid stimulating hormone (TSH)	stimulates development and secretion in the thyroid gland
adrenocorticotropic hormone (ACTH)	promotes development and secretion in the adrenal cortex
follicle stimulating hormone	female: promotes development of ovarian follicle[1]; stimulates oestrogen secretion male: promotes development of testis; stimulates sperm production
luteinizing hormone (LH)	female: triggers ovulation; promotes development of corpus luteum[2] (the tissue left behind after the cells encasing the released egg are ruptured) male: stimulates production of testosterone
antidiuretic hormone (ADH)	promotes water retention by kidney tubules
oxytocin (OT)	stimulates uterine contractions; stimulates ejection of milk into mammary ducts

Pineal

Hormone	Function
melatonin	forms part of the system that regulates the circadian/daytime, night time cycle; enduces drowsiness and sleep

Thyroid and Parathyroid

Hormone	Function
triiodothyronine (T3)	increases rate of metabolism
tetraiodothyronine (T4)	increases rate of metabolism
calcitonin (CT)	increases calcium storage in bone, lowering blood calcium levels
parathyroid hormone (PTH)	increases calcium removal from storage in bone and produces the active form of vitamin D in the kidneys, increasing absorption of calcium by intestines and increasing blood calcium levels

Adrenals

aldosterone	stimulates kidney tubules to conserve sodium which in turn triggers release of ADH and the resulting conservation of water by the kidneys
cortisol (hydrocortisone)	influences metabolism of food molecules; in large amounts it has an anti-inflammatory effect
adrenal androgens	exact role uncertain but may support sexual function
adrenal oestrogens	thought to be physiologically insignificant
adrenalin (epinephrine)	enhances and prolongs the effects of the sympathetic division of the autonomic nervous system
noradrenalin (norepinephrine)	enhances and prolongs the effects of the sympathetic division of the autonomic nervous system

Pancreatic islets

glucagon	promotes movement of glucose from storage and into the blood
insulin	promotes movement of glucose out of the blood and into cells
somatostatin	can have general effects in the body but primary role seems to be regulation of secretion of other pancreatic hormones
pancreatic polypeptide	exact function uncertain but seems to influence absorption in the digestive tract

Ovaries

oestrogens	promote the development and maintenance of female sexual characteristics, with other hormones responsible for breast development and the proper sequence of events in the female reproductive and menstrual cycle
progesterone 'pregnancy promoting steroid'	secreted after the rupture of the follicle during ovulation, maintains the lining of the uterus necessary for successful pregnancy (regulated by FSH and LH)

Testes

testosterone	growth and maintenance of male sexual characteristics and sperm production (regulated by gonadotropins, especially LH)

[1] ovarian follicle – the egg (oocyte) and its encasing cells, at any stage in its development
oocyte (egg) – the immature female reproductive cell prior to fertilization

[2] corpus luteum – yellow glandular mass in the ovary, formed by an ovarian follicle that has matured and discharged its (egg) oocyte